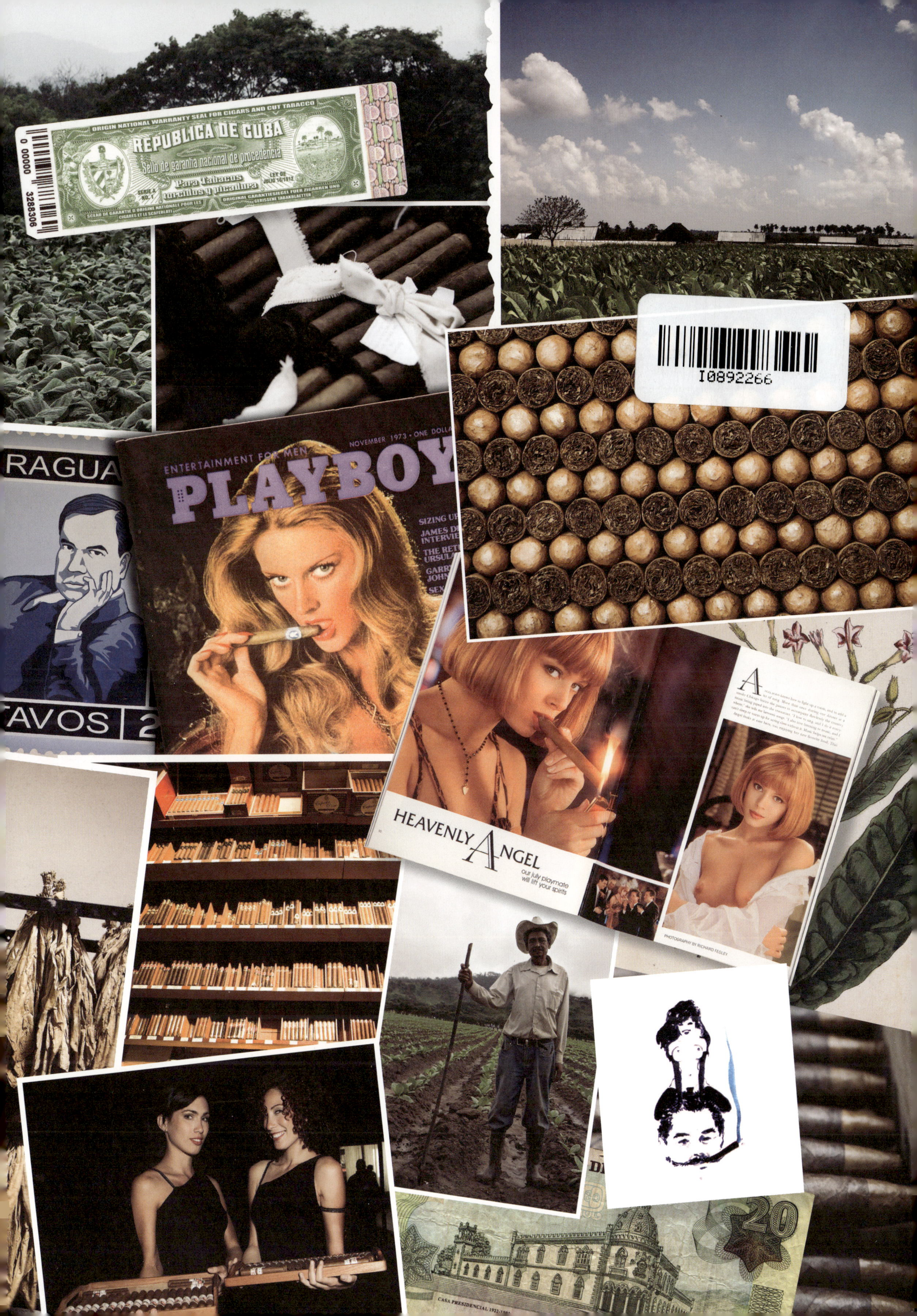

ORIGIN NATIONAL WARRANTY SEAL FOR CIGARS AND CUT TABACCO
REPUBLICA DE CUBA
Sello de garantia nacional de procedencia
Para Tabacos torcidos y picadura
RAGUA
AVOS 2
NOVEMBER 1973 • ONE DOLLA
ENTERTAINMENT FOR MEN
PLAYBOY
I0892266
HEAVENLY ANGEL
our july playmate will lift your spirits

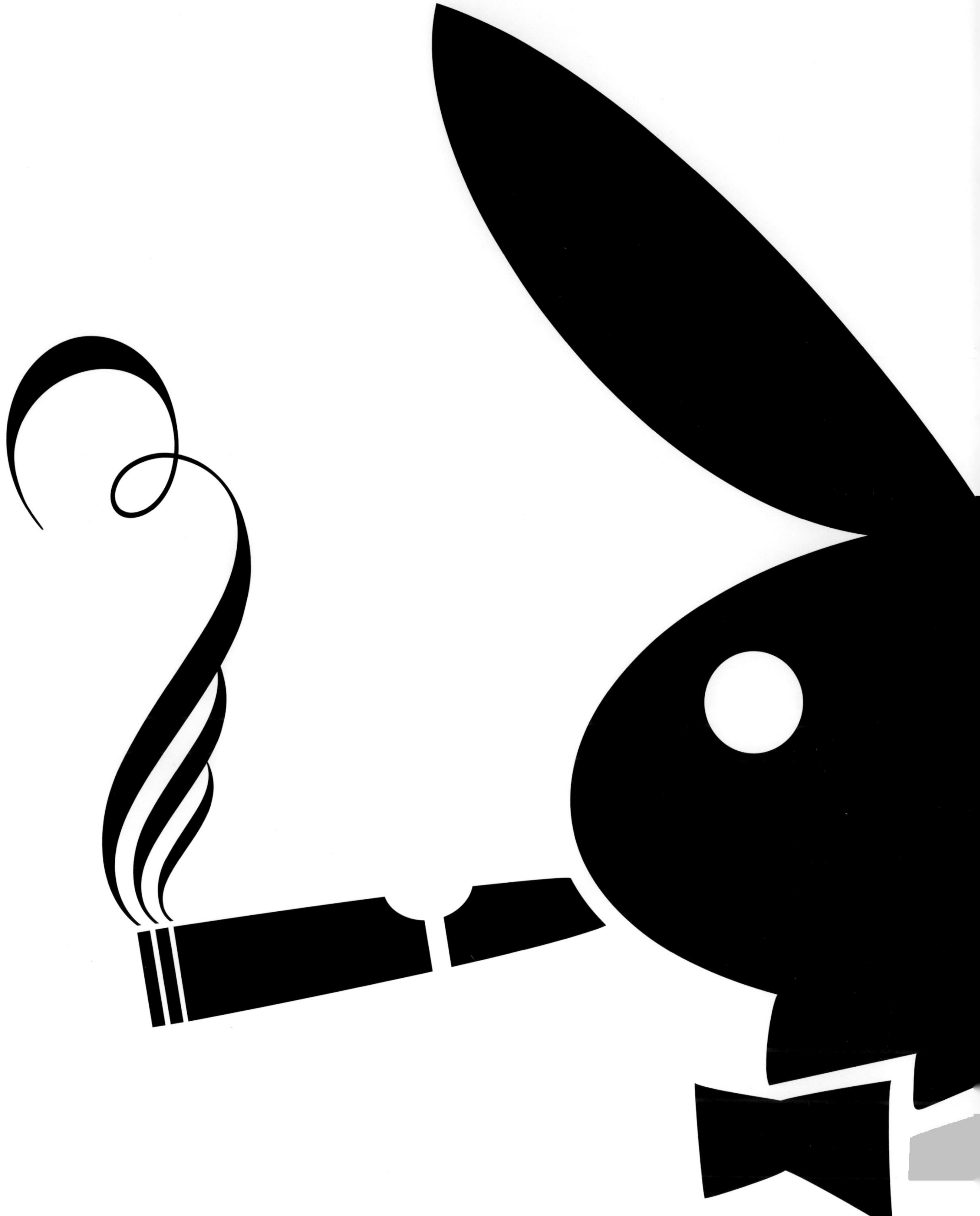

MORE PRAISE FOR AARON SIGMOND'S *THE PLAYBOY BOOK OF CIGARS*:

"A most elegant book proving indeed that wise men love . . . and smoke cigars."

—Peter Weller
Actor
RoboCop I & II, Naked Lunch, 24

"Aaron Sigmond is as passionate about fine cigars as he is about enjoying all of life's adventures to their fullest—the ideal connoisseur to finally bring to life Playboy's long overdue modern tome on one of man's last great male bastions. It's everything you ever needed to know about cigars, with a blow-out-the-cobwebs *Playboy* twist."

—E. Edward Hoyt III
Editorial Director
Smoke and *SmokeShop* magazines

"Finally . . . a sexy, stylish entrée into the lifestyle of handcrafted cigars. An exciting and accurate read as only Aaron Sigmond could deliver."

—Victoria McKee-Jaworski
Director of Public Relations, General Cigar Co.
Macanudo, Partagas, La Gloria Cubana, and Punch

"Every generation of cigar enthusiast seems to have a book to call its own—Sigmond's *Playboy: The Book of Cigars* is unequivocally a book for a new generation, as well as a great read for the seasoned cigar lover—an instant classic of the genre."

—Jim Colucci
EVP Sales & Marketing, Altadis U.S.A.
Montecristo, Romeo y Julieta, H. Upmann

"My new Bible!! I expected nothing less from 'the man' that creates lifestyles!!"

—Paolo Garzaroli
President, Graycliff Cigar Co.

"Like the magazine itself, *Playboy: The Book of Cigars* is smart, funny, and provocative—certainly the best book on the subject to come along in years."

—Keith K. Park
Founder and CEO, Prometheus
God of Fire and Angelenos

"Cigar smokers will enjoy this easy-reading, entertaining book. A definite must have for all cigar lovers."

—Nestor Miranda
CEO and Co-Founder, Miami Cigar & Co.
Nestor Miranda's "Special Selection" & Don Lino

PLAYBOY

The Book of Cigars

Foreword by **LEROY NEIMAN**

By **AARON SIGMOND**
& **NICK KOLAKOWSKI**

Photographed by **IAN SPANIER**
Celebrity Illustrations by **RISKO**

Afterword by **JOE MANTEGNA**

Art Direction and Design by **WARREN MASON / Measure-Design**

Skyhorse Publishing

Playboy The Cigar Book is a collaboration between Playboy Enterprises Inc. (PEI) and Mad/Dash LLC.

All photographs, unless otherwise noted, copyright 2009 © Ian Spanier Photography
Photograph of Mr. Hugh Hefner on page XVII courtesy of and copyright © Lockwood Publications (*Smoke* magazine winter 1996/'97)
Paul Rand papers courtesy of Yale University Library
A Very Brief History chapter photo credits Pages 2-9
General Grant: © Michael Nicholson/CORBIS
Che Guevara: © Madeleine Répond/Corbis
Planet Hollywood: © SIEMONEIT RONALD/CORBIS SYGMA
Winston Churchill: © Bettmann/CORBIS
King Edward The Peacemaker: © Hulton-Deutsch Collection/CORBIS
Sigmund Freud: © CORBIS Mark Twain: © Bettmann/CORBIS
Christopher Columbus's Discovery of America by Theodor de Bry: © Stapleton Collection/Corbis
Tobacco Plant: © Stapleton Collection/Corbis
page 20 (small photo) : © Jimmy Nicol
page 21 (man smoking cigar): © Jimmy Nicol
page 42 : © Matt Furman
page 45 (middle photo) : © Matt Furman

All celebrity illustrations copyright © Risko Inc.
All vector and photo illustrations copyright © Measure-Design

Mad/Dash LLC and Skyhorse Publishing
New York, NY

Playboy Enterprises, Inc.
Chicago, IL

10 9 8 7 6 5 4 3 2

Library of Congress Cataloging-in-Publication Data

Sigmond, Aaron.
Playboy : the book of cigars / by Aaron Sigmond and Nick Kolakowski ; foreword by LeRoy Neiman ; afterword by Joe Mantegna.
p. cm.
ISBN 978-1-61608-023-5 (hc : alk. paper)
1. Cigars--History. 2. Cigar smoking--History. 3. Tobacco--History. I. Kolakowski, Nick. II. Title.
TS2260.S55 2010
679'.72--dc22
2009051680

Hardcover ISBN: 978-1-61608-023-5
Ebook ISBN: 978-1-62914-828-1

Printed in China

This book is dedicated to my father, David Sigmond and Stanley Epstein—two lovers of the leaf who taught me far more about life than they did about cigars.

And to Robert Graham. Bob was a true cigar devotee and an iconic artist, and is a missed friend.

CONTENTS

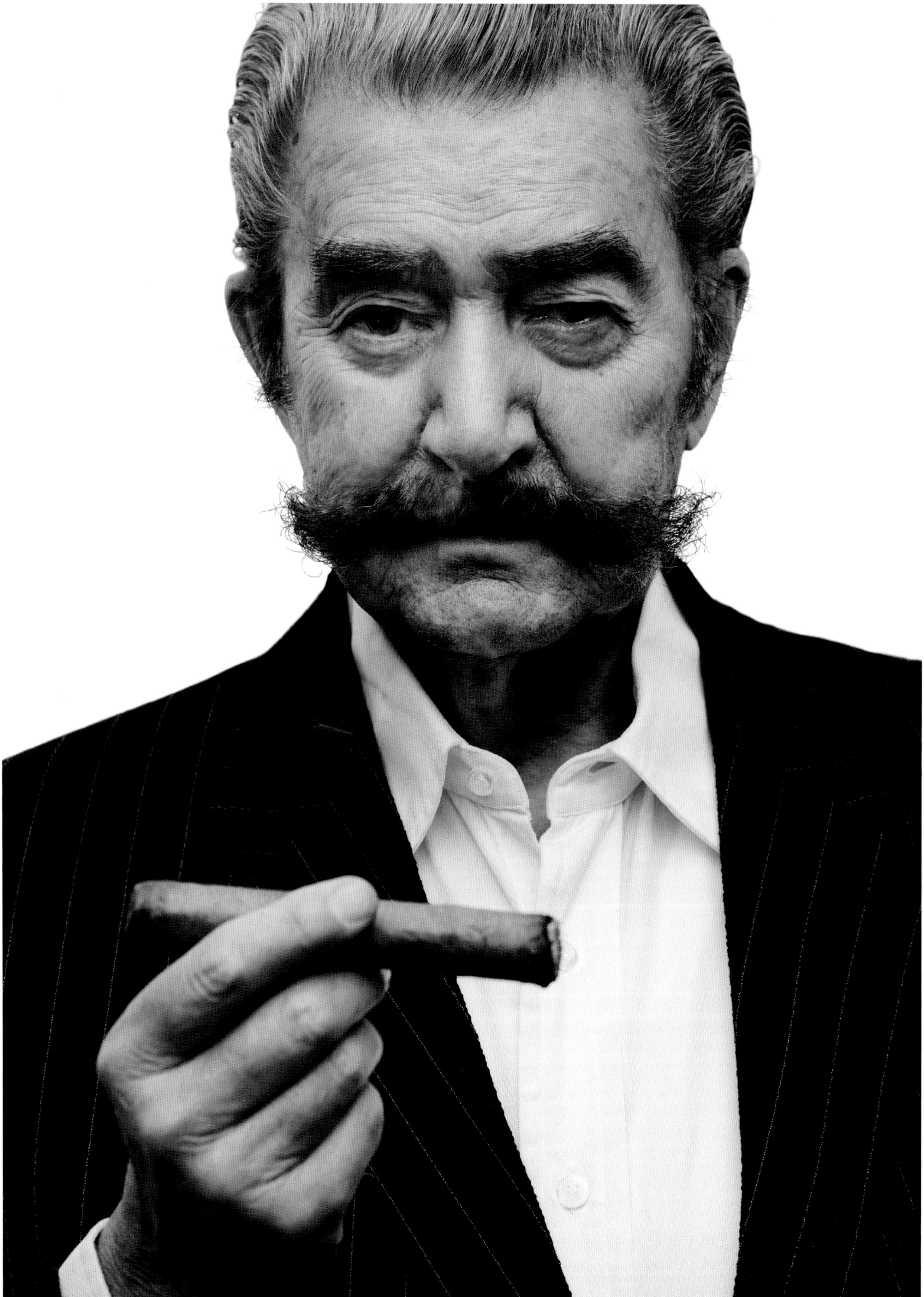

FOREWORD >

By LeRoy Neiman

In the last forty years or so I've become known as a kind of bon vivant—traveling around the world for *Playboy,* staying in first-class hotels, drinking the best wines, and eating in four-star restaurants. I suppose you could say I've led the good life for quite some time. Naturally, cigars were always a major part of that experience for me. I even had my own line of cigars, put out through Playboy and Don Diego, and that's been tremendously satisfying as well.

But then, cigars have always been an important part of my life, regardless of my so-called status. When I was about 15 years old, I started smoking cigars: Harvesters and other five-cent cigars (a ten-cent cigar from Dutch Masters was a big smoke for a kid like me). My father was poor, all our fathers were poor, but everyone I knew then smoked cigars. We did it because guys like Clark Gable and Edward G. Robinson and Al Capone did . . . guys who were conspicuous, who were action-oriented, take-charge figures. I wanted to be part of that, to be like them.

There's a certain kind of man who looks better with a cigar. My father was one of them, and I believe I am, too. As a result, the two most dominant props that I've used throughout my professional existence were developed from those experiences I had as a kid—my cigar and my moustache. I started both as a teenager, and I've never been without them. They were part of my upbringing, part of my development in deciding what I wanted to do and who I wanted to become.

Then, after I got out of the army and began my life full-time as an artist, the cigar became something more for me: an elegant symbol and a companion to each of my successes. When I began traveling in better circles, writing and illustrating the "Man at His Leisure" pieces for *Playboy,* my cigar served as just the right tool for allowing me to feel comfortable and confident in any situation: something to hold, to enjoy, to relax with.

I'm not a big aficionado. I don't get myself all worked up in the ceremony of smoking cigars, but I do know a good smoke. Of course, as you move along in life, you start tasting the better stuff and you develop more and more as a person with a wealth of experiences and a wider scope of knowledge. And the best part of that is that cigars can grow right along with you. Although I was a maduro fan for many years, when I designed my cigar I insisted on a mild, easy smoke—something comparable to a Panama hat: very light and very comfortable.

Throughout my life, cigars have played different roles for me. They've fit easily and well into the various stages and experiences I've had—like a companion, almost. If you've smoked a long time, as I have, they become part of you, a public prop that holds up in private as well. You can look at your humidor and your box of cigars as something that's always there, filled with your selections, your preferences. That's kind of a romantic notion, like the way you'd pick a wife or girlfriend (but of course, they're a lot less trouble).

Nowadays, my favorite form of relaxation is to smoke a cigar and have a glass of champagne. My tastes have mellowed a bit, from Bordeaux to Beaujolais, from Cuban cigars to my own from the Dominican Republic, but I still remain in the world of people seeking pleasure, finding fulfillment in their efforts and their work, whatever that may be. Good food, great cigars, and beautiful women—I enjoy all of those things. It's a good world if you paint the things that you enjoy, and it's a better one with a good cigar.

LeRoy Neiman

Puffing with Playboy

From the very first page of the very first issue, *Playboy* magazine has promoted the art of smoking. In the premiere December 1953 edition, the inside front cover features an illustration of the rabbit in a very Hef-like ensemble of pajamas and a smoking jacket, hoisting a highball while enjoying a puff. From that point onward, *Playboy* has maintained steady editorial coverage of both smoking and the accessories that accompany a well-appointed cigar devotee. Hef, of course, had his custom Dunhill black billiard pipe, but contributors like LeRoy Neiman and the ubiquitous Playboy Jazz Festival host Bill Cosby clung ferociously to their cigars.

Up until the early 1980s, the phrase "cigar media" was reserved for a hodgepodge of dusty trade journals that few cared about and even fewer read. Then the world started to change. In his noted 1997 *New York Times* article on the history of cigars, Tom McNichol touched upon the three most obvious contributions to cigar journalism up to that point, and all three were magazines: Al Goldstein's *Cigar* (1981), Marvin Shanken's *Cigar Aficionado* (1992), and my own *Smoke* (1995).

These magazines fed off a rising trend: a "cocktail/cigar culture" juggernaut that would later be dubbed the "cigar boom" of the mid-'90s. They would be followed by several late-to-market publications, including Jonathan Scott's *Cigar Smoker, Cigar Friendly* and *Cigar Lovers* (to name a few). The boom even spawned two national radio shows: "Lighten Up! Cigar Radio with Magic Matt Alan" and the "Cigar Dave Show." There was also a slate of feature-length documentaries: *The Art of the Cigar,* directed by John Talamini; Brett Mayer's *The Havana Cigar*; and my personal favorite, *Nude Cigar Smoking,* directed by Bert Rhine. The still-infant Web also eked out its first cigar-related sites.

However, surrounding a reemergence of artisanal cocktails, hand-rolled cigars, and big-band music were a number of media carpetbaggers and opportunists—and when the boom went bust, they simply pulled up stakes, leaving behind only two endemic titles: *Cigar Aficionado* and *Smoke.*

Today, in the midst of another resurgence (what some have dubbed a "mini-boom"), some new glossy titles have come to market, all launched in 2007: *The Cigar Report* (my second contribution to cigar periodicals), the lad mag–esque *Florida Cigar Snob,* and *Cigar Press* ("the voice of the next generation"). If *Cigar Aficionado* is geared toward the late-boomers and *Smoke* was Gen X's contribution to all things cigar, then *Cigar Press* is the Millennial Generation's take on the subject. There are some international offerings, too, most notably *Cigar Clan* (with English, Russian, and German editions), the European *Cigar Cult Journal* (German and English, one bilingual edition) and *Cigar Ambassador* (Chinese).

What McNichol oddly overlooked (as almost everyone else did, too) is that one media outlet has indeed kept cigars on the forefront of the men's lifestyle frontier for the last fifty-seven years. That publication, of course, is *Playboy.*

From its inception, *Playboy* offered covers, snippets, and features that cover and celebrate cigars. (Simply turn to the "*Playboy* Archives" chapter of this volume to see what I'm referring to, or check out *The Playboy Guide to Bachelor Parties,* by James Oliver Cury (2002) with its "Cigars 101" section.)

The magazine's traditions of smoking run so deep that it even resulted in an actual cigar launch in 1996: the Playboy by Don Diego, which eventually proved so successful that a second line (simply called Playboy) was released in 2007. Both cigars, produced by Altadis U.S.A., capitalize on a fifty-seven-year belief that a man should enjoy not just anything and everything, but really only the best that life has to offer.

6° of Separation

I. My entire career as a cigar journalist (yes, there is such a thing) is a direct result of my being, in fact, a failed *Playboy* cartoonist.

As a young teen, I chanced across a small storefront gallery in Corona del Mar (a small village just south of Newport Beach) entirely dedicated to original comics and animation. The owner, Jerry Muller, was an influential and pioneering art dealer in the medium, and much to my mother's chagrin, I befriended him (or rather, latched on to him) much in the way that Dennis the Menace glommed onto Mr. Wilson. While doing so, I attended gallery openings and lectures that Jerry gave, which in turn facilitated introductions to some of *Playboy's* most legendary cartoonists: Virgil "VIP" Partch, Phil Interlandi, John Dempsey, Bernard "Hap" Kliban, and others.

Meeting these unique and creative individuals nailed a single notion into my mind: "I will be a *Playboy* cartoonist." Once I moved back to Los Angeles as a student at USC, I started drawing in earnest, and upon graduating, dropped off my portfolio at *Playboy*'s Sunset Strip offices with a cover letter to the late Michelle Urry, *Playboy's* longtime cartoon editor. Urry rejected all of them.

Like many young people with broken dreams, I fled to grad school. Classes were at night, and to earn some pocket change, I spent days working at the newly opened Davidoff of Geneva boutique (which also housed The Keep, a private cigar club) on Via Rodeo, a faux-cobblestone tributary of Rodeo Drive.

That was when my (usually elusive) pragmatic side kicked in to high gear and prompted me to write a business plan for a trilogy of men's niche, glossy publications: *Smoke, Drink,* and *Eat.* I must have sounded like I had a vague clue as to what I was doing, because I rather quickly found business partners in New York willing to back my efforts to launch *Smoke*—which went on to become one of the most successful independent publications of its day. *Drink,* the sequel to Smoke, also came to fruition—though it achieved far less success—and *Eat* just never materialized (though my expanding waistline would indicate that I didn't suffer too terribly from the fact).

Magazine publishing was the perfect gig for me at the time; it combined my love for the visual arts, writing, and the good life: libations, fine dining, luxury travel, fashion, men's accessories . . . and (of course) cigars.

While at *Smoke,* and in one of my imitation-is-the- sincerest-form-of-flattery moves, I became dedicated to preserving two truly original American art forms: comics and cartoons. Basically, I hired all the cartoonists and illustrators whose ranks I had sought to join a few years before. By the end of my run at *Smoke,* the likes of Arnold Roth, Sam Gross, Danny Shanahan (who would also draw for *The Cigar Report*), John Dempsey, and Gahan Wilson had drawn gags for me . . . and cigar gags at that.

Rather early on in my publishing career, a mutual acquaintance who knew I loved all things *Playboy* introduced me to Chris Napolitano, who was slowly-but-steadily working his way up *Playboy's* editorial ladder (eventually, he would do a long stint as editorial director, and is now editor at large). After our first meeting, I threw him some freelance work, and over time he reciprocated the favor by having me write some cigar-related pieces for *Playboy.* Our friendship grew and endured over the rollercoaster ride of my career in print and online publishing.

So, Michelle had rejected my cartoons, but in the end Chris accepted my words. My cartoons may never reach the pages of *Playboy*—a fact I would nonetheless like to hug and thank Michelle for—but twenty years and two cigar magazines of my own later, my journey has brought me to *Playboy: The Complete Guide to Cigars.*

II. Cigars and *Playboy* have been part of my life ever since I started sneaking peeks at dad's magazine collection (I decidedly was *not* reading the articles) at around age ten. In combing through the library at the Playboy offices here in New York for the archival chapter of this book, I was struck by how many issues I recalled; in fact, while doing research, I felt as though I relived my entire childhood while flipping through those pages.

Growing up, I was also surrounded by a select and passionate group of cigar devotees, including my father and a great uncle. Cigars were always around . . . and not always just the good ones. My formative years were great for the sexual revolution and women's rights, but one could rightly classify the 1970s and early 1980s as the Dark Ages for cigars in the U.S.

Though the domestic premium cigar market back then was synonymous with the Canary Islands–produced Montecruz and Mexican-made Te-Amo (of course, Europe and the rest of the civilized world still enjoyed fine Havanas), it didn't seem to matter; even if you were smoking a Dutch Master (followed by some Mateus Rosé–yes, my friend, the '70s were ugly that way), their effect remained the same: cigars were (indeed, are) a social activity, so much so that someone once said, "Cigar smoking is a social experience . . . even when I do it alone." That same sentiment is one I've touched upon countless times in writing and lecturing about cigars.

The fraternal nature of cigars is one reiterated time and time again by other devotees and statements such as "cigars are social," "a symbol of camaraderie," "they bring out amity and promote social discourse far beyond what would have transpired without their presence," etc.

Or, in the words of my good friend Adrian, "The mere presence of wispy plumes of blue smoke that curl lazily in the languid air above one's head seems to inspire a person to attain wisdom and quiet sophistication, coupled with gruff charm."

Adrian's statement may wax a bit too poetic, but the idea behind it is universal; cigars are a hobby, not a habit, and a noble and gentlemanly leisurely pursuit—one that carries on from generation to generation.

At the height of the cigar boom, and while editing *Smoke* magazine, I was asked to pen the foreword to Mark Stucklin's concise cigar digest, *The Cigar Handbook* (Apple, 1998). The book itself was rather diminutive, with a foreword that (unlike this one) fell on the side of brevity. It recounted my first fond and pronounced memory of cigars, and I've excerpted it here because I still believe that it represents a shared memory. Oh, perhaps not identical to your own; but any dedicated cigar-smoker has their own version of this recollection:

I couldn't have been a boy of more than eight years old on the day that my father steered up our drive in his new XJ6 Jaguar, with its midnight blue lacquer and deep navy interior. The late afternoon sun sent a cascade of glimmering rays off its concupiscent bonnet, and for that instant, the XJ6 seemed like a sailfish, taut against a line, skirting the watery surface of our steep driveway. With all the curiosity that eight years bestow upon a child, I hurried over to the passenger door and climbed over to greet my Dad. I will never forget the intoxicating mélange of aromas I encountered as I climbed on to the seat: the Connolly leather hides, walnut trim, the wool carpet—and a Montecristo No. 2. It wasn't as if I'd never smelled a cigar before, but that day was different, magical. Just like that sailfish, I was hooked!

By the age of 17, I began pilfering my old man's cigars. One of the drawers of the solid oak partners desk in his office had been converted to a humidor, and it held two boxes. One day, my buddies and I skipped out of school at lunch and cruised over to his office in the Mustang convertible I had received for my birthday. I knew my father would be at the club or somewhere else for lunch, so I darted inside and grabbed four sticks (one for each guy in my posse) and peeled out of the parking lot as though I had just looted Fort Knox. We made a beeline for the Pacific Coast Highway and the beach, where we would sun-soak and puff away the rest of the afternoon.

Now, Newport Beach, CA was still a very small town in the early '80s, and a colleague of my father's had spotted both my questionable driving (never give a teenage boy a 5.0 liter V8) and that we were smoking. He promptly went to my dad and said, "David, I think I just saw your son and three of his cronies tearing down PCH at some ungodly speed with the top down—and they were all smoking your cigars!" Needless to say, Pop and I had a wee bit of a chat that night.

Curiously, he was far more upset about my speeding than the pilfering and smoking of his cigars. That night, I had a second cigar—with him. He taught me a how to cut, light, and smoke properly. And that was the end of the beginning.

The next significant cigar influence in my life is a man who was and remains a gentleman, in fact the first true gentleman of whom I had the pleasure to make acquaintance. His name is Edward Sahakian, and to this day he continues as the proprietor of Davidoff of London. I first met Edward in the late summer of 1986, when I was attending Selwyn College, Cambridge, on sojourn for studies in English Lit. I made a habit of taking the train from Cambridge to London on Saturday mornings to tour cigar stores, and sampled everything I could afford on a student's stipend. On my first expedition, I found my way to Edward's shop, where he greeted me with both a brilliant smile and a form wrapped in impeccable sartorial splendor.

During our first afternoon, and as I peppered Edward relentlessly with query after query, he effortlessly fired back answers that never seemed to satisfy my endless curiosity about Cuban cigars. At the end of what was undoubtedly an exhaustive hour and a half, I purchased one meager five-pack of Davidoff No. 2, then still made at the El Laguito factory, just on the outskirts of Havana in Miramar.

You would have thought, though, that I was purchasing a dozen boxes instead of that five-pack, given Edward's level of attention and respect. He still imparts the same intimate experience to everyone, whether princes or passersby. This is another thing about cigars at which I simply marvel: they bring out the best in men.

Years later, after the launch of *Smoke,* I visited Edward with a number of fresh copies in hand. We were in the midst of catching up when who should stroll in but Sylvester Stallone (a client of Edward's) with his stunning wife, Jennifer Flavin, by his side.

Before I go any further, I should probably mention that I was experiencing a terrible allergy attack during the trip, and had downed a handful of pills to stem the, er, river flowing from my nose. Of course, the side effect of all those wonderful medicinal chemicals was I felt as if I'd been partying for days.

Such was my mental state when Edward introduced me to Rambocky. I shook Stallone's hand and gave him a copy of the magazine. Stallone, in return, wanted my ear—and the answer to a burning question:

"Why do you think cigars have gotten so popular again?"

I stood there in my altered state, desperately trying to ponder with a head that felt detached from my body. After what seemed like (and probably was) an eternity, I responded . . .

"I simply don't know."

All three of them looked at me like I was madder than the proverbial hatter. Sly, having decided that discretion was probably the better part of valor, wished me good luck and walked out. Edward, too much the gent to ask me why my brain had shut down in the face of Rambocky, probably felt as if his years of tutorials had gone asunder.

They hadn't.

My real cigar education didn't begin, though, until I was working at the Davidoff of Geneva shop in Beverly Hills. And, as luck would have it, my indoctrination to the cigar industry was right when the first rumblings of the approaching cigar boom could be heard over the horizon. It would be impossible for me to articulate what my time at the House of Davidoff taught me; between the store, my first treks down to the Dominican Republic and Honduras and engaging in conversations with industry leaders—some still here today, some gone—I was well on my way.

Keep in mind that there were very few outsiders entering the cigar business prior to the boom, which blazed from 1993–98. Not having a last name that appeared on one of the eponymous cigar brands that dotted the smoke mise-en-scène relegated you to be viewed as a curiosity at best. (Not that the industry was xenophobic, per se; it's just a very tradition-based group, not unlike the families and individuals that work in other artisanal industries.) Slowly, though, I was accepted.

I earned my stripes working in the store, but *Smoke* is where I made my mark. Only the second publication of its kind, this glossy cigar-lifestyle and corresponding Web site (one of the first magazines to have one) came on the scene strong and never let up...that is, until my partners and I split, and it spiraled down. For a time, though, we were Avis to *Cigar Aficionado*'s Hertz, and I traveled around the world, hosting cigar dinners and lecturing on the topic (including my being the keynote speaker at the Washington Press Club's annual cigar dinner, back when such a thing existed). Along the way, I sharpened my cigar acumen and collected all manner of smoke-related accoutrements, accessories and memorabilia—and memories.

Celebrities have always been part of the cigar world, whether gracing the cover of magazines like *Smoke,* attending high-profile cigar dinners or having their own lockers at the country's more exclusive lounges. However, my all-time favorite story about cigars and celebs actually involves . . . not smoking.

When *Independence Day,* starring Will Smith and Jeff Goldblum, was released in 1996, I lined up for it like everybody else in the Western hemisphere. At the end of that popcorn-flick magnum opus, Smith and Goldblum celebrate blasting the alien invaders into itty-bitty particles by lighting up cigars. Upon seeing that, I immediately wanted Smith (then working on *Men in Black*) for the cover of *Smoke*. So my then–power publicist, Julie Nathanson, arranged a dinner with Mr. Smith at The Ivy, the steadfast see-and-be-seen L.A. eatery.

Smith and his two managers were already at the table when I arrived; I sat down and made some small talk. You could smoke on the patio at The Ivy then, but I refrained, in favor of cutting right to the chase, asking Smith to be on the next cover. He replied that, while flattered, he found cigars "nasty," so he demurred.

In addition to my surprise that he had agreed to take the meeting (knowing, after all, that I was from *Smoke*), I also felt somewhat foolish—just as a table-hopping Chris Rock sauntered over and sat down next to me. (He and Smith knew each other; Rock had even appeared in an episode of *The Fresh Prince of Bel-Air* way back when.)

Rock introduced himself to me: "Since you're the only white man at this table, I gotta assume you're *somebody*." Smith just laughed. I smiled and introduced myself, explaining that I ran a magazine and was trying to convince Smith to be on the cover. When Rock heard that Smith had passed on the opportunity, he quipped, "I'll be on your cover—I'll be on anybody's cover!"

Everyone at the table chuckled again. I said, "The only problem is, I still have no idea who you are." After all, it had been years since he played Pookie in *New Jack City,* and I'd never seen his first HBO special. At that juncture, we were fortunate enough to be getting A-list stars for the covers, and so I passed on him. Smith had already passed on me. I did enjoy a cigar on the drive home, but that was little consolation.

In the end, Kurt Russell (then releasing *Escape from L.A.*) graced that particular cover with his longtime friend and collaborator, film director John Carpenter. And, needless to say, I came to regret the decision with regard to Rock, who in my humble opinion is one of the funniest entertainers ever—whether he actually likes cigars or not.

Then it all stopped for me. Just like that.

Not my love for cigars, mind you; that remained stronger than ever. But my *Smoke* partners parted, and I went on to, as they say, "pursue other interests." Even as I did, the cultural wave that brought cigars to such a pinnacle began to temporarily dip.

Which brings us to today. The leap that transformed cigar aficionados in the waning years of the twentieth century to social pariahs in the beginning of the twenty-first has been a remarkably short one. Despite the omnipresent propagation of draconian antismoking legislation, however, there has (ironically) never been a better time than now to be a cigar enthusiast.

Recent years have heralded the arrival of complex blends (not to mention stellar packaging) as well as the rise of cigar "speakeasies": a proliferation of smoke-friendly rooftop bars and outdoor cigar festivals. In tandem, these developments have lead to some record sales years, proving that you can't snuff out a five-centuries-old gentlemanly pursuit, especially one that symbolizes amity the way cigars do.

This new landscape has fostered a contemporary breed of cigar crafters (and related accessory makers) who are bringing vitality to a once-stale industry. It is a welcome change. That second wave of cigar media, including *The Cigar Report, Cigar Clan, Cigar Magazine,* and *Cigar Press,* has firmly entrenched itself as well. Throughout all this, the amusing thing is that *Playboy* never lost its beat, continuing to cover the subject with aplomb.

The following pages highlight *Playboy's* dedication to cigars. Not unlike *Playboy's* original mission of guiding America from its puritanical iciness to sexual liberation, *Playboy: The Complete Guide to Cigars* emphasizes, if nothing else, one thing: you cannot legislate morality. So, have a drink (or even two), light up the biggest cigar you can, eat a juicy steak, have incredible sex, and remember that anything as satisfying as these things is worth fighting for and learning more about.

I hope you enjoy the book.

Sig
New York City
2009

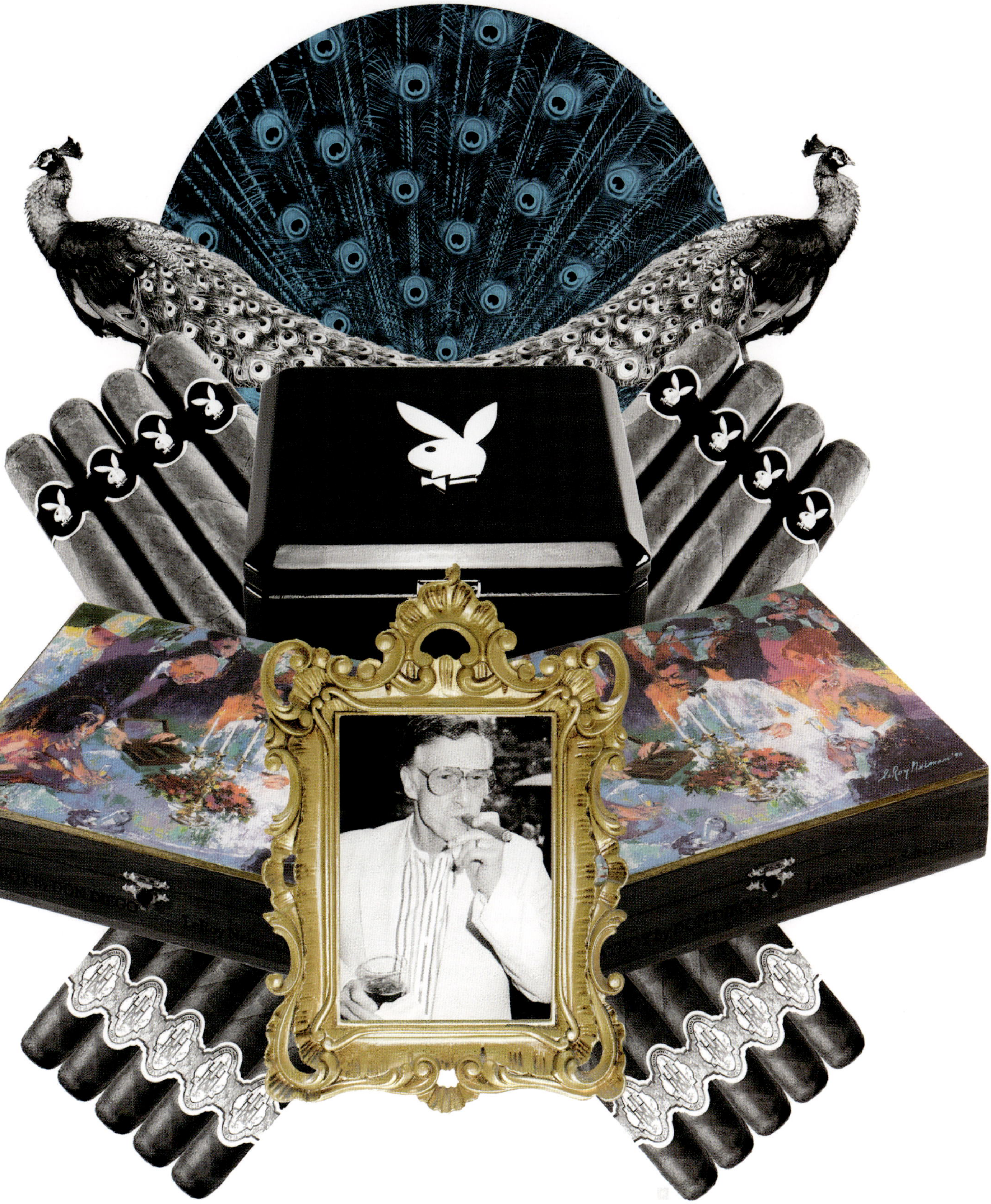

Hugh Hefner, a dedicated pipe smoker for many years, on one of the rare occasions he smoked a cigar—at the Playboy Mansion West party celebrating the launch of the Playboy by Don Diego cigar. Other Playboy-related cigars include the limited-edition LeRoy Neiman and *new* Playboy cigar.

PART I

A VERY BRIEF HISTORY

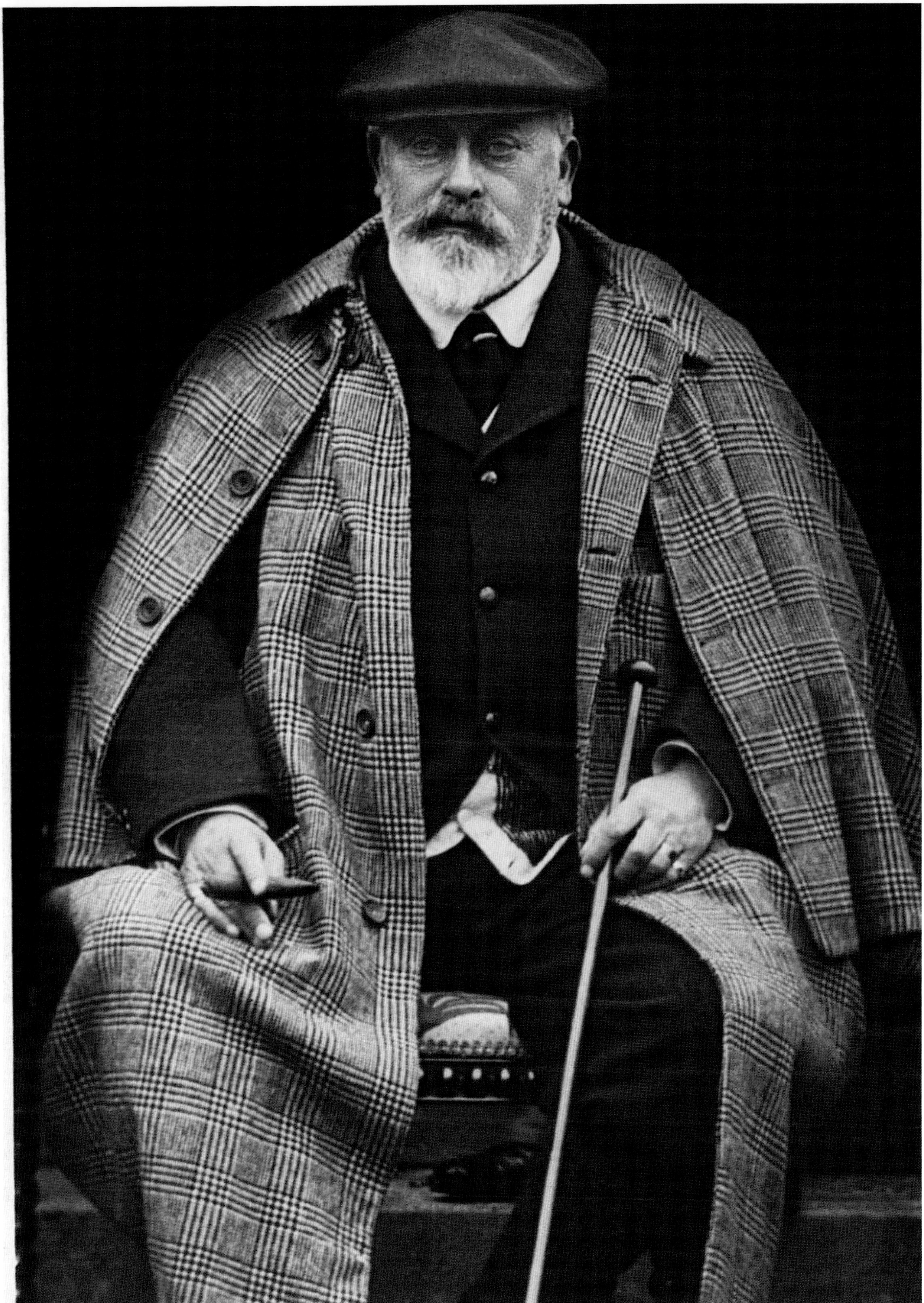

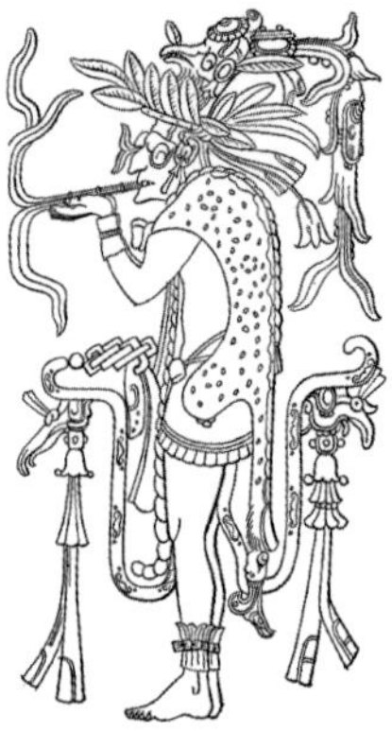

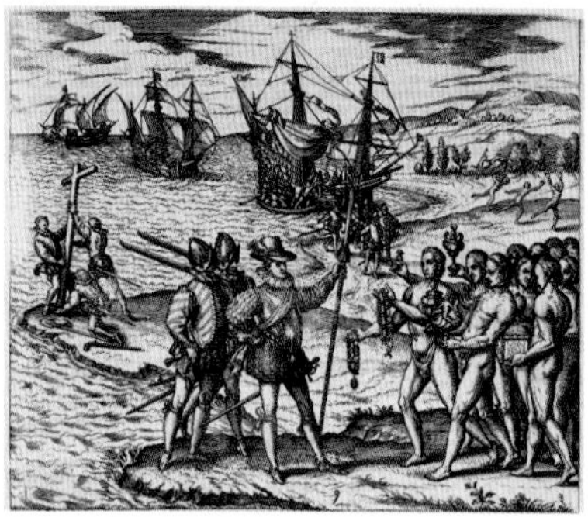

(Previous page) King Edward VII of England; (this page) Mayan jaguar priest; (opposite page, left to right) Ulysses S. Grant, portrait of Stéphane Mallarmé by Edouard Manet.

Ancient Times–1492

> Holy Smoke in Mesoamerica

"Son, bring me the firefly of the night. Its odor shall pass to the north and to the west. Bring with it the beckoning tongue of the jaguar."
—Book of the Chilam Balam (jaguar priest)
of the Chumayel people

Cigars, like beer, wine, and most of the world's great pleasures, find their origins rooted in religion. The Mayan Indians—who at the height of their culture occupied a vast swath of modern-day Guatemala, Belize, El Salvador, Honduras, the Yucatán Peninsula, and southern Mexico—smoked tobacco as part of their religious rituals (in addition to developing a written language, a 365-day yearly calendar, and vegetable cultivation—no slackers, they).

Artifacts from the period portray both nobles and Mayan deities puffing away. Their verb for smoking, *sikar,* would eventually be co-opted by the Spanish into a noun, *cigarro.*

Nor were the Mayans alone in their enjoyment of smoking: from the tribes in Mexico and North America puffing on pipes to the Aztecs setting fire to tobacco-stuffed reeds, it was something enjoyed by a broad swath of cultures in the Americas.

1492

> Meet The Tainos

In 1492, Columbus sailed the ocean blue. After a five-week journey from the Canary Islands, one involving epic waves, huge distances, and likely increasingly awesome body odor on the part of all involved, the explorer's crewmen dropped anchor within sight of the Bahamas. From there, it was another sixteen days' sailing before they arrived off the coast of Cuba on October 28, 1492.

Once ashore, two of the explorers named Luis de Torrès and Rodrigo de Jerez came upon an unusual sight: indigenous people puffing away at lit "catapults" (most likely rolled plant leaves) stuffed with tobacco. These were the Taino Indians, who inhabited not only Cuba but also Hispaniola (modern-day Haiti and Dominican Republic). One can imagine how the Spaniards, still stressed from the most cramped and terrifying Atlantic crossing prior to the invention of the 747 and coach class, responded to the sight of people calmly drinking smoke:

"We'd like some of that. Now."

In the first recorded case of "bumming" a smoke, Jerez took a deep puff of the natives' catapult, and promptly became the Old World's first hardcore connoisseur. (And in the first recorded case of antismoking regulations, the Spanish Inquisition would later condemn his new fixation and toss him in prison for seven years.)

Over the next several years, Columbus would visit most of the region's prime tobacco-growing spots, including Hispaniola and Honduras, collecting leaves along the way, but he himself largely abstained from smoking. Instead, other famous figures of the next few centuries became linked with tobacco's spread to the Old World.

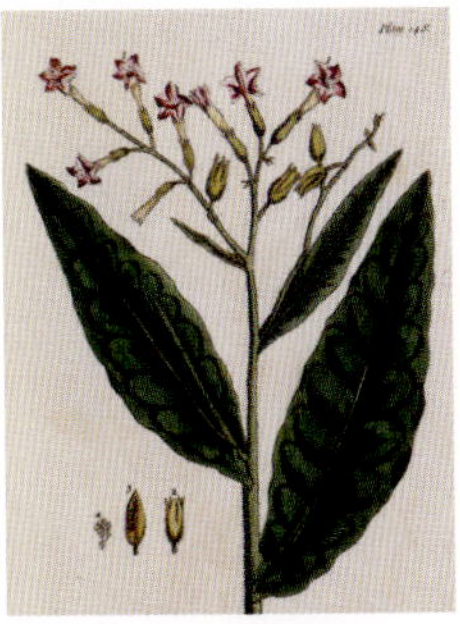
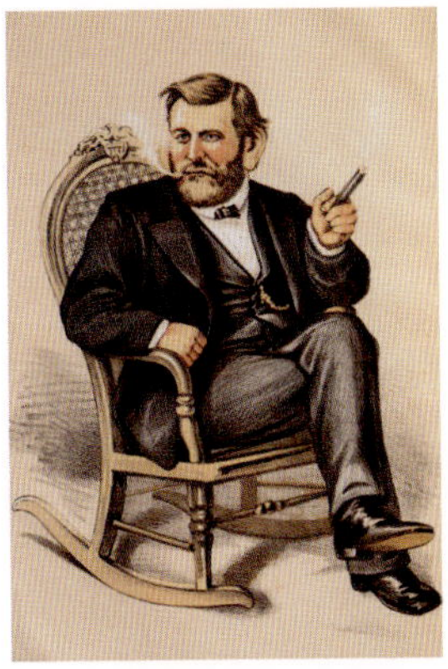
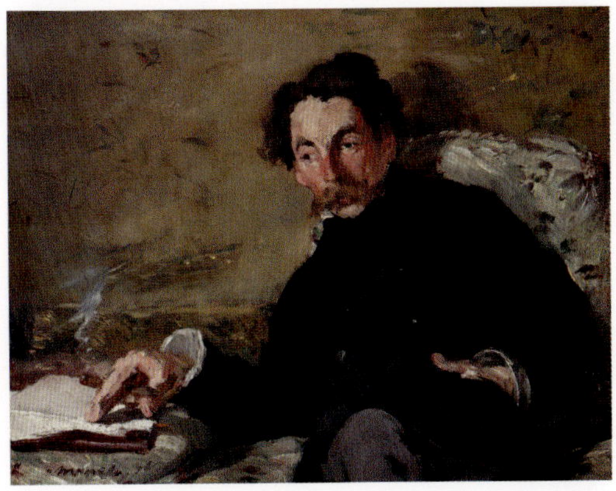

1518–1901

> Europe's New Thrill

One circle of historians credits Hernán Cortés with bringing the first actual tobacco seeds back to Spain in 1518. The Portuguese and Dutch argue that their own heroes were the first to import the plant. Another good story has pearly colonist-poet-adventurer Sir Walter Raleigh introducing tobacco to Jolly Ol' England, although chances are better that it came overseas from France after ambassador Jean Nicot brought the plant there from Portugal. Although tobacco started as a medicinal cure (Nicot wrote in 1573 that the plant, which he named "nicotiane," was "an herb of marvelous virtue against all wounds, ulcers, noli me tangere, herpes, and other such like things"), smoking it evolved into a pastime of note among the French and Spanish, and spread from there to other European nations, endlessly fascinated by novelty. Backed by its growing popularity, a farmer's potential earnings from growing an acre of tobacco soon outraced that of staple crops by a healthy multiple, and tobacco plantations sprouted throughout the Americas, from Virginia to the Caribbean.

England's King James I, along with a variety of continental monarchs ever anxious to appear as moral stalwarts, may have railed against its supposed evils in decree and print—but none seemed too concerned with taxing the plant to fill the royal coffers.

How Europeans of various nationalities smoked was largely dependent on where in the New World their colonists had stumbled on tobacco. The natives encountered by the British largely smoked pipes, and so pipes initially became standard-issue in England. Spain, in contrast, took its influences from the Caribbean basin, and thus smoked the precursor of the modern cigar.

When Napoleon decided to overcompensate for his lack of tallness by invading Spain, and the British decided that fighting him there (from 1808 until 1814, in the Peninsular War) was preferable to that miniature megalomaniac controlling yet another chunk of Europe, returning soldiers on both sides brought Spain's cigars home with them.

Cigars soon became a hit in Britain, and even more à la mode in France. Factories started up to fuel the fad, and Edward VII (who would later make the famous pronouncement, "Gentlemen, you may smoke," after the death of his mother Victoria), even took up puffing—a fact that must have left his predecessor, James I, spinning in his crypt.

Ulysses S. Grant (1822–1885) often smoked a cigar while considering his next strategic or tactical maneuver. During the Battle of Shiloh in April 1862, after the Union Army had taken a particularly brutal beating, General William Sherman found Grant sitting under a tree, puffing away.

"Well, Grant, we've had the Devil's own day, haven't we?" Sherman said. Considering the previous hours' casualties, this statement qualified as one of the great understatements of the century.

Grant remained unperturbed. The cigar (an item whose calming effects have been noted since its discovery) may likely have helped his quiet.

"Yes," Grant replied, breathing smoke.
"Lick 'em tomorrow, though."

And so they did.

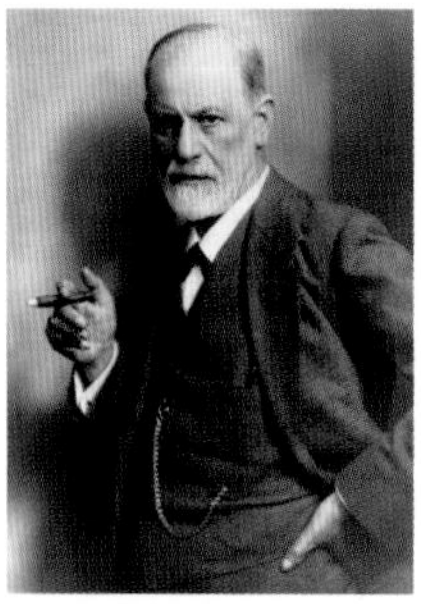

One historical figure was particularly famous for smoking while thinking: Sigmund Freud (1856–1939), who puffed over a dozen small sticks a day and once proclaimed cigars "one of the greatest and cheapest enjoyments in life." Although the Austrian-born father of psychoanalysis spent his days parsing his patients' deepest fantasies and the subtexts of their dreams, he also famously said, in response to others trying to seek deeper meaning in his favorite lifestyle accoutrement: "Sometimes a cigar is just a cigar."

1518–1901

> Meanwhile, Back in the Americas

Colonization and invasion continued to drive the cigar's expansion on both sides of the Atlantic. In 1762, after the Brits made a saucy attempt to wrest Cuba from the Spanish as part of the Seven Years' War, soldier and future American patriot Israel Putnam brought Cuban tobacco seeds to New England, perhaps launching the proud tradition of Connecticut-grown leaf.

In the decades following the American Revolution, cigar production along the Eastern Seaboard reached into the tens of millions of sticks, with factories springing up from New England to Florida. Indeed, cigars became intensely popular in the United States from the early nineteenth century onwards. Many a gentleman carried their cigars around in a pig's bladder (the preferred conveyance in the days before cedar boxes). Authors including Mark Twain praised the virtues of the stogie. General Ulysses S. Grant kept one smoking in his mouth while surveying the battlefields of the Civil War.

The nineteenth century was also the beginning of Cuba's moment in the sun, cigar-wise. A decree by King Ferdinand VII in 1821, allowing Cubans to not only grow leaf but also roll cigars, turned the island into a production powerhouse. No longer would Cuban tobacco merely be shipped to the world's factories.

Even as their cigar prestige increased, the Cubans themselves launched a fight for independence from the mother country. Readers in Florida's cigar factories read the latest revolutionary news from the island to the rollers, who in turn funneled cash to plotters such as Cuban philosopher and political thinker José Martí. When the time came, many also ventured with Martí to Cuba to fight the Spanish.

Eventually, the battles on the island grew to such intensity that the United States stepped in, igniting the Spanish-American War in 1898—the conflict perhaps most famous for its iconic image of Teddy Roosevelt and the Rough Riders charging up San Juan Hill on their way to a resounding American victory.

By 1902, Roosevelt had become president, and ceded Cuba its independence, with caveats: The U.S. would maintain a base at Guantánamo Bay and an ability to intercede in the island's affairs, which it did in 1906, reoccupying Cuba for another three-year stint before again ceding independence. The U.S. government, along with business interests and La Cosa Nostra, would keep their fingers deep in the island's affairs until the rise of Castro.

1901–1973

> World on Fire

Politics and cigars have always had some common ground. You need a cloud of carbonized tobacco, after all, to fill those rooms where the big decisions are made. In contrast to today's politicians, who like to appear as if they live off nothing more than distilled water and a daily 10K, many of the early twentieth century's leaders smoked and drank quite openly (whether that chemical boost helped them generate ideas is an open question; but it likely made their jobs more endurable.)

A few politicians became as famous for their cigars as they were for policy decisions. During Woodrow Wilson's presidency, his unassuming and now largely-forgotten vice president, Thomas Marshall, uttered for a senate clerk's amusement the most oft-quoted quote: "What this country needs is a good five-cent cigar." (Historians have asserted that Marshall, rather than dreaming up that zinger himself, was merely repeating a joke from a popular newspaper comic.)

And, of course, the twentieth century also saw the rise of Winston Churchill, that cigar enthusiast par excellence who kept several thousand sticks at his country home, Chartwell Manor, and smoked between eight and ten of them daily. Having first acquired the smoking lifestyle while visiting Havana in late 1895, the prime minister developed a lifelong attachment to Cuban cigars: one so strong that, during World War II, he had the pilots of an unpressurized plane modify an oxygen mask so he could continue to puff away while in flight. Unsurprisingly, a truly massive cigar size, the Churchill (generally seven inches long, with a 47 ring gauge), was named after him.

Perhaps influenced by the constant presence of cigars in the hands of the famous and powerful, everyday people continued to smoke sticks in mass numbers through the postwar period. By 1973, some 11.2 billion cigars—a substantial portion of them machine-made—were sold annually in the United States (up from 9.9 billion in 1964). Thomas Marshall would have approved.

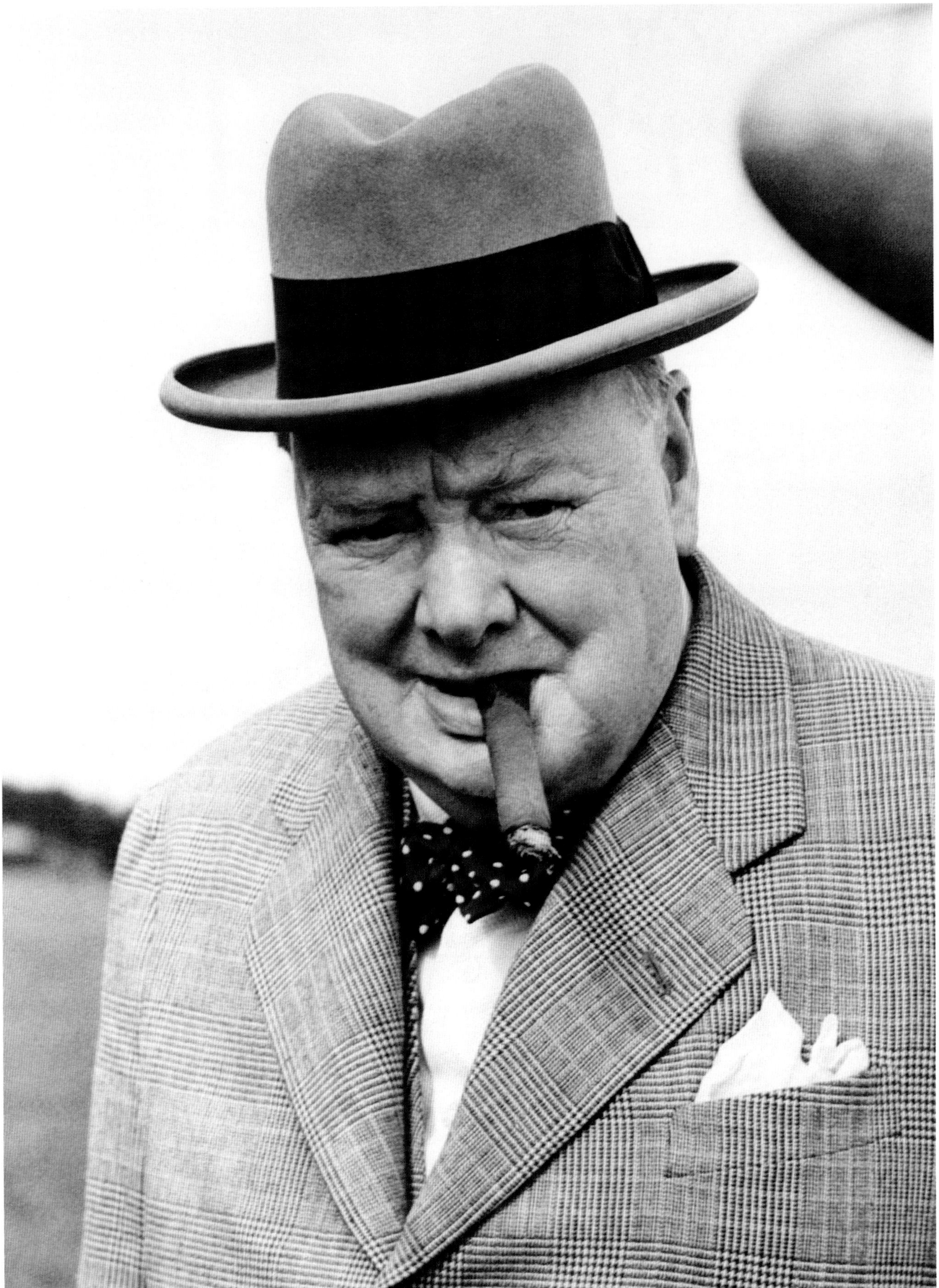

Winston Churchill: statesman, author, painter, cigar superstar

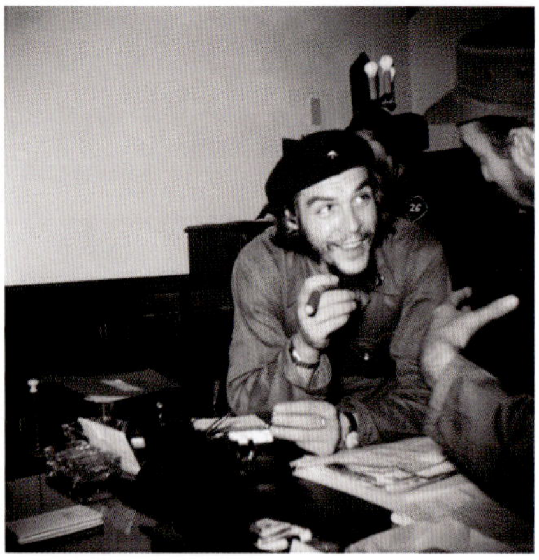 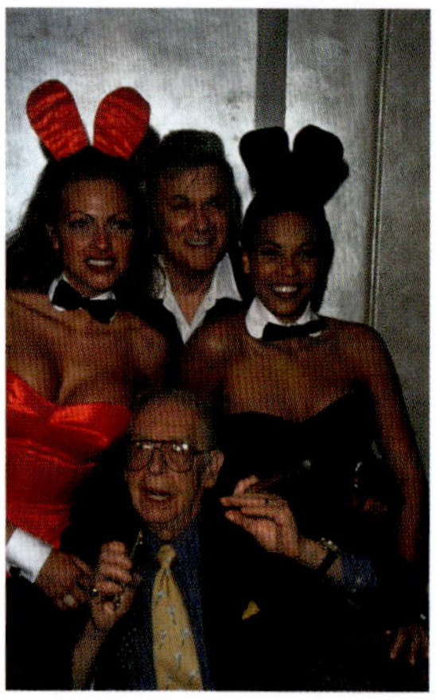

Thanks to Mark Twain and others, cigars achieved a prominent place in the literature of the nineteenth century. In the twentieth, as paper gave way to film as the mass-entertainment medium of choice, cigars became a mainstay of movie stars and their iconic characters. Groucho Marx, Orson Welles, and John Wayne were just a few of the cinematic legends puffing away while doing what they did best and Hollywood titans such as Jack L. Warner and Darryl Zanuck torched up as they mulled what they'd have the American public watching next year.

Perhaps unsurprisingly, cigars became a mainstay in macho genres such as crime flicks and Westerns. Something about a smoking stogie, cocked at a rakish angle, made Edward G. Robinson or Al Pacino that much more subtly menacing—not to mention Clint Eastwood's Man With No Name, whose Toscano (also useful for lighting the fuse of badman-exploding dynamite bundles) seemed almost as much a part of his persona as his six-shooter.

1973–2008

> From Boom to Bust to Boom 2.0

"Ah, cigars . . . the ponytail of the nineties."
—Dana Gould

In the years following the Cuban Revolution and the U.S. embargo (more on that in our Cuba chapter), the island's exiled cigar makers fled to the Canary Islands and Miami before scouting out new countries in which to resume their rolling. Soon, cigars from the Dominican Republic, Honduras and Nicaragua began to fill the void in American humidors left by Kennedy's embargo.

Despite this diversification, fewer Americans smoked cigars throughout the 1970s and 1980s, and by the early 1990s the number of premium cigars imported annually had fallen to the 100 million mark (cigar consumption itself had dropped to 3.4 billion per year for both premium and machine-made sticks). Cigars as a viable lifestyle seemed as doomed to marginality as the suit styles worn by Edward G. Robinson in *Little Caesar.*

Then came the cigar boom of the mid-1990s. By 1997, 417.8 million cigars were imported into the U.S., and the average cigar price rose precipitously. Across the Caribbean basin, hundreds of new cigar factories sprung up as smoke entrepreneurs (some legitimate and quality-minded, others mere carpetbaggers looking to ride the wave to a quick buck) set up their own labels and scrambled to hoard as much quality tobacco as they could find. Glossy cigar magazines became huge sellers.

What goes up, though, must come down. As U.S. and foreign markets flooded with inferior product, sales figures for premium cigars went flat after 1998. Cigar producers who stuck to creating high-quality sticks largely weathered the dip; those willing to flood the street with anything for money packed up and went on to exploit the next big thing.

The smokers left behind had boom-educated palates, and they started seeking out both their old favorites as well as new cigars. By 2007, despite smoking bans in many American cities, imports had climbed again to 335.1 million sticks, the third-best (after 1997 and 1998) since the figures were first tabulated.

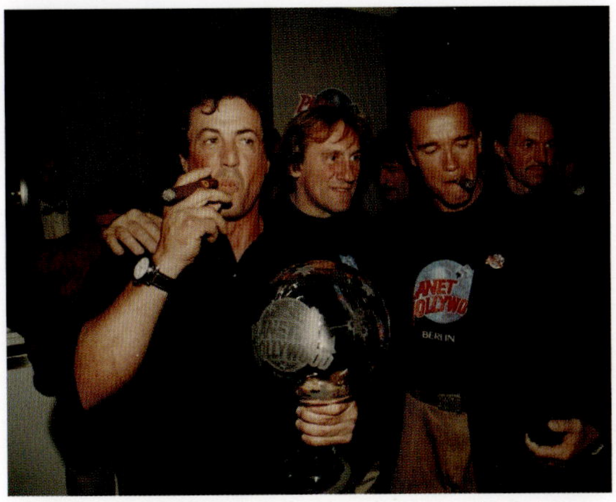

(From left) Mid-century: Ernesto "Che" Guevara and Milton "Mr. Television" Berle (with Tony Curtis and 1996 Playmate of the Year Stacy Sanches); late twentieth century: Sly and Arnold puffing away with Gérard Depardieu.

2008 and on . . .

> The Best and Worst of Times

Some cities have instituted the strictest possible bans on smoking (as in Chicago, where the number of cigar stores and lounges has dwindled to near-zero, and the California town of Calabasas, where torching up is forbidden not only inside, but also in public common areas such as parking lots and sidewalks), while others such as New York remain somewhat unimpeded—although smoking that Montecristo on your way down Fifth Avenue now comes with a slight thrill of the forbidden, like slugging from a pocket flask on the bus in 1928.

Not so in many other countries around the world, which have greeted their new rise in wealth (not to mention the appearance of a middle class) with cigar booms of their own. In Hong Kong (China) and mainland China, sales of cigars (mostly Cuban) have increased along with that nation's increasing industrialization. In Russia, the rise of an ultra-wealthy class has led to the appearance of cigar bars all over Moscow, where oligarchs can torch up in a style not seen since the days of the tsars.

Nonetheless, this new landscape has fostered a contemporary breed of cigars and makers—as well as related accessories—that is bringing vitality to a once stale industry . . . a breath of fresh air (though perhaps not in the form of sweet breath) to cigars. The blends, quality, and availability of handmade, long-filler premium cigars have all reached a point unrivaled in history. Best of all, instead of relying on the pig's bladders of yesteryear, modern man can keep his prized smokes in an actual box.

TERROIR

TOBACCONIST

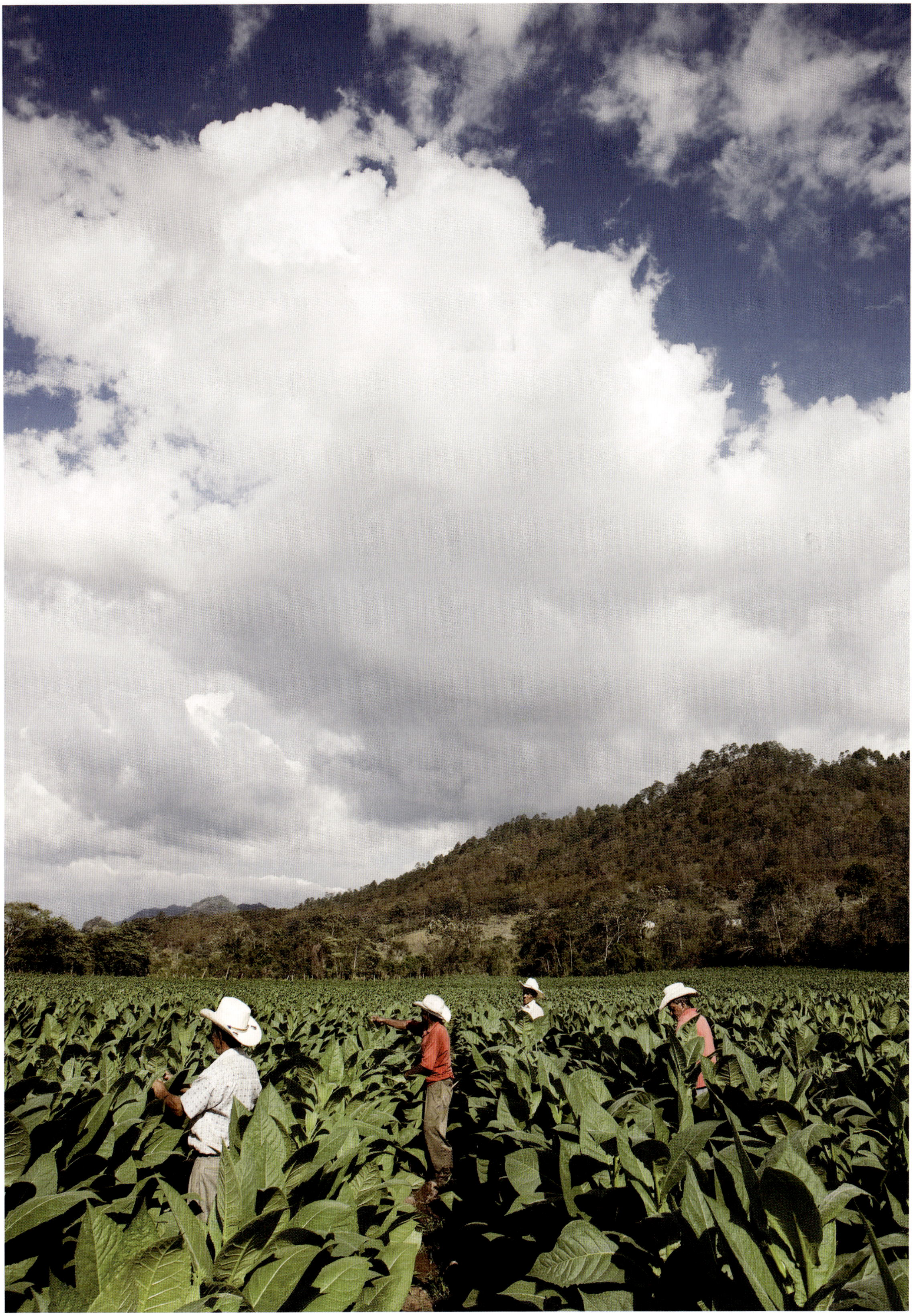

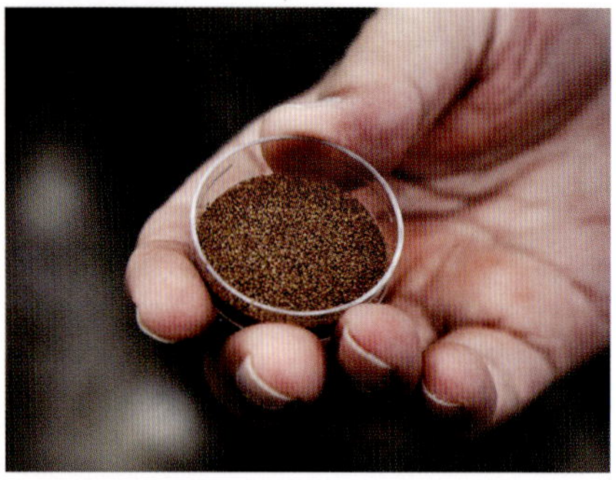

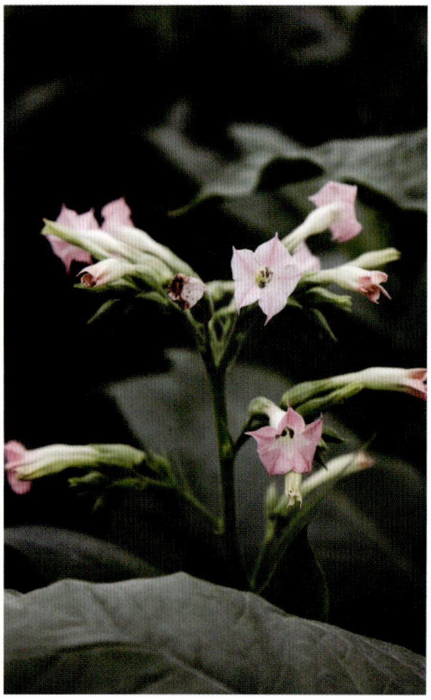

(Clockwise from bottom left) From the flower of *Nicotiana tabacum*, to seed, to seedling, to 30-day growth, to mature plant (opposite page) to harvest, to curing barn

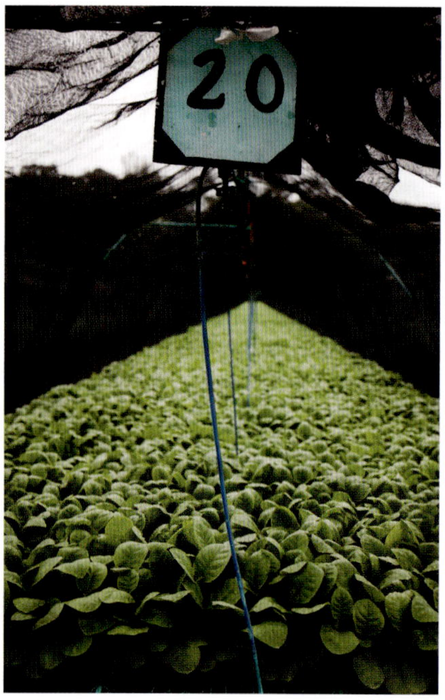

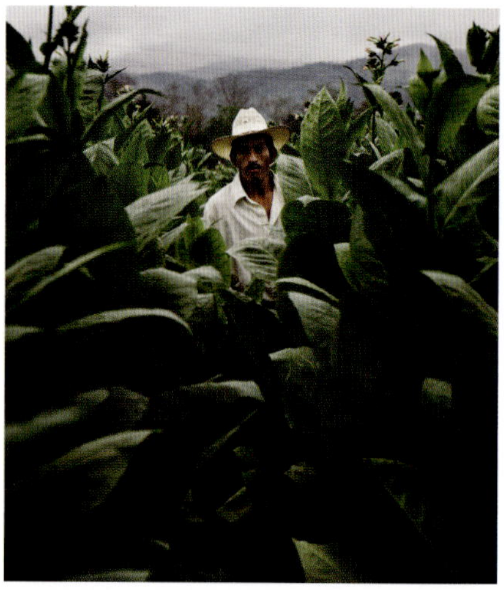

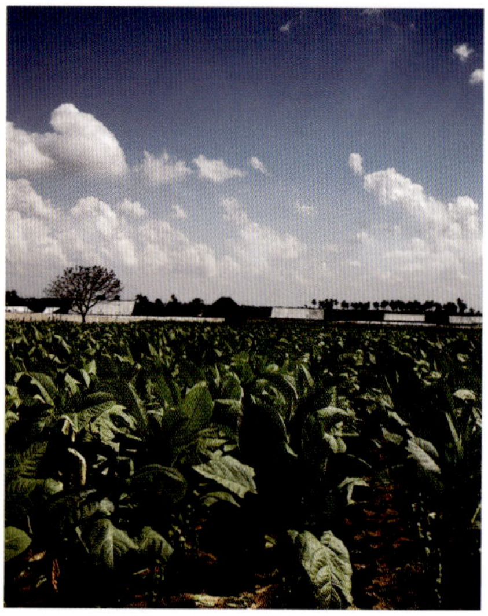

IN THE BEGINNING > What ends in your humidor starts in the soil—and not just any soil. The best tobacco for cigars relies on a finely tuned mixture of earth, temperature, and sunlight. Whether in Cuba's Vuelta Abajo, the Dominican Republic's Cibao Valley, the highlands of Nicaragua, or growing areas even further afield (such as the Sumatra or Cameroon), geographical differences influence tobacco's taste.

Whatever the species of tobacco being planted (though all fall under the genus *Nicotiana*), the seeds themselves are barely larger than grains of sand, and thus planters take particular care to nurture them in the initial stages. Within the cigar compounds that dot Central America and the Caribbean Islands, the first green buds sprout from specially prepared dirt trays inside Plexiglas-and-mesh nurseries. These are then field-planted near the end of October, covered with cloth or straw to block sunlight, and monitored constantly by teams of *vegueros,* or planters. After a certain point, the covering is taken away to expose the growing plants to the full blast of the sun. For shade-grown wrapper, cheesecloth tents (called *tapados*) are erected over the fields to block the light.

Whatever the technique used, the time between transplant and harvest generally takes around four months (there is variation in growing time, depending on the tobacco's ultimate purpose; wrapper leaves tend to be left longer before cutting). Cooler temperatures and moderate rain are most conducive to growth: Many a farmer's season has been wrecked by excessive rainfall. In Vuelta Abajo, temperatures during the dry season (when tobacco is customarily grown) rarely drift north of 75°F, and the land receives less than two inches of rain per month.

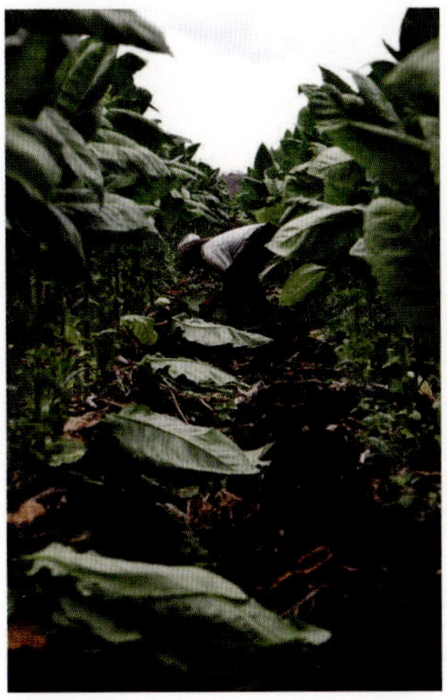

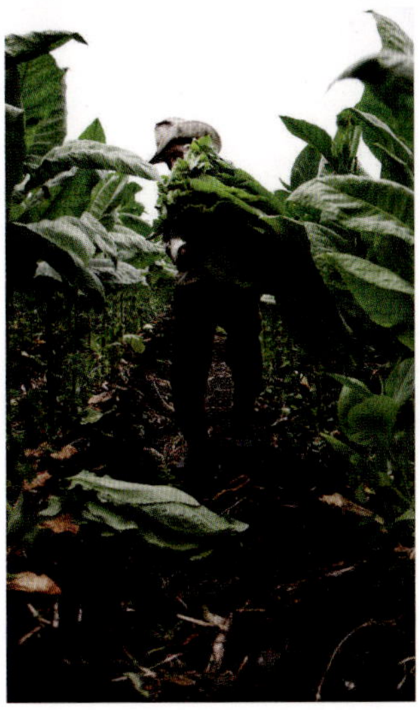

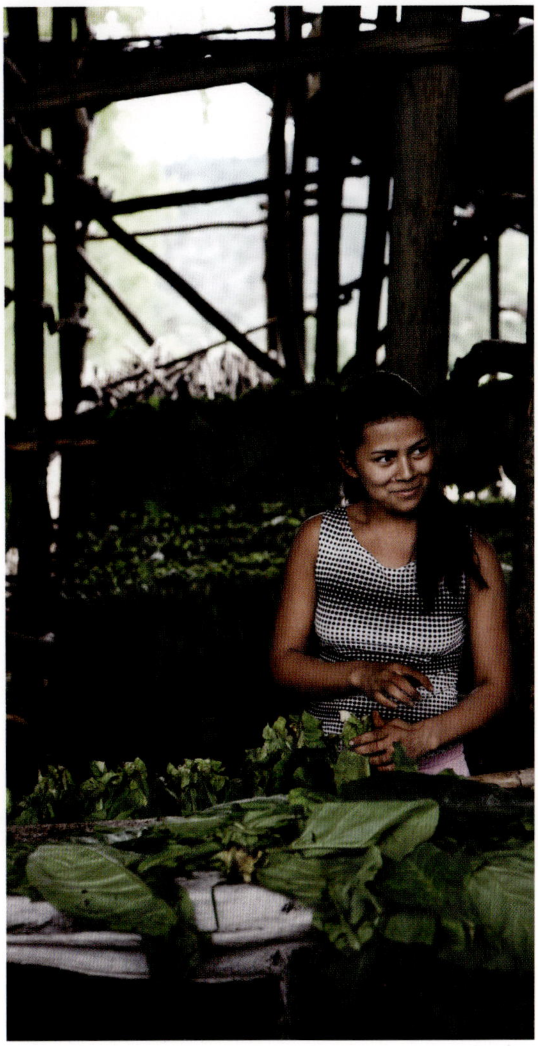

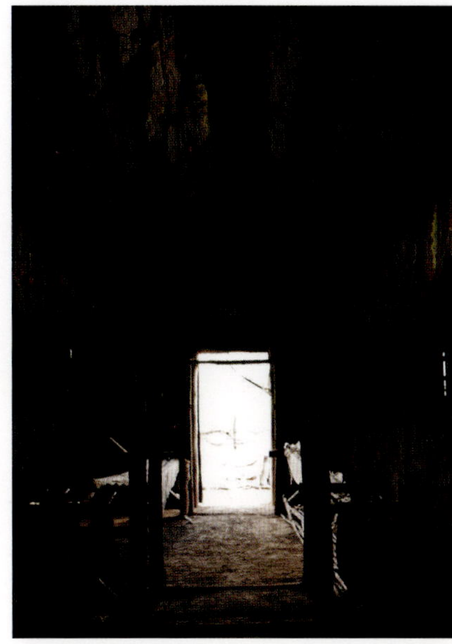

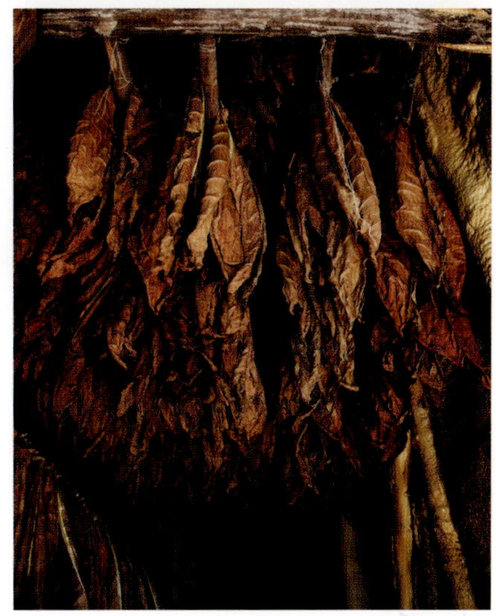

Then harvesting begins. Workers move through the fields, taking the bottom leaves of each plant first. Once collected, the tobacco is taken to the *casa de tabaco,* where other workers string them by the hundred onto long poles and lift them into the building's rafters, to cure for twenty-five to forty-five days. Across the cigar world, the *casa de tabaco* has remained in its centuries-old form: a multistory wooden shack with dirt floor and narrow windows whose shutters can be opened or closed to control temperature and humidity levels. However, many farms (such as those run by Mexico's Turrent family, producers of Te-Amo cigars) have constructed ultramodern curing barns using metal sheeting and massive machines to control those variables.

The length of the curing varies according to the type of tobacco and the leaf-color desired at the end of the process (occasionally, a grower will light fires in pits beneath the tobacco to help them achieve the necessary tint), but eventually the air circulating through the *casa de tabaco* leeches the sugar and water from the leaf until it adopts the familiar brown hue.

PARTS OF THE PLANT

The amount of sun a leaf receives will determine its amount of oils; more oil translates into a stronger taste. When it comes to selecting tobaccos used for filler, those top portions of the plant, exposed full to daylight, known as *Ligero*, will be stronger and slower-burning than those from the middle (lighter-colored, and known as *Seco*), and they are more powerful than the mildest leaves found near the bottom (*Volado*). Stronger cigars will feature a higher portion of Ligero as filler; milder cigars may be virtually all Volado inside the wrapper.

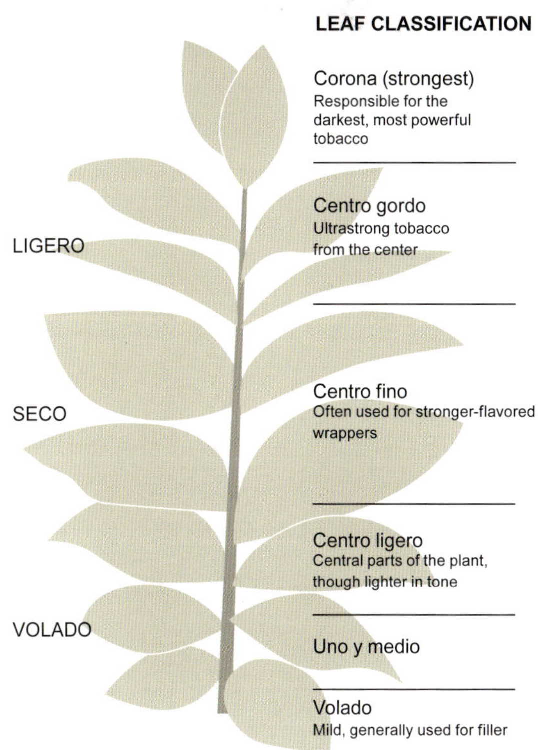

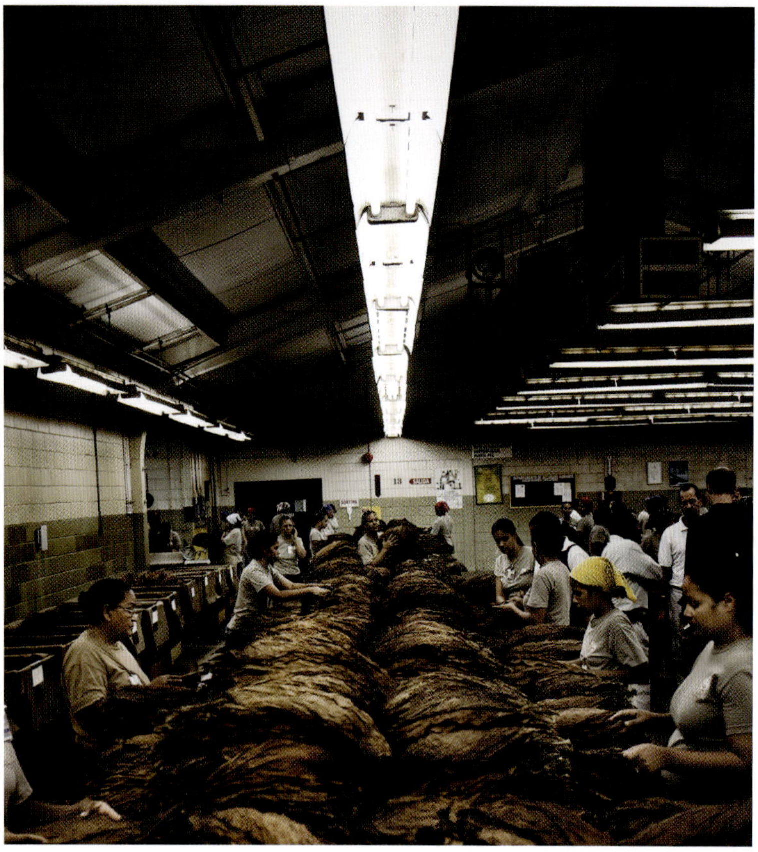

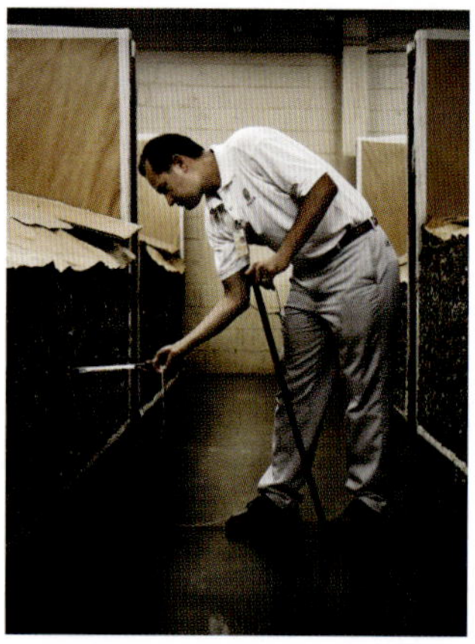

(Clockwise from left) Sorting, *pilon* temperature check, compressing a bale of short filler

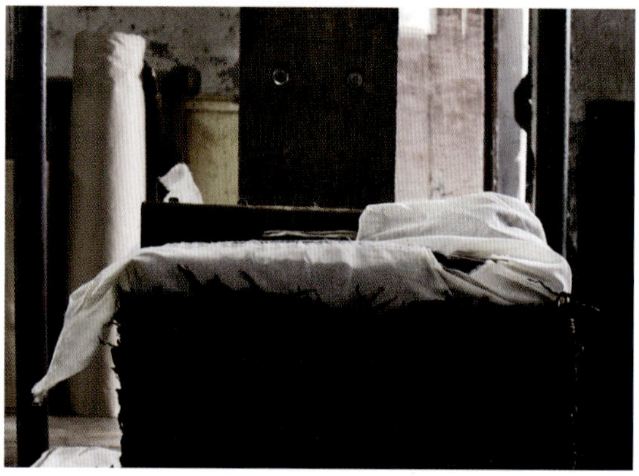

THE NEXT STEP > Now comes fermentation. Most cigar makers consider aspects of their fermentation process proprietary; in truth, no two cigar manufacturers have identical processes, though the end result of "finished" tobacco remains the constant. As such, what's described here is a more traditional method.

The cured leaves will be taken down from their racks and moved into a warehouse. Then—after being sorted—they'll be stacked into waist-high rectangular piles called *pilones*. With so much nitrogen-rich tobacco pressed tightly together, the pilones rapidly heat up, a carefully monitored process. If the pile's temperature reaches a maximum threshold (110–130°F depending on the tobacco's texture), the workers rotate the pile, moving the inner leaves outward to cool. Otherwise, the pilones are rotated every two weeks, ensuring even fermentation for all leaves—during which each pilon may be rotated up to twelve times. This initial fermentation takes between sixty and seventy days, after which the pilones are broken down and the leaves cooled. But that's far from the end—after this first fermentation is complete, some of the tobacco will undergo two more rounds before it is deemed ready for use in a rolled cigar.

Before the next round, however, the cooled leaves undergo yet another sorting, as they're divided with an eye toward their eventual use. Walk through the cavernous rooms of a typical cigar factory and you'll see workers at long tables carefully sorting leaves according to size, color, texture, pliability, and a variety of other factors under the watchful eyes of inspectors.

Afterward, the tobacco is sent deep into the factory for a second round of fermenting, this time in stacks known as *burros*. For more than two months, the fermentation rooms will fill with nearly overpowering ammonia fumes as the leaves expel their impurities.

Once finished, the wrapper, select binder, and long filler leaves are packed in *tercios* (traditional bales made of palm bark and hemp rope) for an additional one to two years of aging. The tercios provide a soft maturation—one without any sudden changes in temperature—which enhances the flavor and aroma of the tobacco.

All tobacco, after being stripped of its stem and sorted, is dried out and packed in burlap for additional aging.

Tobacco not placed in traditional palm-bark tercios is packed straight away in burlap bales or wooden crates, where the leaves wait (sometimes for years) for rolling to begin.

LEAF DESTINED FOR CERTAIN CIGAR BLENDS UNDERGOES ADDITIONAL AGING SPECIAL PROCESSES > All the shade wrapper leaf intended for General Cigar Co.'s famed Macanudo cigars is hand-picked in New England (in the picturesque Connecticut River Valley), processed in the Dominican Republic, then sent to Hatfield, Massachusetts, for one winter. During that season, the tobacco dries out slowly, its humidity level dipping below 10 percent. As spring comes, sustained moisture returns to the tobacco leaves, enhancing the aroma and flavor of the resultant cigars.

Another manufacturer, Aurora S.A., the oldest cigar maker in the Dominican Republic uses seasoned oak barrels that once held Dominican rum to further age tobacco for four years. The principle behind barrel aging is not to impart flavor to the cigar (the rum has long been leached out of the staves). Rather, barrel aging keeps the leaves in a nearly sealed environment, concentrating the heat and the maturation. The result is the tobacco used in the coveted La Aurora Barrel Aged cigars.

After all these myriad fermentation and aging processes comes the actual rolling of the cigars.

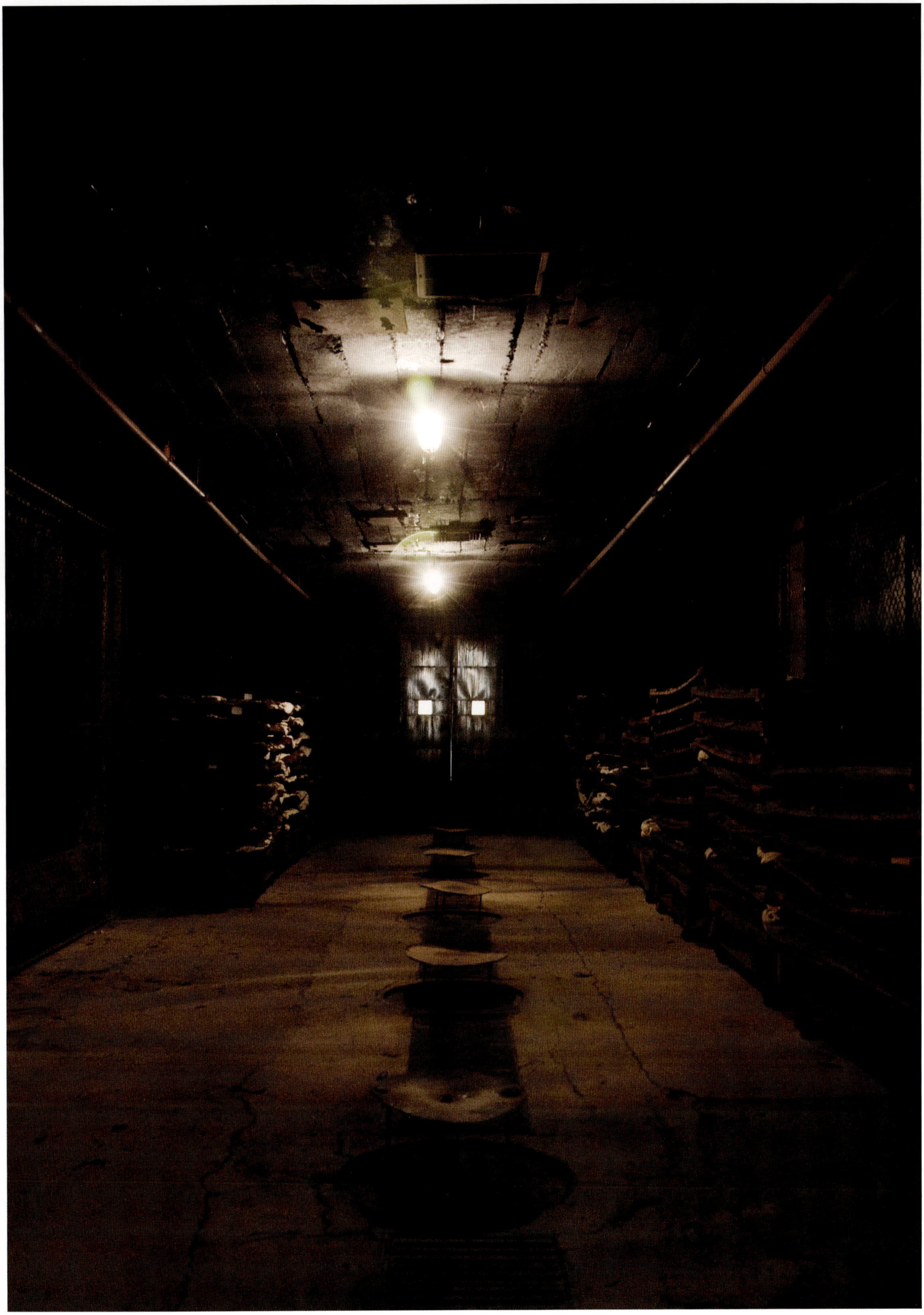

FILLER & BINDER

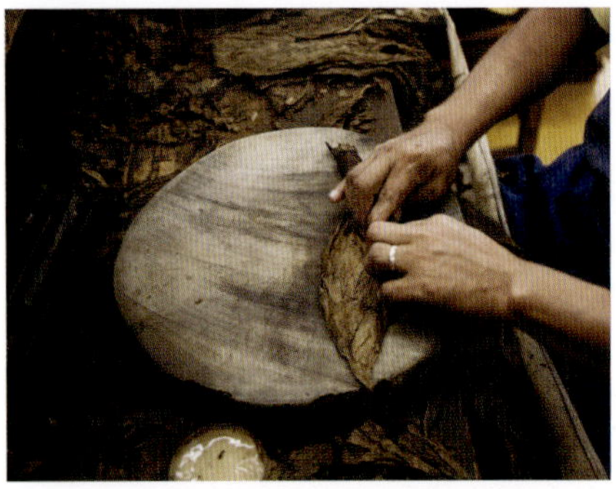
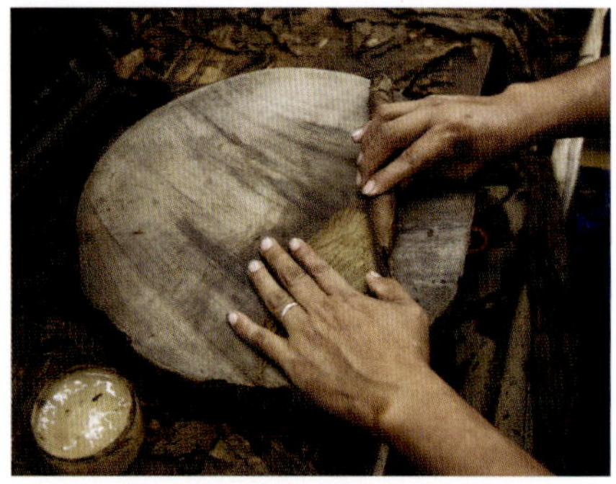
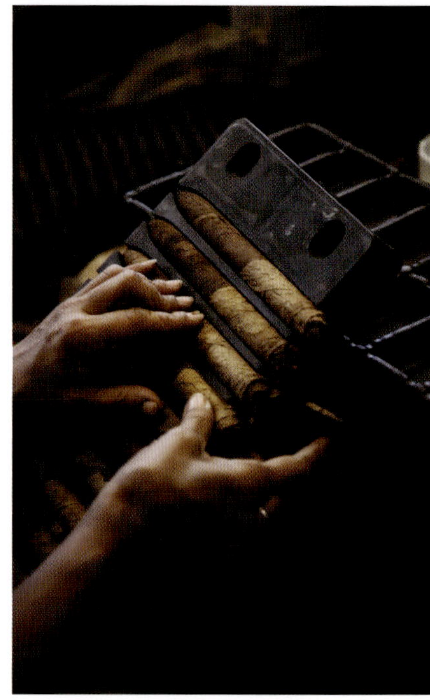
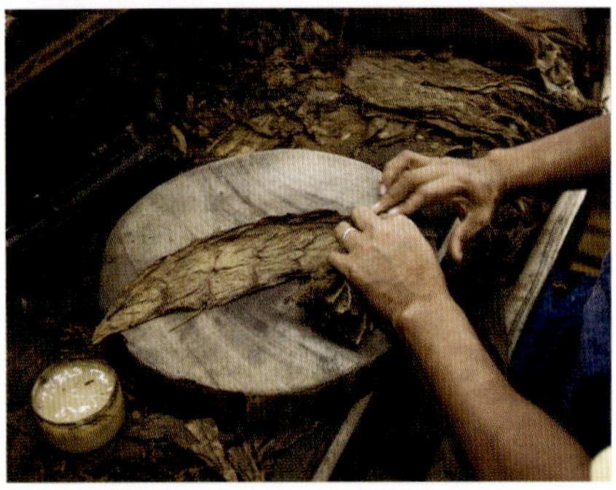
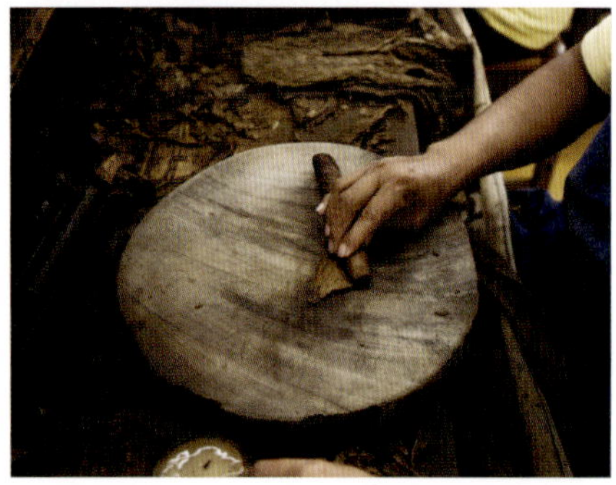
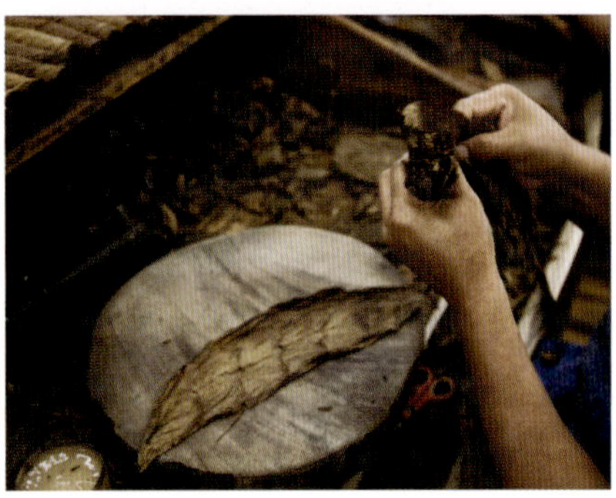
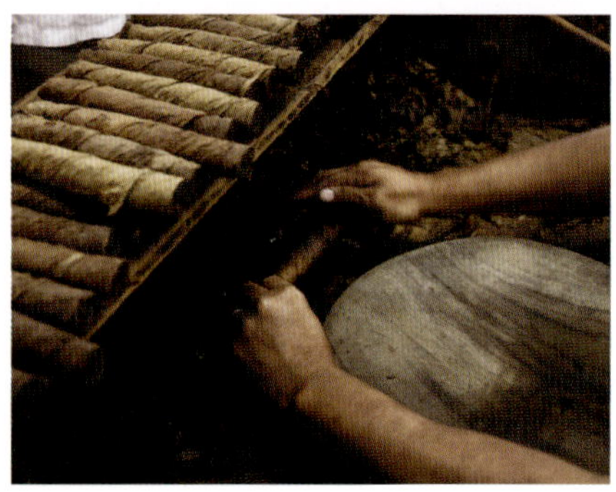
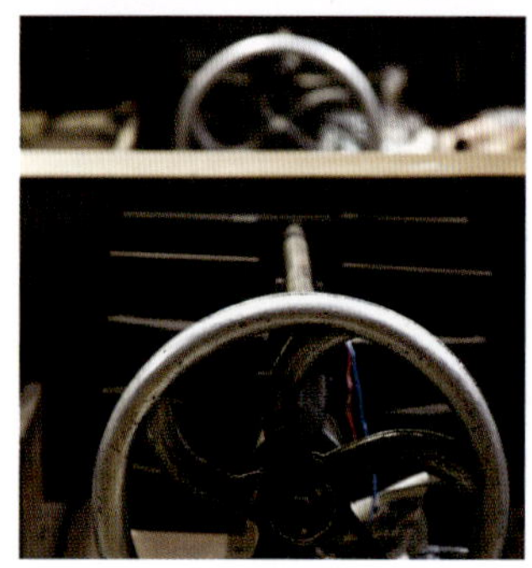

(This page) A roller starts with bunching the filler leaves, before moving on to the binder leaf and mold. After the press, (opposite page) the wrapper is fixed around the already formed shape/size. Lastly, the cap is applied.

TAKING SHAPE > The morning sun has barely risen over the hills, but already the workers' bicycles line the front of the cigar factory like a chrome snake. Inside, the day is underway. A radio blares American or Latin pop, or else the lector (in an ever-shrinking handful of *fábricas*) has cracked open the newspaper or book and begun to read—in sonorous tones—over the *clack-clack-clack* of *chavetas* slicing leaf in preparation for rolling. In the main rolling room, pairs of rollers sit at two-desk wooden tables with all the tools of their trade at hand.

From an office window set into one wall, the rollers exchange a ticket for a bundle of leaves large enough to produce fifty cigars. Such is their skill that little of this tobacco will be wasted in the making; and of those made, only an exceedingly small percentage will fail to pass the factory's rigorous quality-control standards.

To become an expert roller is a process that takes years, and cigar company owners will only let the most experienced handle their most prestigious brands.

A fermented-and-ready tobacco leaf is uniformly colored, virtually spotless, and elastic. It is not, however, the most forgiving material with which to work. It takes delicate but quick precision to wrap the two to four leaves' worth of filler into the binder. Joined, the two parts together are referred to as the bunch. Each bunch is placed into a ten-count wooden or plastic mold, which will force it to keep that round shape. The mold is pinned beneath a clamp- or screw-press for up to two hours, removed once at the halfway mark so the bunches inside can be turned in their chambers.

After this pressing, the bunches are removed and handed to the second member of the rolling team, who has spread a damp wrapper leaf, across his or her wooden block and sliced its ends into shape with the *chaveta*.

In the time it takes to read this sentence, the roller takes the bunch from its mold, places it at the edge of the wrapper-leaf and rolls the two together, using one hand to keep the remaining wrapper stretched out (an incorrectly applied wrapper will pucker or peel away, ruining the whole endeavor). With one quick motion of the *chaveta*, the roller takes the nearly completed cigar and slices away the head, then fixes a cap over the cut using a small tab of tobacco (cut from a scrap of wrapper) daubed with vegetable glue. Using the hand guillotine, the roller makes a clean cut across the cigar's foot.

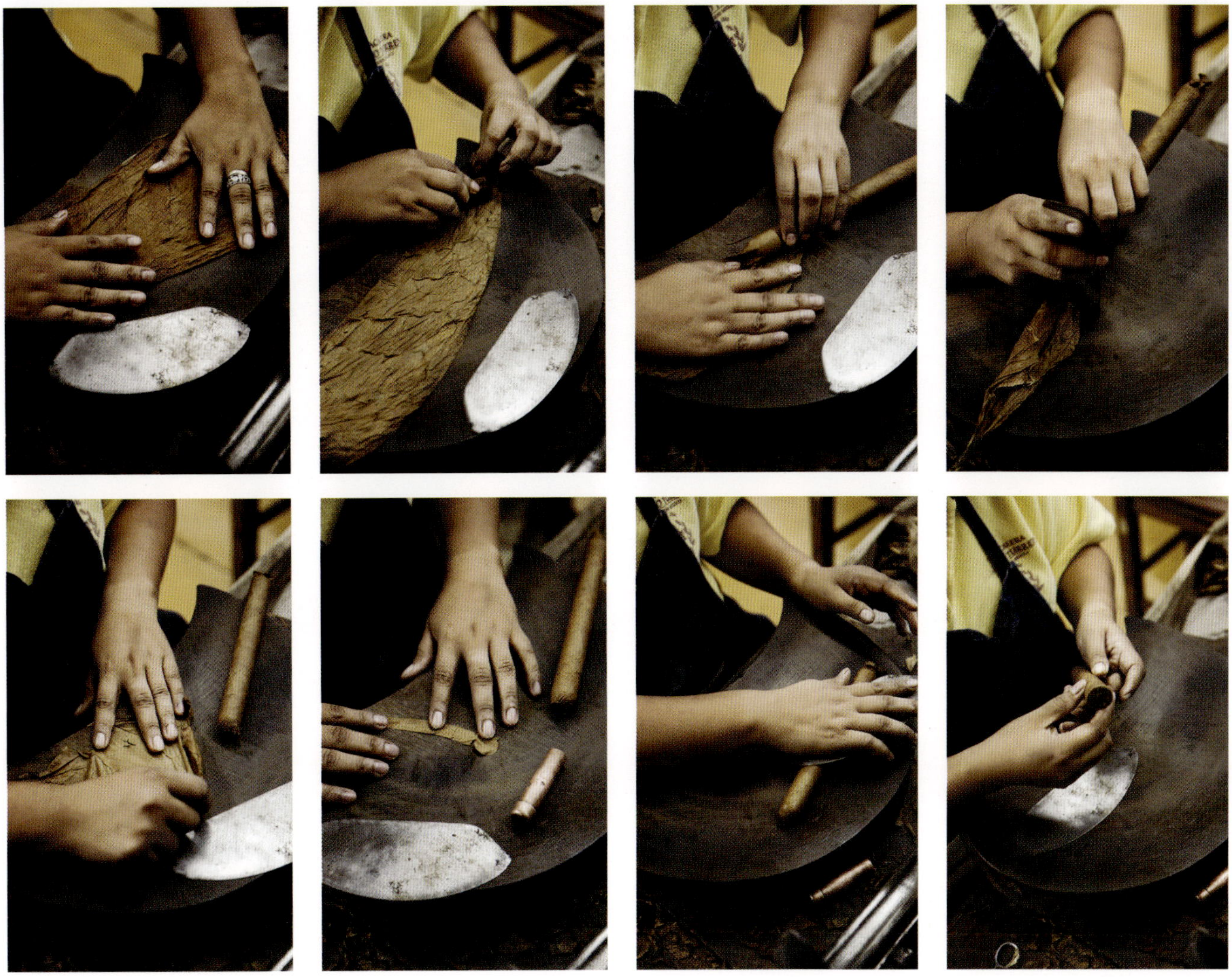

The almost-ready cigar is given a quick roll back-and-forth along *la tabla,* the roller's board, and slid through a ring to ensure the gauge is correct, before being placed into a wooden bin atop the roller's desk for one of the roving floor inspectors to examine. An experienced roller can roll nearly 150 cigars per day, depending on the cigars' size and shape; some factories will limit the number rolled per day in order to keep focus on quality.

ROLLERS' TOOLS OF THE TRADE

1. *Chaveta*: The crescent-shaped cutter used to slice tobacco leaves in preparation for rolling into a cigar.

2. *La Tabla*: The wooden cutting board on which rollers do their work.

3. Hand Guillotine: To ensure a cigar with a cleanly cut foot, cigar rollers use a desktop hand guillotine (also known as a cigar cutter or tuck cutter).

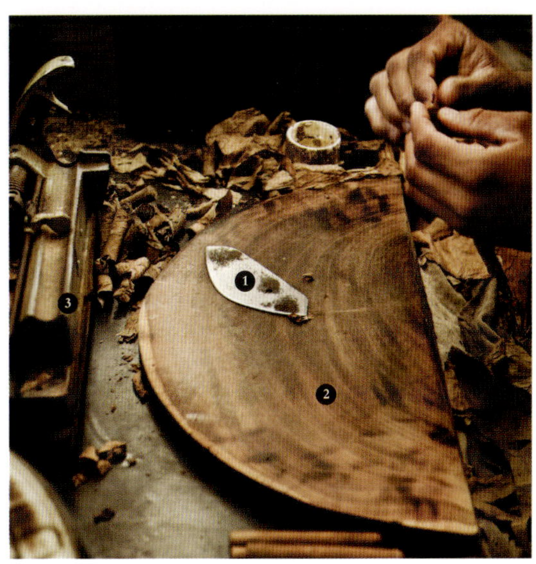

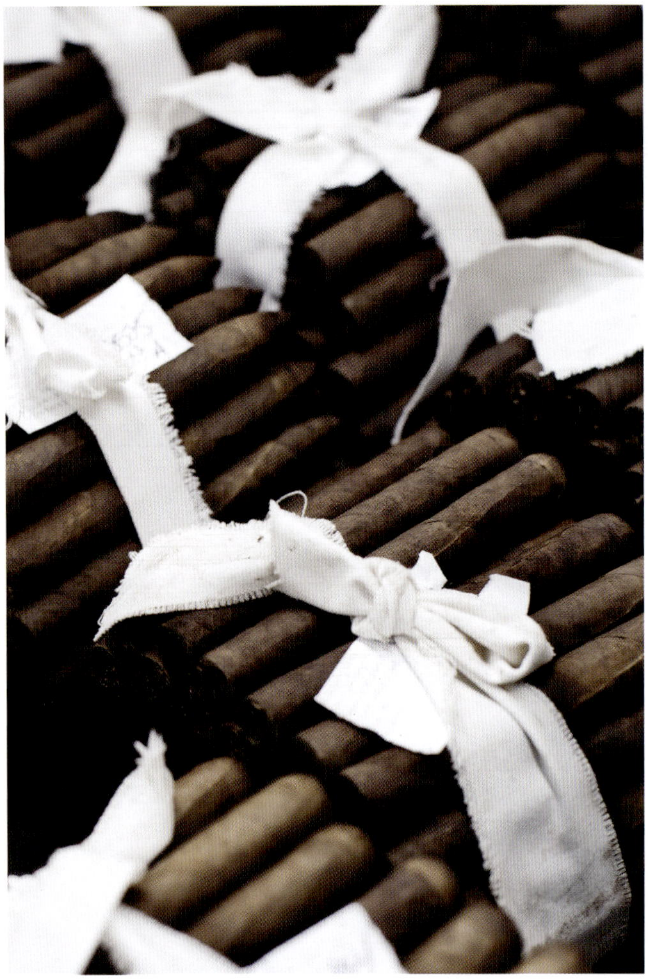

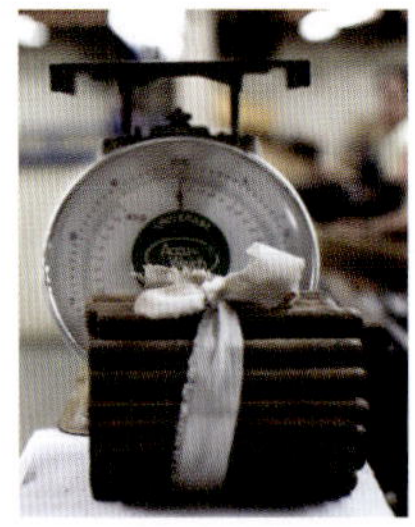

Quality control, attaching the band, (opposite page) boxing the cigars

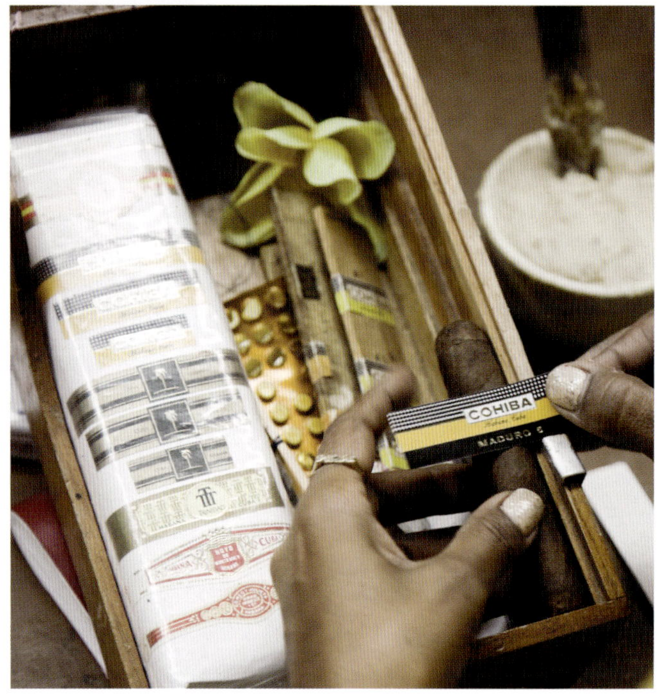

FINAL STAGES > The rolling teams' cigars are then wrapped into circular bundles of fifty, known as *media ruedas,* and bound with string. From here the cigars are subjected to the factory's quality control procedures. Many factories use a Drawmaster, a machine that checks the pull of each stick. Many weigh the finished product to determine whether they hold the right amount of tobacco. Random selections of cigars are judged for proper length, color, texture, smoothness, and other factors; many factories maintain a team of tasters who sample an inch from selected cigars to determine whether the draw, strength, and aroma are acceptable.

Those cigars that survive inspection head to storage in the factory's bowels, where they sit in cooled chambers, called *escaparates,* for a few weeks or even longer. Then comes shipping time, when the cigars will be removed, examined again, and then sent to a fluorescent-lit room for the last test. This cinderblock cube is far quieter than the rolling floor, but its workers move with no less speed, sorting the cigars according to color—making sure, down to the finest gradient, that the gross destined for each box are the exact same shade of Claro, Colorado, Colorado claro, Maduro, etc.

The cigars that pass this final inspection then receive their bands, placed with care at the exact same spot on each stick, and are placed in the waiting cedar box, with bands facing upward. The boxes are sealed, stickered, and sent to the loading dock, ready for final shipment to your local tobacconist.

According to legend, H. Upmann was the first to start packing its cigars in cedar boxes. The new containers' durability soon made them a favorite among the industry at large, although many companies still offer bundled cigars, sans box. As time went on, cigar makers began to color and design the boxes in increasingly elaborate ways, frequently using sultry women, historical or literary figures, or the company's corporate logo (such as the silver bunny on Playboy cigar boxes).

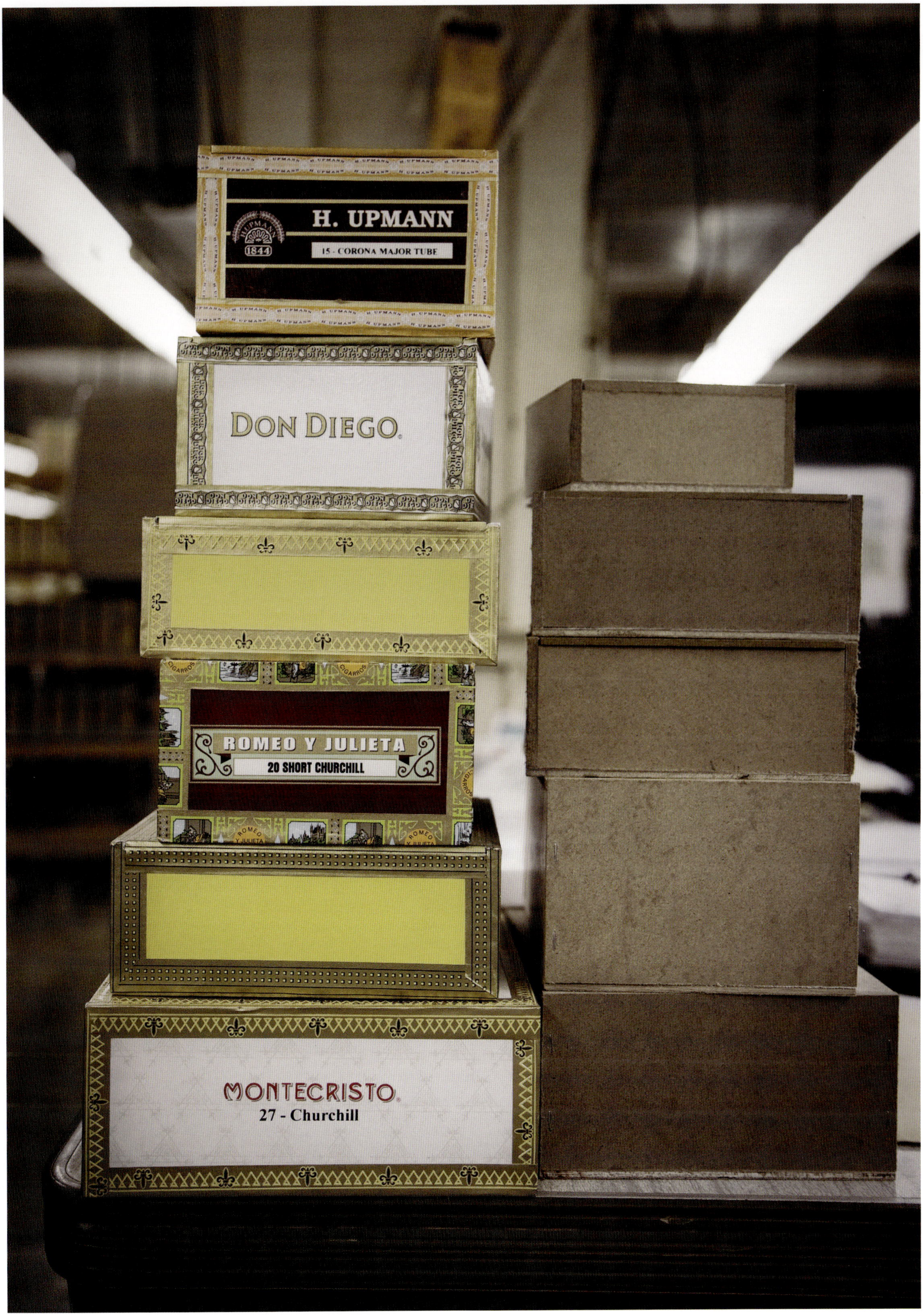
H. UPMANN
1844
15 - CORONA MAJOR TUBE
DON DIEGO
ROMEO Y JULIETA
20 SHORT CHURCHILL
MONTECRISTO
27 - Churchill

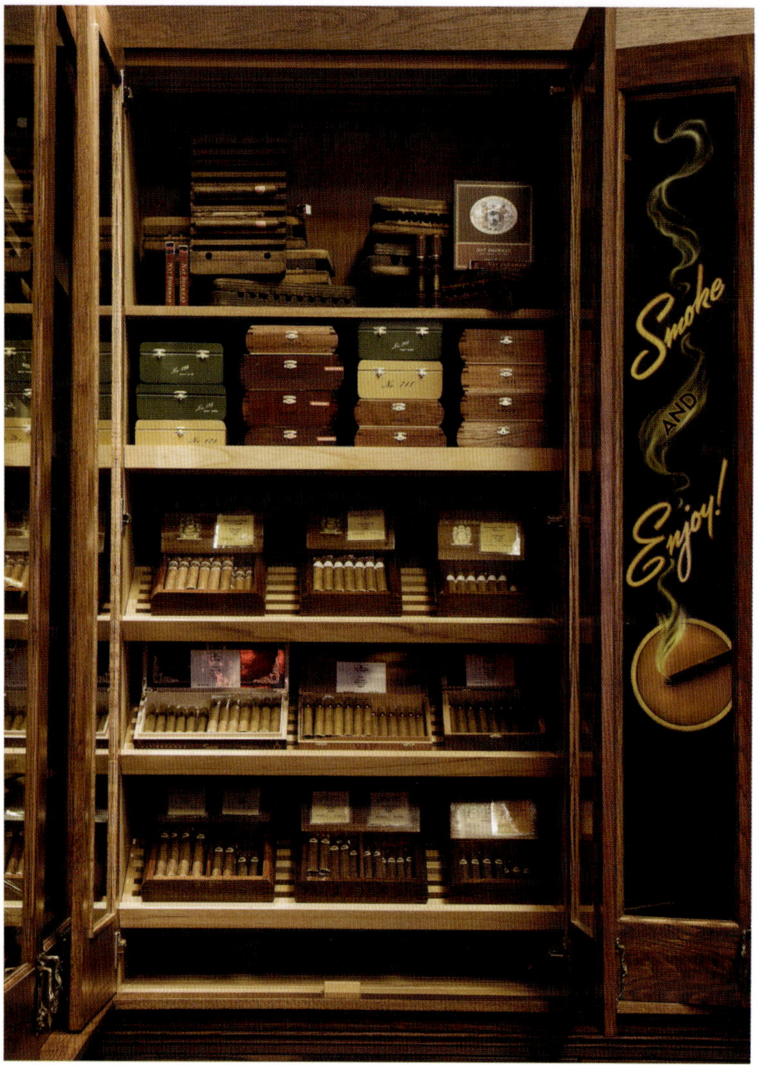

Different tobacconists' shelves. The key is to take your time when selecting.

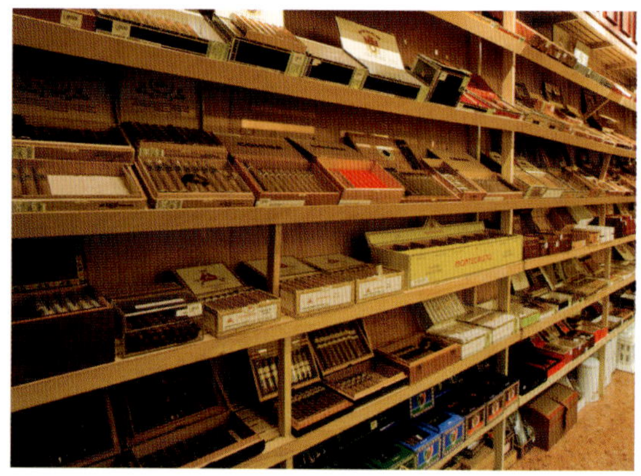

CHOOSING YOUR CIGAR > The box of cigars has arrived at your local shop, where you stand, cash burning a hole in your wallet, practically aching to purchase some fine smokes. Before you can partake, however, there are a few simple guidelines to ensure that the sticks you choose are of proper quality, and are right for you.

If you are a beginner on the cigar scene, you may benefit from starting off with smaller, simpler-tasting sticks. Larger cigars are filled with more tobacco and thus have a tendency to be more complex. Good advice is to start small and work your way to the Churchills and Double Coronas as you become more of a connoisseur. (The next chapter provides a comprehensive chart of cigar sizes; it may take some experimenting to find the one right for you.)

The neophyte should also take the cigar's components (filler, binder, and wrapper) under consideration. Cigars with Dominican filler and binders and those with Cameroon wrappers often provide a milder taste (that said, there are many exceptions to these broad guidelines.) Cigars with Nicaraguan filler and binder, however, as well as those with Cuban and Ecuadorian wrappers, may be more suited to those who enjoy complex blends with pronounced flavors (though again, exceptions abound), such as Dominican *puros*. Cigars in which the filler, binder, and wrapper all come from the DR one would think of as being mild, when in fact all are either medium- or full-bodied.

This is why your local tobacconist versed in such things is always happy to let you pick his brain about all things cigar. Trust him, but be sure to ask any burning questions you may have about the box in your hands. After all, those cigars have taken quite a journey to reach this point. Pay them the proper respect by making sure they're ideal before you take them home.

True beginners should dip a toe into the water, so to speak, by purchasing single sticks; once you become used to the lifestyle and have a better idea of what you like, you can graduate to purchasing full boxes.

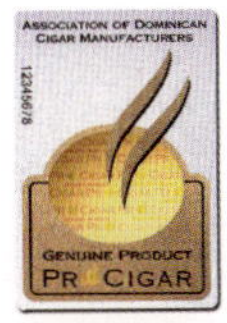

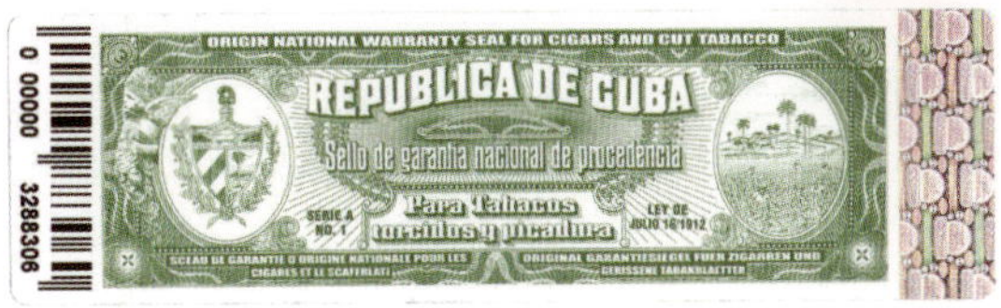

SIGNS OF QUALITY

Cigar counterfeiting is a major issue facing the industry, and one that's being met aggressively by cigar makers the world over. Often, you're protected before you even enter the store; reps from cigar companies big and small have eagle eyes when it comes to scanning proprietors' humidors for potentially counterfeit product. Should they find some, their relationship with that store will end.

It almost goes without saying that, should you be vacationing in the Caribbean or Central America, a dubious eye should be cast upon anyone trying to sell you an "authentic and cheap" box of cigars on the street. Of course, fake cigars often lack the superior quality of the real deal in ways that are patently obvious: think peeling wrappers, amateur capping, and bands that look like they came fresh from a photocopier.

Your box of cigars should be sealed, cellophane-wrapped, and bear few signs of wear and tear. Make sure, too, that the logo on the box matches the actual manufacturer's mark. Cigars from the Dominican Republic will have a sticker that reads "Genuine Product ProCigar" on the back, along with a number code and a hologram. Once you open the box, make sure the cigars are of uniform color and consistent to the eye and touch.

Cuban cigars are some of the most notorious counterfeiting targets in the world, and thus their boxes feature several marks of authenticity:

Each box should feature a "Republica de Cuba" seal on the front; this seal contains a UV-visible watermark.

Check for the distinctive red-and-gold "Habanos" label with the tobacco-leaf logo in either the top- or bottom-left corner.

On the underside of each box there should be a branded factory/date stamp, along with the words "Hecho En Cuba," "Habanos S.A.," and "Totalmente a mano."

Look for the region-specific distributor's sticker on the packaging.

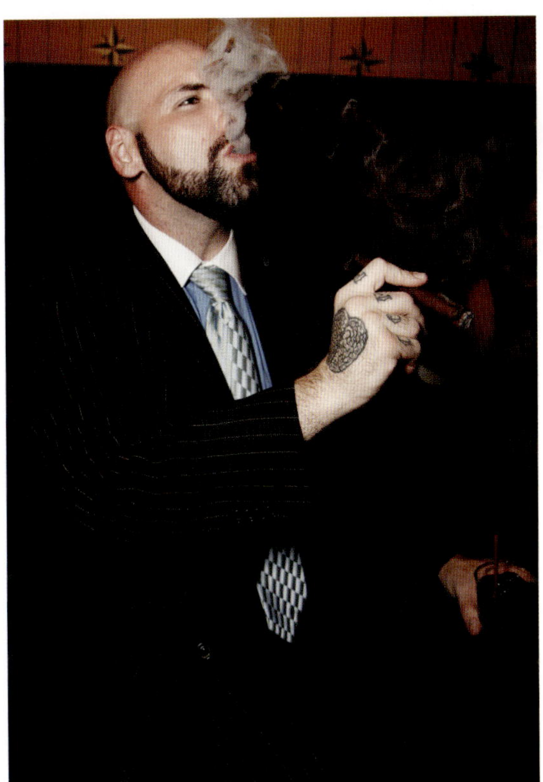

(Above) The ever-evolving Hologram seals/labels are a mark of quality from ProCigar (Dominican Republic) and Habanos S.A. (Cuba), and also serve to deter counterfeiting. (Right) Once chosen, the cigar is savored.

EXAMINING THE GOODS

When purchasing cigars, it always helps to do a little quality control of your own:

Touch: Pick up the cigar and squeeze gently. The stick should spring back to shape instantly. If the cigar feels like rock, or a bit too "spongy," chances are it won't provide a decent burn.

Listen (rarely): In the old days, it was customary for people to roll the cigar by their ear to check for the crumbly sound of loose tobacco that would indicate the stick was too dry. The last person we actually saw doing this, however, was Denzel Washington in *American Gangster.*

Smell: An important test. Press your nose close to the cigars and breathe deep. The scent should instantly appeal to your sensibilities.

Check the Box: Make sure the box has structural integrity, and looks right. You won't have to worry about well-cared-for boxes in reputable, big-name cigar stores, but it can be an issue when purchasing from airports or a few smaller dealers; some don't hold the same level of regard for cigars as you do.

Many boxes come factory-sealed in cellophane; if you're purchasing an un-plasticized box, you can always ask the proprietor to open it up so you can check the cigars inside. Make sure the sticks are of uniform color and have been properly humidified; apply your touch and smell tests to a randomly selected one or two.

CIGAR

FUNDAMENTALS

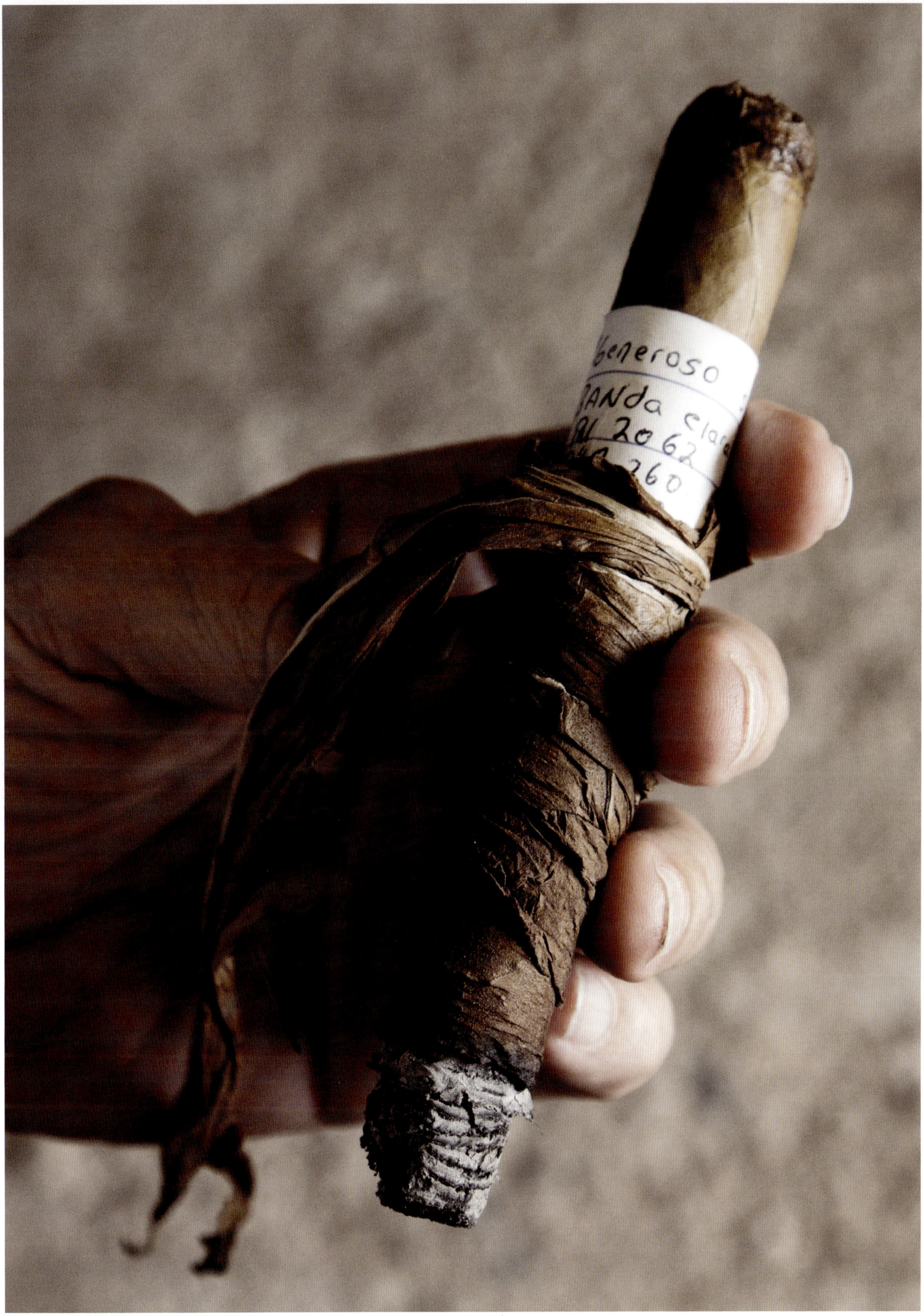
Generoso

If I've said it once, I've said it a million times: between the lexicon, protocol, accessories and accoutrements, clubs, cliques, dinners, sites, blogs, magazines, and (of course) books, cigars are a bona fide hobby. What this chapter will hopefully do is provide you with a solid introduction to the rather intricate world of cigars. For those who already know the joys of a fine stick, it will hopefully offer some tidbits you didn't previously know. How deeply you wish to delve into the hobby beyond these basics is entirely up to you—though if you bought this book, there's likely at least a bit of curiosity on your part.

Aside from the actual cigar, one needs only two things to become a cigar smoker: A cutter. And fire. While your teeth or fingernails can substitute for a proper cutter, and a disposable plastic lighter (or freebie drugstore matchbook) will provide all the flame you need, the person who resorts to these misses out on the ritual and nuances of enjoying a fine smoke. Once you've made a commitment to exploring cigars, you will inevitably fall into one of four broad categories:

Part-time Puffer: Some guys (my old man, for instance) smoke a few cigars a week and on special occasions (bachelor parties, weddings, bar mitzvahs, etc.). They know what they like (a country of origin, a particular brand, a flavor profile) and along the way have acquired a respectable humidor and lighter—as well as some cigar jargon from years spent going to their local store. If you grilled them, though, they would be hard pressed to tell you the difference between a Ligero and Seco . . . or care, for that matter.

Dedicated or Daily Dabbler: These are your one- to two-stick-a-day guys (maybe a few more while on vacation). They have a solid grasp of cigars and perhaps either have (or had) a private cigar locker and a subscription to a magazine or three. Any newbie who familiarizes themselves with this chapter will have close to the same degree of cigar fluency as these guys. The rest you can pick up on the street, just as you did sex. Actually, knowing how well that went at first, it's probably better to learn at fine tobacconists, cigar bars, and special cigar dinners and other events.

'Gar Ganster: These guys pound five to ten sticks a day. They eat, sleep, and possibly you-know-what cigars. They go to every cigar dinner, belong to every cigar club in town, read every blog, and contribute to every chatroom. Personally, these guys scare me.

'Gar Geek: A fanatical cigar zealot that could tell you the number of cross-breed generations it took to create a new binder leaf, for instance. As a mission of mercy, consider hooking them up with one of your single friends, just so they get out of the humidor once in a while.

In time you will find the category that's right for you. I myself fall squarely in to the Dedicated Dabbler category. Cigars can be a wonderful facet of a man's life, creating camaraderie and guiding one to become a little bit more contemplative, but too much of anything isn't good.

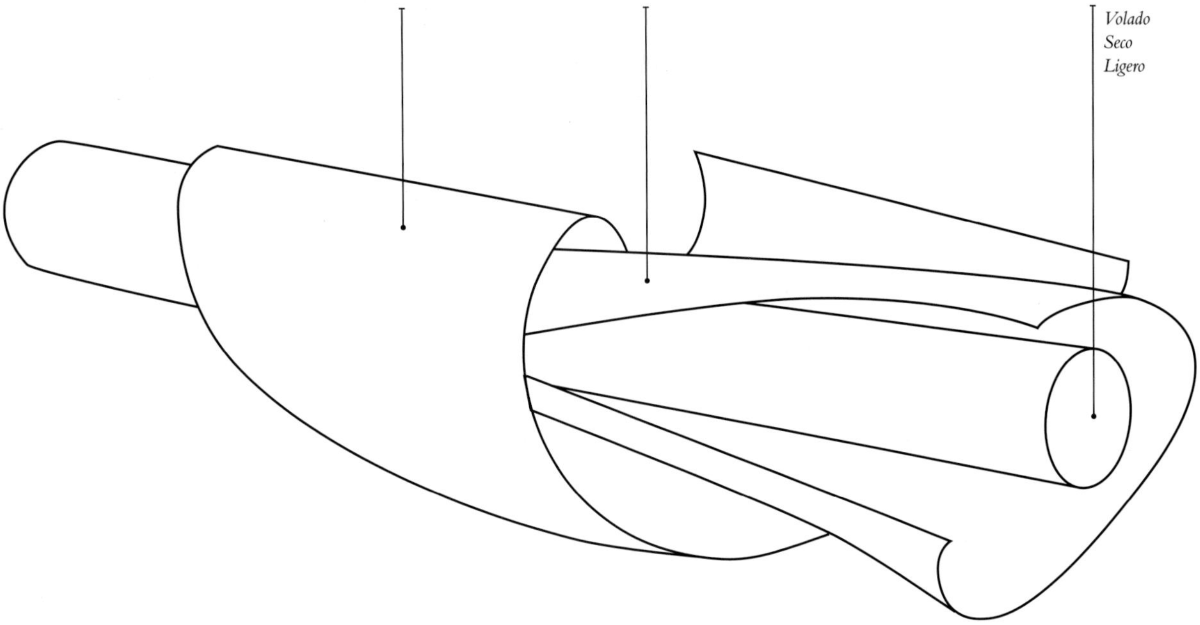

PARTS AND PARTS OF PARTS

Many cigar books sport a rather impressive glossary of terms, but the fact is that there are really rather few terms or words you will ever actually use (and if you come across one that stumps you, well, that's why Google was invented), but here are the basic terms you will need to be somewhat conversant:

Blend: Even though they are a solid, cigars are nonetheless "blended" artisanal products, in the mode of nonvintage meritage wines, Champagnes, or blended sprits such as cognac. The cigar's blend is made up of the tobaccos selected for its three components: wrapper, binder, and filler. All tobacco leaves contain natural oils, which over time mix together. Coupled with the way the cigar itself is rolled, these oils give a cigar its blend and yield its flavor.

Filler (Tripa): The tobaccos bunched in the core of the cigar. These leaves form the bases of the blend and provide much of the flavor.

Volado, Seco, and Ligero: The basic types of filler tobacco. The lower leaves of sun grown plants (Volado) are used for lighter flavored fillers, while the middle leaves (Seco, "dry" in Spanish) are used for medium flavored fillers, and the top leaves (Ligero, "light" in Spanish) for full-flavored.

Binder (Capote): The leaf wrapped around the filler, beneath the wrapper, that binds the cigar together

Wrapper (Capa): The outside leaf of a cigar. The wrapper not only determines the color category designation and aesthetic of the cigar, but it is a huge component of the cigar's flavor and body. Opinions vary as to how much the capa actually contributes to this, but thought runs somewhere in the 35 to 70 percent range.

Puro: A Spanish double-entendre for "pure." In, cigar parlance, a cigar where the binder, filler, and wrapper are all grown in the same country that it's rolled.

Long Filler (Tripa Larga): Filler tobacco leaves that run the length of a cigar.

Short Filler (Tripa Corta): Filler composed of leaf trimmings and chopped tobacco, but rolled inside full-size binders and wrappers.

Body: The body—or strength—of a cigar is not tantamount with flavor, though people often use the terms interchangeably. You can have a very flavorful but still light- or medium-bodied cigar, but you can also smoke a bland cigar whose strength will nonetheless knock you on your ass. If someone says that a cigar is "full-bodied," it is a complex or flavorful blend.

Tobac in the Box: Is not a term, but rather a reference to how cigars come packaged. A tobacconist will offer you cigars in any number of ways: as individual sticks, packs of three to five cigars, or in boxes, which traditionally hold twenty-five cigars. 8-9-8 boxes hold twenty-five cigars as well, however, instead of the twelve on the bottom/thirteen on the top configuration of packaging, they have three sequential rows of 8-9-8. Cabinet boxes hold fifty cigars and traditionally come unbanded.

VITOLAS SIZES & SHAPES

"With a cigar, like in life," the comedian D.L. Hughley once said, "you got to have some length, and some girth." Indeed.

It can be a little confusing to discuss the "size" and "shape" of cigars, because size and shape are often referred to synonymously. For instance, if I say, "I'll have a Monte 2," that one word and number convey the size, shape, and brand. The following terms will help clarify matters:

Length: A cigar's length is either listed in inches or centimeters, or both. Since Americans never learned the metric system, all of our cigars will be listed in inches.

Diameter: The basic unit of measurement of a cigar's diameter—or girth—is the ring gauge, which is based on increments of 1/64 of an inch. For example, a standard toro size is "6 by 50", which means it is six inches long and 50/64ths of an inch thick.

Shape: If you're searching for common denominators to use as a starting point for shape, consider that all cigars can be divided into two categories: parejos, or the straight-sided cigars that everyone thinks of when they conjure up a mental image of a cigar; and figurados, or irregular shapes such as a torpedo or perfecto.

Box-Pressed: Parejos all start out rounded and straight. However, some become square-ish cigars known as box-pressed. Originally box-pressed cigars achieved their namesake shape by being placed into a tight-fitting box. Today various techniques, including the traditional one, are employed to achieving this squaring-off.

Pigtail Cap: Both parejos and figurados can be finished off with the flourish of a pigtail cap—i.e., a twisty tobacco tail. There are many variations of this, as master rollers can do fans, beehives or other fancy finishes. It's nice for roughly a second . . . right before you twist or lop off the cap.

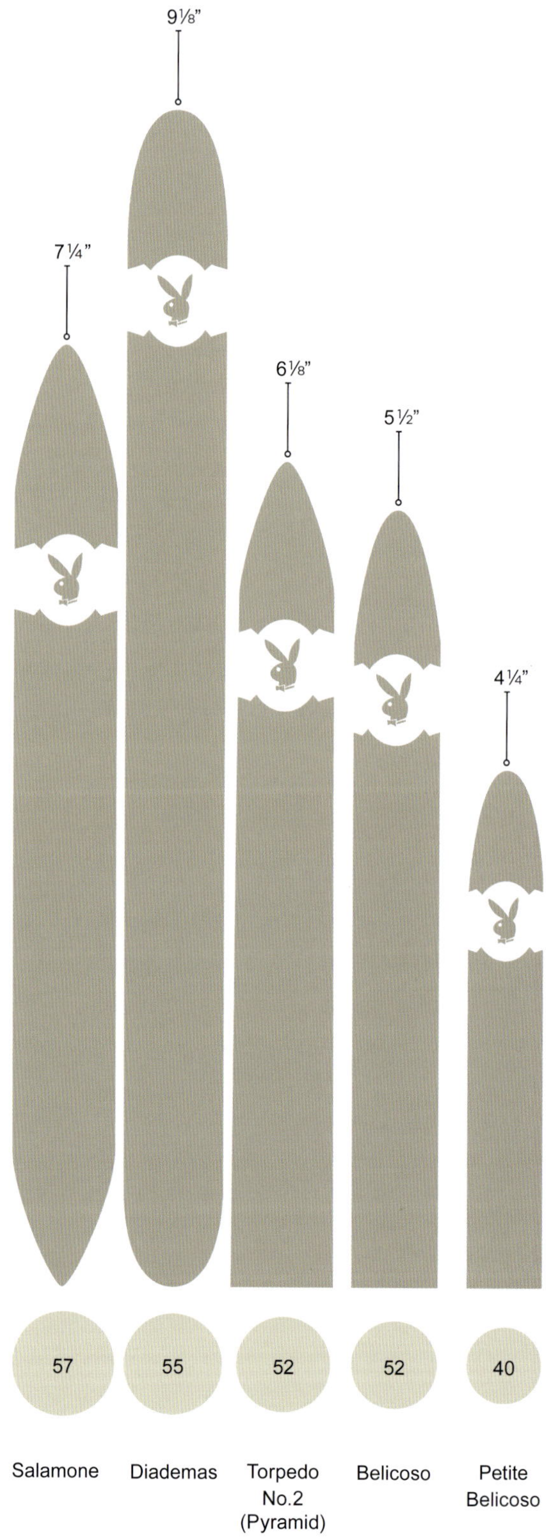

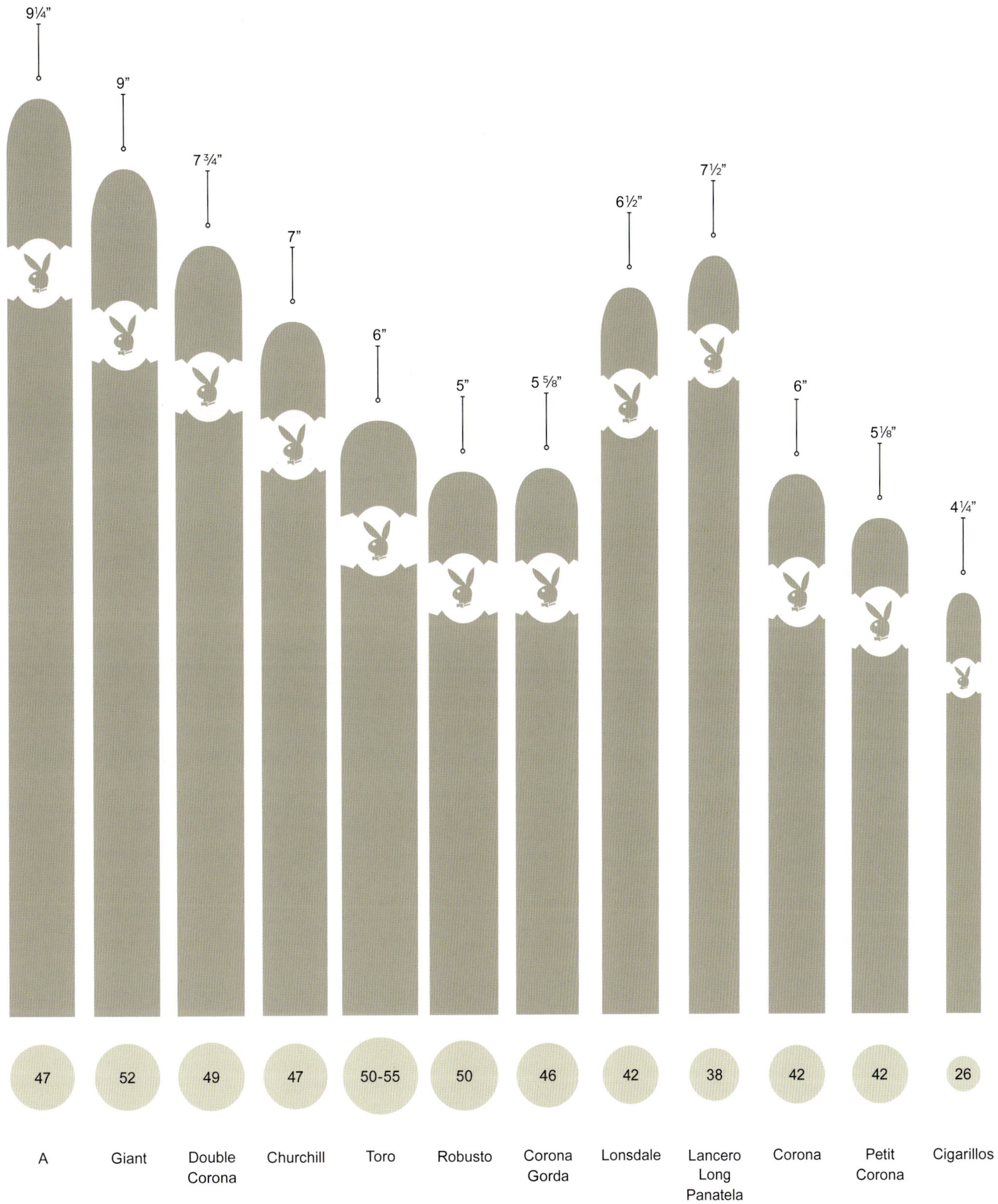
9¼" 47 A
9" 52 Giant
7 ¾" 49 Double Corona
7" 47 Churchill
6" 50-55 Toro
5" 50 Robusto
5 ⅝" 46 Corona Gorda
6½" 42 Lonsdale
7½" 38 Lancero Long Panatela
6" 42 Corona
5⅛" 42 Petit Corona
4¼" 26 Cigarillos

SHADES OF COLOR & VARIETALS OF WRAPPERS

Cigars are graded and referenced to by their respective wrapper (capa). This is only fair, since, aside from the band, the wrapper is the only part of the cigar that the smoker really sees. Some espouse the rule of thumb "the lighter the color, the milder the taste." This is true with regard to the candela-Colorado Claro spectrum, however, after that, one really has to look at the wrapper varietal and/or country of origin. You can have two leaves with the Colorado color designation, one grown in the Connecticut River Valley (also referred to as Tobacco Valley) and one from the Vuelta Abajo in Cuba, and the odds of them falling in the same range of taste or flavor is nada.

CIGAR TOBACCOS, FROM LIGHTEST TO DARKEST:

Candela: Ranging anywhere from a greenish-tinted blond to a light green, achieved by harvesting the plant before it fully matures and then drying it quickly, often with exposure to fire as opposed to air. Flavor tends to be extremely mild, and generally lacking in depth. Also known as Double Claro, Jade, and American Market Selection (AMS).

Claro: A blond or tawny color, resulting from being cut before full maturity (and well before maduro leaves are harvested). Also known as Natural.

Colorado Claro: A light brown color.

Colorado: A medium brown leaf. It can also have reddish hues, sometimes referred to as *Capa Roja*.
Also known as English Market Selection (EMS).

Colorado Maduro: a full brown color.

Maduro: Dark brown in color, though it can also have some red tints. Strong, by virtue of them being taken from the top of the plant, these dark-brown leaves wrap many Cohiba Maduro 5 (Cuban) cigars, as well as brands such as the Dominican Montecristo Reserva Negra. Occasionally referred to as Spanish Market Selection (SMS).

Oscuro: This is as close to black as a tobacco leaf gets. This leaf is often left in the field the longest, exposing it to the maximum sunlight; it is also matured longer than other tobaccos. Also known as Double Maduro.

WRAPPER VARIETALS

Like wine grapes, there are multiple varietals of cigar-wrapper leaves. And as in viniculture, where the plants are grown (country, region, and microclimate—also known as *terroir*) results in a diversity of favors and aromas. The Romeo y Julieta and Montecristo cigars made for the U.S. market, as well as the La Aurora Preferido range, are all fine examples of cigar lines that experiment with and vary blends with multiple wrapper varietals. While there are many wrappers out there, these are the most-encountered:

Cameroon: Grown in the Bertoua region of the West African country of Cameroon, as well as the neighboring Central African Republic, this sweet, thin, and somewhat fragile leaf is favored among many cigar connoisseurs for its spiced flavor and sweet aroma. It is easily recognizable from its "toothy" texture, and is covered with countless fine bumps.

Connecticut Shade: Harvested in the Connecticut Valley, this golden- and gold-red-hued tobacco is among some of the most expensive and sought-after in the world. Connecticut Shade wrappers, which have a mild- to medium-flavor, have a silky/elastic quality that makes them a friendly leaf to roll.

Connecticut Broadleaf: Also grown in Connecticut, U.S.A., this very thick, oily, and veiny wrapper leaf is none too pretty, and often is treated as a poor relation to the famed Connecticut Shade; however, it remains popular and is full of flavors and aromas.

Cuban: Many cigar boxes from all around the world feature the words "Cuban Seed." However, when one speaks of Cuban cigars, Cuban seed is a given, though the exact variety of that seed is often treated as a national secret. The most recent wrapper leaf is from a seed known as Habano 2006 (a hybrid of Habana 2000 and Criollo 1998), its forerunners in chronological order were: Habanensis (1907), Criollo (circa 1940), Habana 2000 (1992), and Criollo 98 (1998). All Cuban cigars range from medium- to full-bodied, with a Colorado Claro to Colorado Maduro color, although occasionally you will see a rosado (reddish-hue) leaf.

Dominican Shade: It was said for decades that wrapper-quality leaf could never be grown in the Dominican Republic, until Carlos "Carlito" Fuente Jr. proved the world wrong by cultivating a piloto cubano on the farm now known as Chateau de la Fuente. Fuente the man, of course went on to use this wrapper on his cult cigar, the Fuente Fuente OpusX (the first Dominican puro). Subsequently, a number of other Dominican puros have been released by other manufacturers; all are medium- to full-bodied smokes.

Ecuador Connecticut Shade: Connecticut seed shade wrapper grown in Ecuador; similar to the actual Connecticut Shade, but slightly more flavorful and richer in color.

Ecuador Special Sun Grown: A thick, dark wrapper leaf with a unique medium- to full-bodied flavor and a hint of sweetness. Unlike shade wrappers, sun-grown wrappers are left exposed to the elements. Ecuador's consistent cloud cover acts as a natural sun protector and buffers the leaves from the sun. Ecuadorian Sumatra: Sumatran seed wrapper grown in Ecuador; mild, with almost a neutral flavor.

Habana 2000: A Cuban crossbreed seed wrapper—and grown in both Nicaragua and Honduras—it is a very attractive, oily, dark wrapper with light veining. It has rich and peppery notes and a toasty aroma. Sadly, it also has some combustion issues, which means you will probably be relighting your cigar more than once.

Nicaraguan Habano Corojo: A Cuban seed wrapper leaf originally grown in the 1930s, reborn in Nicaragua in the nineties. The Cuban standard for decades, this wrapper makes for beautiful, full-bodied leaves. Because of its temperamental and fragile nature, however, it is also a mercurial plant to work with. With only the top set of its leaves typically possessing enough quality to become a wrapper, yields are low and cost high.

San Andres Morron: Grown in the San Andres Valley of Mexico, this thick and flavorful wrapper leans toward the higher end of the medium-bodied spectrum. Aesthetically beautiful, it, sadly, has fewer fans than it rightfully deserves. More than worth sampling.

HOW TO SMOKE WITHOUT DROWNING

My approach to writing this book is the same one I use with my two cigar magazines: keep everything simple and convivial, not bombastic (a tone unfortunately common to other publications). In that spirit, and given that this chapter is titled "Cigar Fundamentals," let us post the simplest query possible:

How does one actually smoke a cigar?

For those so inexperienced they don't even qualify as "Part-Time Puffers," this is a recurring inquiry arising far more often than a seasoned cigar lover might expect.

Beginners are perplexed by the technique of smoking without inhaling. (Trying to smoke a cigar like a cigarette or a spliff is what we call bad. Try it, and you will be what we call unhappy.) But hey, if President Clinton could smoke without inhaling, so can you.

My good friend—and tobacconist extraordinaire—Michael Herklots offers the best smoking lesson I've ever come across:

To learn how to smoke a cigar without inhaling, you will need the following: two water glasses, a small bottle of water, a straw, a cigar, a cigar cutter, and matches or a lighter.

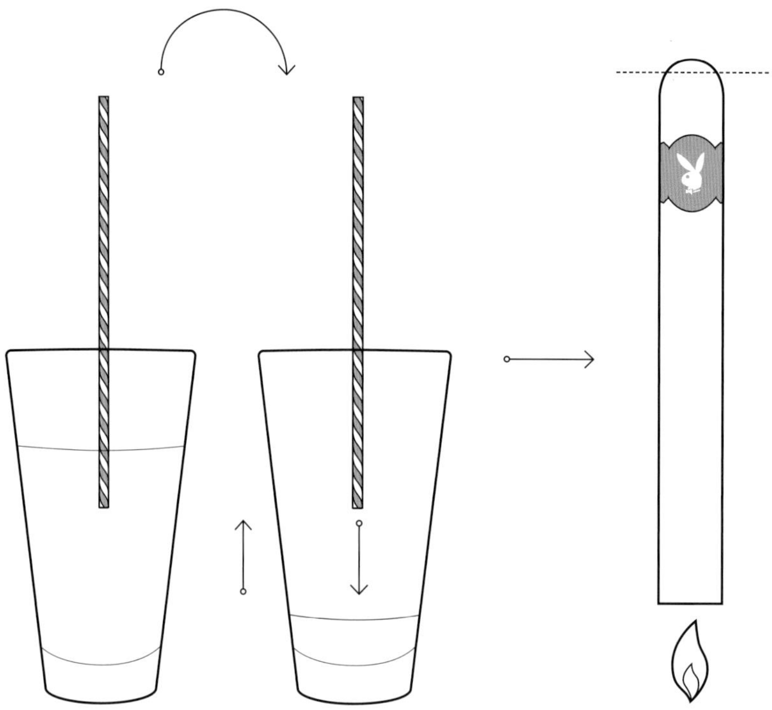

STEP ONE:
Fill one of the drinking glasses between halfway and two-thirds full. Leave the other glass empty. Place the straw in your hand as you would a cigar.

STEP TWO:
Placing the straw between your lips, draw off a partial strawful of water from the first glass (swallowing none) and expel it into the second glass. Repeat this process at a comfortable pace until the water from the first glass has been transferred to the second.

STEP THREE:
Have a cocktail. Hey, it can't hurt.

STEP FOUR
Cut and light a cigar.

STEP FIVE
Bring the smoke onto your palette, letting the body and flavor work on your tongue. Then eject the smoke. It's that simple.

If you accomplished steps one and two without drowning, you can achieve step five without inhaling.

CIGAR TASTING 101

Now that you know how to smoke, the next question is: What are you actually tasting?

Cigars break down into two primary components that make up their overall flavor profile: taste notes and body.

Taste notes are simply the flavors generated by the tobaccos in the cigar's "blend" (see the previous section, "Parts and Parts of Parts"). Cigar magazines, websites, and books assign numerous descriptive words and phrases to convey a cigar's flavor notes: almond, berry/fruity, cinnamon, hint of coco, trace of coffee, earthy, floral, grassy, leathery, nutty, peppery, spicy, woody—the terms go on and on (and on and on).

These tastes come not from a cigar having been infused with artificial flavors, but are in fact organic notes found in the tobacco itself. Does it really taste of coco/cacao? Yes. Does it taste like biting into a Hershey chocolate bar? No.

Tasting cigars is akin to tasting Cognac, Champagne, premium coffees, and the like; the adjectives used to describe the resulting sensations are simply a guide that will let others determine if a cigar will appeal to them and their favored flavor profile. Your preferred flavors are determined by your taste sensory palate. All mammals, man included, taste numerous compounds, yet the sensory palate consists of only five (not four) basic tastes: bitter, salty, sour, sweet, and umami (the taste of monosodium glutamate).

Contrary to popular belief, these basic tastes and the resulting labyrinth of flavor compounds and notes they yield are not detected by specific regions on the tongue. This common misconception stems from what's often referred to as the "tongue map," based on a German paper written in 1901 and later mistranslated by Edwin Boring, a Harvard psychologist. This "map" purportedly shows that the back of one's tongue registers "bitter," the rear left and right sides "sour," the front left and right sides "salty," and the front region "sweet."

Some regions of the tongue are indeed more sensitive than others, but those supposedly segregated taste areas are in fact distributed fairly evenly over the surface of the tongue.

Body, the other primary component of the overall flavor profile (also referred to as the cigar's "strength"), falls into three categories: mild, medium, and full-bodied. A new smoker may require some time to determine which cigars' strength best suits his personal comfort zone. Think of body the same way you think about the alcohol content of a wine: some wines are as low as 9 percent; others are as high as 15 percent. The flavors you experience as a result of the fruit and tannins in a wine are the "notes."

A true cigar enthusiast will judge his puro by evaluating a number of criteria: construction, aesthetic and condition of the wrapper (smooth, veiny and oily, matte), draw, how the cigar lights, aroma, ash, and aftertaste. Ultimately, however, there is one undeniable truth: the difference between a "good" cigar and a "bad" cigar is something only you can determine—it's an entirely subjective observation. (Keep in mind that ratings, reviews, and blogs are, like the terms they coin, merely guides.) The one exception to this rule is the cigar's construction; it is either well-made or not.

{70 - 72% *RH*}

[70°F]

SELECTION & CONDITION

At this juncture, you know all about the three components of a cigar: how blends are achieved, how cigars are rolled, and more than you ever wanted to about wrapper leaves. Now what?

Time to select a cigar. Keep in mind not only everything touched upon in the "From Terroir to Tobacconist" chapter, but one other crucial element: condition.

When examining the goods, the primary condition to look for is proper humidity level.

In pursuit of perfect humidity, it's instructive to, again, bring up the similarities between assessing a fine wine and a good cigar. If this book makes hay of these similarities, it's because, while some have an understanding of cigars, most have a fundamental comprehension of wines.

In much the same manner that oxygen and temperature influence a wine's ability to open up and express its bouquet and balance, moisture is the active element in determining how well a cigar will smoke. This is chiefly why maintaining a desirable level of humidity is so critical—and the need for every serious cigar-smoker to own a suitable humidor.

To carry the earlier analogy a bit further, as with the major wine producing regions of the world, the major cigar-producing areas are located in two comparable climate zones, one in the Northern hemisphere, another in the Southern—this is known as the "Latitude Effect."

And again, as with wines, cigars need to be stored in an environment that reflects the regions of the world where they are grown and produced.

For cigars (primarily grown and made in tropical and subtropical climates/microclimates), the superlative range of stasis exists at 70–72 percent relative humidity (RH) and 70°F/21°C—or, as many simply refer to it, "70/70." (If you're ever on *Jeopardy!* and need to know the wine target numbers, they are 70 percent RH and 55°F/12.5°C.)

Any reputable tobacconist with a proper working humidor room and/or set of humidor cabinets maintains that desirable 70/70 environment to keep their inventory—and your impending purchases—in exceptional condition.

ACCESSORIES

Buying a single stick—or even a single box of cigars—is kind of like a kid getting just one G.I. Joe for his birthday, without a tank or plane or a Cobra dude to try and kick Joe's ass. Sure, you might get a cheapo plastic cigar cutter and a small box of wood matches when you purchase your box, but even novices to the smoking art will soon know that pleasure deserves better.

I've often said that the psychographic of a cigar smoker is a simple one: a cigar guy is a watch guy, is a pen guy, is a single-malt scotch guy, and so on—all the same guy. Smoking cigars is a hobby that appeals to men who are interested in gentlemanly pursuits that require a certain connoisseurship and epicurean knowledge, and appeals particularly to those predisposed to collecting.

So, it comes as no surprise that brands closely associated with cigars, such as Montecristo, Davidoff, Elie Bleu, and S. T. DuPont, as well as luxury houses such as Asprey, Hermès, Louis Vuitton, Goyard, and many more all make accessories for cigars and their smokers.

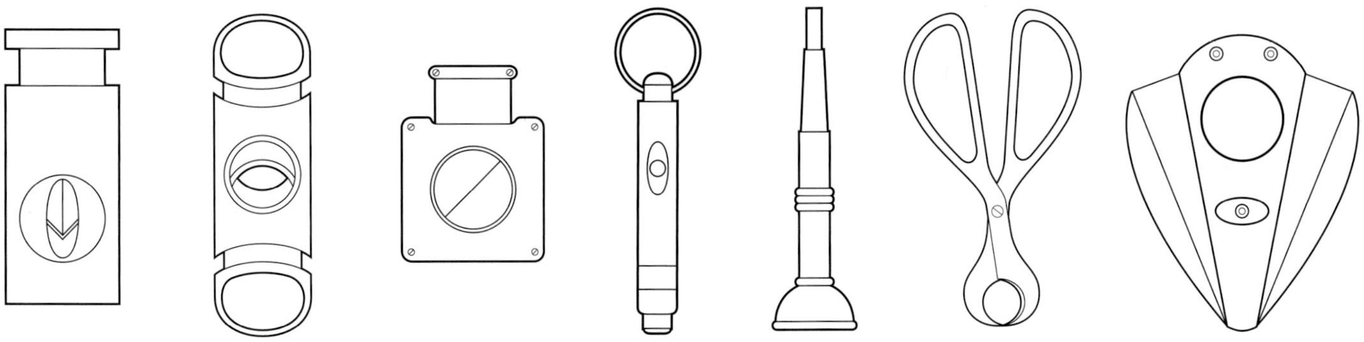

I. V-CUTTER · II. ZINO DOUBLE-BLADE GUILLOTINE · III. ELOI SINGLE-BLADE GUILLOTINE · IV. BULLET/PUNCH · V. PIERCER · VI. SCISSORS · VII. XIKAR XI BUTTERFLY GUILLOTINE

CUTTERS AND CUTTING > To smoke a cigar, part of the cap must be removed to allow air to flow evenly through the stick's body. Each of the six basic types of cutters will make this happen; the one you choose is dictated merely by personal preference. However, regardless of the style cutter you go for, select with care and keep in mind that as with any blade, sharper is better:

V-Cutter, or "Cat's Eye"
Double-Blade Guillotine
Single-Blade Guillotine
Bullet/Punch
Piercer
Scissors
Butterfly Guillotine

The scissors and guillotine: are the most popular ways to cut a cigar. They produce what is colloquially referred to as a straight cut, eliminating most of the cap of the cigar. This is the only way to cut torpedo, belicoso, or perfecto format cigars.

The bullet/punch and piercer: both pierce the head of the cigar, creating a small hole in both the wrapper and binder. In the case of the punch, the filler is also punctured as the punch drills down a like core sampler. What results is a very narrow, deep hole that creates a very concentrated stream of smoke. The punch is a very esoteric and old-style way to cut a cigar, and is rarely used. The bullet is popular among a certain crowd of cigar enthusiasts, it leaves a shallow slice anywhere from a .25 caliber to 9 mm in diameter.

The V-cutter: (once referred to as a Cat's Eye) was popular throughout the first seven decades of the twentieth century. While a perfectly respectable way to cut a cigar (and for years the version espoused by the Alfred Dunhill stores), it has fallen out of vogue.

FINAL CUT > When cutting a straight cigar, it is important to keep the perimeters of the cap intact; in other words, don't lop off the entire end of the cigar. If you do, the head will start to unravel and the rest of the wrapper leaf will soon follow (the one exception to this rule are tapered-end cigars). Once a cigar is cut, you are ready to torch up.

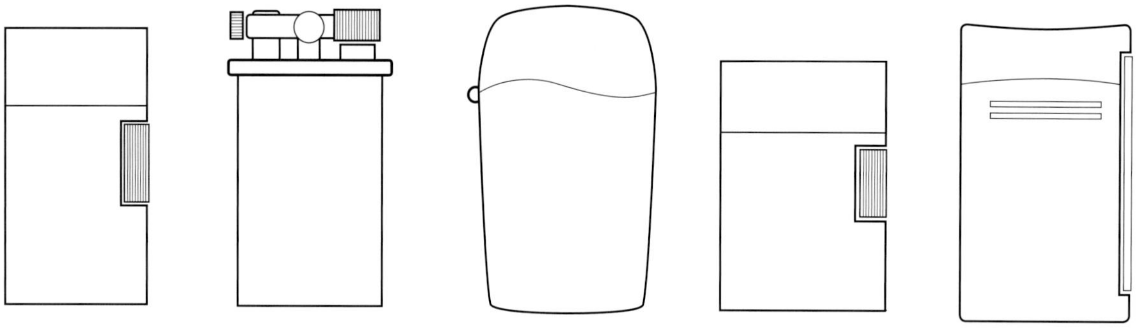

I. DUNHILL ROLLAGAS | II. DUNHILL UNIQUE | III. ZIPPO BLU | IV. S.T. DUPONT GATSBY | V. X.TEND BY S.T. DUPONT

LIGHTING AND LIGHTERS > Many cigar enthusiasts will insist on not having the flame actually touch the cigar, regardless of whether one is using a match or lighter. Whatever. Try as you might, flame will touch tobacco. Some pretentious smokers prefer using a cedar strip (called a "spill" or "split") to light their cigars, but these are messy and hardly practical (although fun for guys looking to unleash their inner pyromaniac).

Those paper matches you pick up for free by the gas-station register are almost as impractical to use as cedar splints, although acceptable in a pinch. For many, long wooden matches are a preferred method of lighting a cigar.

The other method is to use a butane lighter, which burns without producing odor or flavor. Lighters that use kerosene-based liquid fuel, such as the iconic infantry Zippo, are not recommended for cigars; pungent lighter fluid has a propensity to alter the tobacco's flavor.

Once your devotion to the leaf has solidified, treat yourself to a lighter from Alfred Dunhill, S.T. Dupont, Caran d'Ache, or Cartier—all make both flame and torch lighters (the latter produces a very hot and windproof jet of flame).

It is essential to ensure that the entire end of the cigar is afire. First, toast or char the end ("foot") of your cigar to ensure an even burn. Then, place the foot of the cigar at an angle slightly above the flame, and gently draw air through the cigar while keeping the flame going.

In order to make sure your cigar is properly lit, turn the cigar so as to expose the entire circumference to the flame. As my friend Rich says, "Remember to turn and burn, baby."

Think you're done? Turn the cigar around so the foot is facing you and blow gently toward the new ash. If the orange glow is the precise diameter of your cigar, you've finished lighting and are ready to enjoy your smoke. If there are some unlit spots, apply cigar to flame again, concentrating on those unlit areas while drawing in more air. Double-check the foot until the cigar is perfectly lit; an uneven burn will mess up a cigar.

Cut, light, and enjoy!

ASHTRAYS > Along with a handsome humidor, one should really have a proper crystal or porcelain cigar ashtray. How does a cigar ashtray vary from others? Size, for one; they are large, and come with notches of specific ring gauges designed to accommodate cigars.

Most fine crystal design houses, such as Baccarat (which makes the incredible Havana Ashtray) and Lalique (which not only makes cigar friendly ashtrays, but also a crystal topped humidor) offer a range of styles.

Porcelain ashtrays are not only traditional to cigars, but many of the fine porcelain manufacturers have some sort of direct tie-in to them.

Porcelanas Bidasoa of Spain produces all the limited-edition Habanos ashtrays, including the ones that commemorate the annual Festival Habano gala dinners, including the legendary (ashtray and gala) Cohiba 30th Anniversary.

Mottahedeh & Co.'s Tobacco Leaf pattern, originally created circa 1780, is one of its most popular and enduring.

To receive a Hermès porcelain ashtray means you must have done something really right in life. As with their ties and pocket squares, new and vibrant patterns are released periodically. The ashtrays are finished on the bottom with hand-applied suede.

None of these ashtrays come cheap (then again, the best rarely does).

CIGAR STARTER KIT

5 DOMINICAN CIGARS
5 NICARAGUAN CIGARS
5 HONDURAN CIGARS
5 MIXED CIGARS
1 CUTTER
1 CIGAR CASE
1 LIGHTER
1 SMALL ACRYLIC HUMIDOR

ETIQUETTE

Band

Much deliberation and credence has been given to whether to remove a cigar's band or let it remain. There is, however, no right or wrong answer. Do as you please. Keep the following in mind, though: Should you decide to remove it (as I usually do), be careful not to tear the wrapper leaf, which happens upon occasion.

Ash

I am a flicker: not a habitual flicker like cigarette smokers, but a whimsical and playful flicker who likes to dispose of my ash in anticipation of its inevitable fall. Most will tell you to let a cigar ash linger until it falls off into the ashtray of its own volition. This works, but should you be wearing a Kiton suit, my advice is to take preemptive steps and ash when it exceeds an inch and a half or more.

The Considerate Smoker

To some, a cigar's smoke is a perfumed mélange; for many others, it's a malodorous cloud. I have always tried to be a mindful smoker, even more so as it has become a less-public vocation. When in a cigar bar or tobacconist, anything goes; anywhere else, be thoughtful of others (especially the ladies).

The End

Let your cigar rest in an ashtray and extinguish itself. Never, ever, mash it out, or it shall give off an acrid, noxious, and completely avoidable smell.

Some of the details in this chapter might have seemed like esoteric minutiae, but they really were just the basics. However, to reiterate: when all is said and done, all you need is a cigar, a cut, fire . . . and to enjoy.

For anyone whose mind is positively reeling with all this information, jump ahead to the "Archives" chapter (where a few nudie pics will ensure that your brain relaxes) before coming back to the Advanced Course.

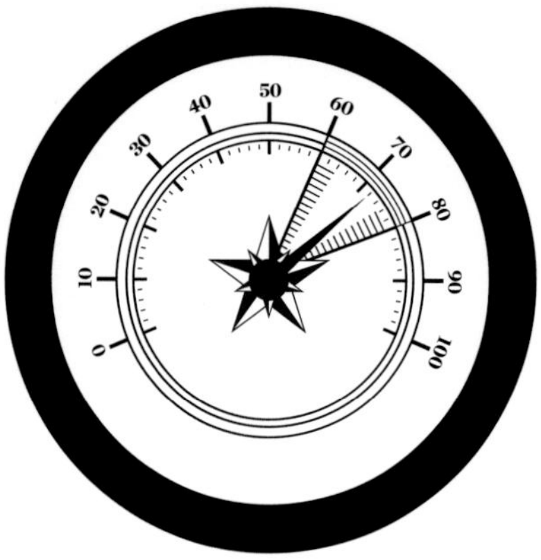

STORAGE

Cigars at home or in the office are stored in desktop humidors, which also need to maintain 70/70 conditions. Without a properly working and maintained humidor, your cigars will be rendered unsmokable, and all hope as you know it will be lost; the compact tropical microcosm you sought to create will become a desert. Humor aside, this means all the money you just spent on boxes of cigars was wasted.

Used properly, a humidor will keep your cigars safe for years. The actual humidification device (called an "element," "unit," or "regulator") in a humidor falls into three categories:

Passive: Passive humidification units are by far the most common. While some are unequivocally better than others, they are nonetheless at their base level nothing more than a sponge filled with distilled or tap water. As such they do not regulate humidity, but rather release it based on rates of evaporation. Maintained properly, they can work however, even if their method is a jot on the crude side.

Bóveda: The Bóveda would best be described as the next generation of passive humidification devices. Created and manufactured by HumidiPak, Bóveda is a two-way humidity control packet designed specifically for desktop humidors. It both emits needed humidity and absorbs excess humidity to maintain cigars at 65 percent, 69 percent, or 72 percent RH, provided the right number of packets are placed inside a given humidor.

Each Bóveda packet contains a specially prepared, saturated solution of pure water and natural salt enclosed in a reverse osmosis membrane. Pretty much idiot-proof, all it requires is replacement once dried out (this takes sixty-ninety days depending on season, outside conditions, etc.).

Active: Active humidification regulators are electronic, and continuously monitor the interior humidity level of a humidor. They are found almost exclusively in high-end cigar cabinets, though the odd active desktop humidor features them as well.

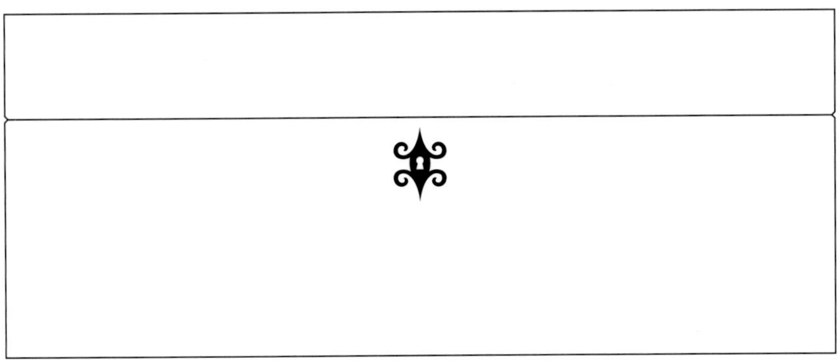

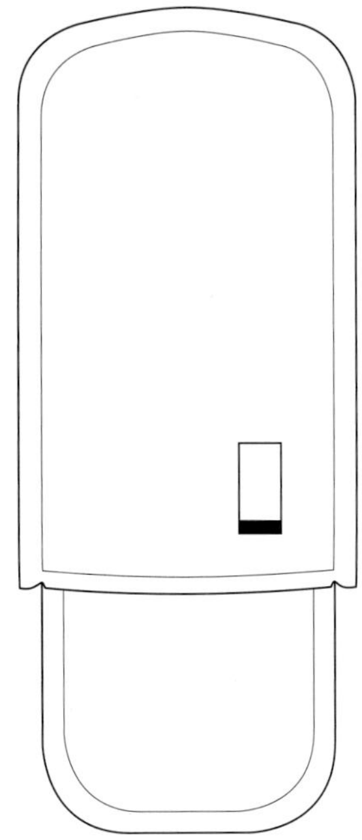

HUMIDORS > Okay, you know what they do, and how they do it, and why they do it, but what does one look for when purchasing one's first (or fifth) humidor—or *cave des cigars,* as they are referred to across the pond?

First of all, know that humidors come in all shapes and sizes, and have primary structures constructed from a great diversity of materials that include wood, stone, carbon fiber, leather, ceramic, and more. Most would agree, though, that the best material for a humidor's frame and exterior veneer is a hard wood.

Then there is the exterior hardware: locks, handles, feet, etc. These range from austere to ornate, and are completely contingent upon the design direction that the maker takes. The interior of any fine humidor is always lined in non-aromatic cedar wood, and has wood (sometimes varnished, sometime unvarnished) shelves and dividers. The interior hardware is limited to a humidification element and a hydrometer . . . nothing else.

The most critical thing in any humidor is the seal. When the lid is shut, it should feel firm and final. All good humidors will have an inside lip which also prevents air from coming in or moisture from escaping.

To check the seal of a humidor, hold it closed up to the light and inspect where the lid and the box meet—it should be uniform all the way around and tight—no warps or gaps. Should you be in a store with minimal dramatic lighting at night, an easy way to test a humidor's seal is to take a dollar bill and close the lid down on it, so that half of the bill dangles outside, then gently pull it out. If the dollar slips out with ease, the humidor has a poor seal; if it comes out with a firm degree of effort then you have a well-constructed and thoroughly sealed box.

When you go to purchase a humidor, the sales associate will tell you that the box you are look at is a "fifty cigar count" or "one hundred" or what have you. That count is based on a traditional Corona-size cigar (6" x 42), which by today's popular sizes such as robusto, toros, etc., is a pretty thin cigar. If you want a humidor that will hold two standard boxes of twenty-five robustos, purchase a seventy-five- or one hundred-cigar humidor.

Be sure to choose with great care. A good humidor, if properly maintained, can last generations, and will probably be the single largest cigar-related purchase over the years, other than the sticks themselves.

VARIATIONS

Humidors come in three basic categories, in size, from smallest to largest:

Travel Humidors: Small humidors that carry six to a dozen cigars, and sometimes more. They are specifically designed with travel in mind. All travel humidors feature a passive system.

Desktop Humidors: The "desktop humidor" is what comes to most people's minds when they think of a humidor box. They come in a wide breadth of sizes, ranging from fifty- to three hundred-cigar count, and are mostly outfitted with either a passive humidification unit or a Bóveda. Many come with hygrometers.

Cabinet Humidors: These also come in a wide variety of shapes and sizes, though the preferred style seems to be an upright cabinet, modeled after refrigerated wine cabinets. All have active systems and are specifically intended to hold a number of whole boxes as opposed to individual sticks.

Cigar Cases: What a travel humidor is for a five-day jaunt, a cigar case suffices for a single day's outing. Most cigar cases are made of molded, hard leather and predominantly come in "two finger" and "three finger" sizes, which to no surprise hold two to three cigars, respectively. I take exception to most two-finger holders, as a cigar smoker should really have three sticks on him—one for himself, one to give away, and one with which to trade. The basic design is a base with a telescoping top that accommodates cigars of different lengths. Some are specifically designed to accommodate wider and/or taller cigars, but most come in just one size. A very few number of cases have small humidification units; however, the majority do not. Have no fear: A few hours—or even a day—outside the humidor will not harm your cigar.

CIGARS

ADVANCED

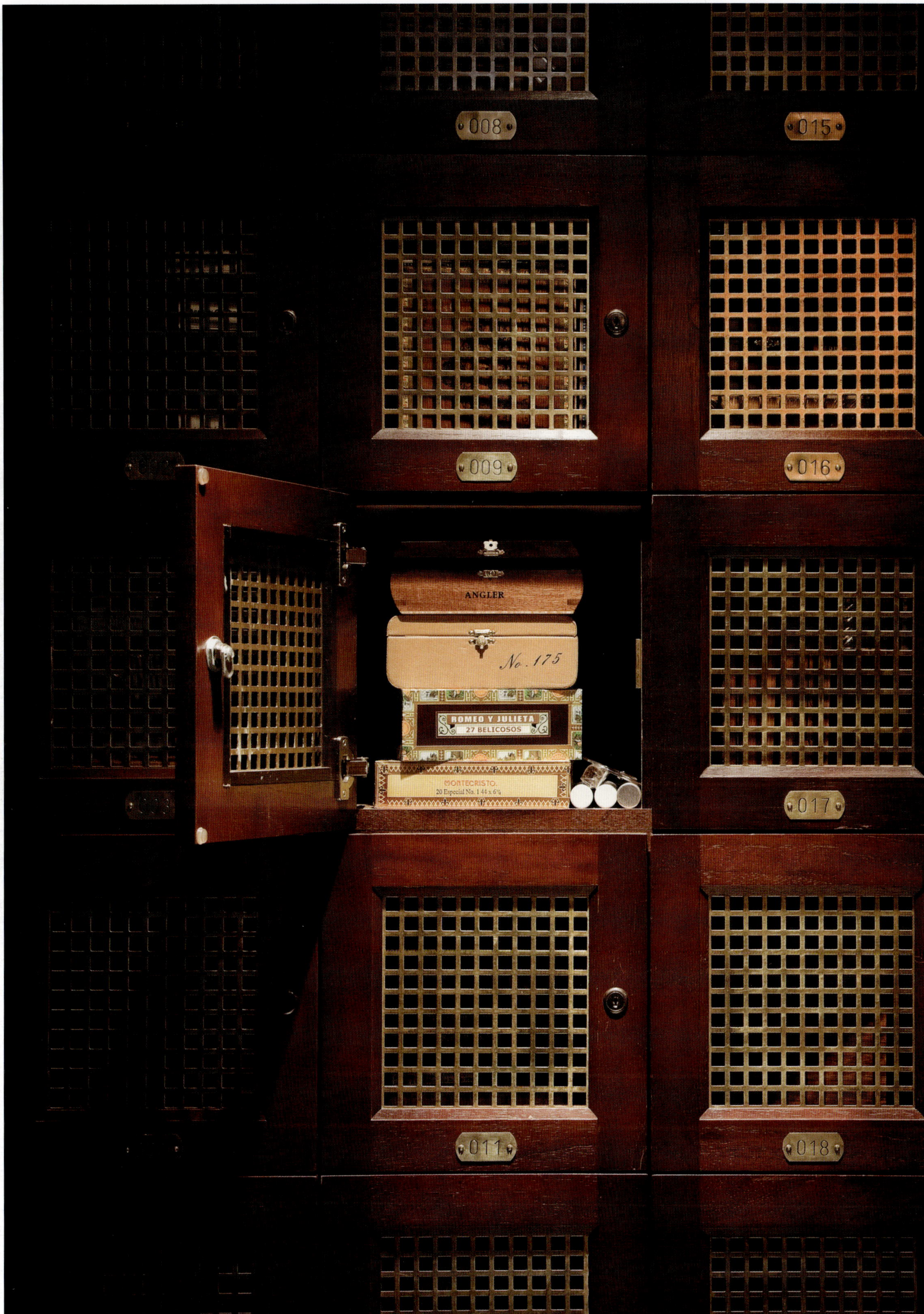
008
015
009
016
ANGLER
No. 175
ROMEO Y JULIETA
27 BELICOSOS
MONTECRISTO
017
011
018

How far would you travel to sample a cigar? What lengths would you go to get there? How long would you age and keep a cigar?

If your answers to the above were: a) the outer reaches of a space-time continuum . . . or at least as far as an international flight will take me; b) absolutely anything, including being stuck alone in a car with Chris Tucker for twelve hours; and c) longer than my momma's been kick'n . . . then this is the chapter for you.

Should cigars have finally become your thing (as they certainly are mine), and you've leaped ahead of "Part-Time Puffer" status, then this is the chapter for you.

And if you're as obsessed with cigars as I am (after all, my smoke mania did lead me to create two magazines, write this book, and roam the world in search of limited edition and prototype cigars, not to mention visit every major cigar growing region and factory), then this chapter is definitely for you.

DINNERS & FESTIVALS > Most people agree that Henry Schielein—the former general manager of the Ritz-Carlton Boston and legendary cigar-zealot—ushered in the contemporary era of cigar salons-cum-dinners in the early 1980s with a black-tie cigar fête in the hotel's tearoom. By the peak of the 1990s cigar boom, literally thousands of such evenings were being held in venues across the country and, indeed, around the world. Though far less frequent these days than during the boom years, cigar dinners are great, not only because of the social and networking opportunities they offer, but also because cigar makers often use them as a venue for launching new cigars.

Some dinners and events are long-standing affairs with a charitable aspect, such as the annual God of Fire dinners, held in New York and Los Angeles to benefit the Cigar Family Charitable Foundation, which provides for children in the Dominican Republic. The Montecristo Cup ProAM golf tournament, held at Casa de Campo in the Dominican Republic, is also a grand affair; it benefits the Montecristo Relief Organization, which provides aid for victims of natural disasters in the Caribbean and elsewhere.

The list goes on and on—here are but a few highlights (keep in mind while perusing that awards season in the U.S. corresponds with cigar festival season in the Caribbean):

Premiering in 2008 as a celebration of "Cigar Country" products, the Dominican ProCigar Festival is a five-day celebration, divided between the towns of Santiago and La Romana, and includes a golf excursion, factory tours, and festive nightly dinners and shows.

La Festival del Habano, a celebration of Cuban cigars, has been held every February since 1998; the concluding gala is now considered a must-attend for true cigar connoisseurs—if only because Cuban cigar monopoly Habanos S.A. now uses the occasion to debut its newest products and unveil its annual Edición Limitadas.

La Festival del Habano began with the far less august Fiesta del Habano, which began in 1994 with the 150th anniversary celebration of H. Upmann. Each of the following successive years also featured a fiesta (the 150th anniversary of Partagas in 1995, the Cohiba thirtieth anniversary dinner in 1996, and so on), and things grew from there. They kept right on growing, in fact, until the three-day party had become a five-day festival featuring a cast of thousands.

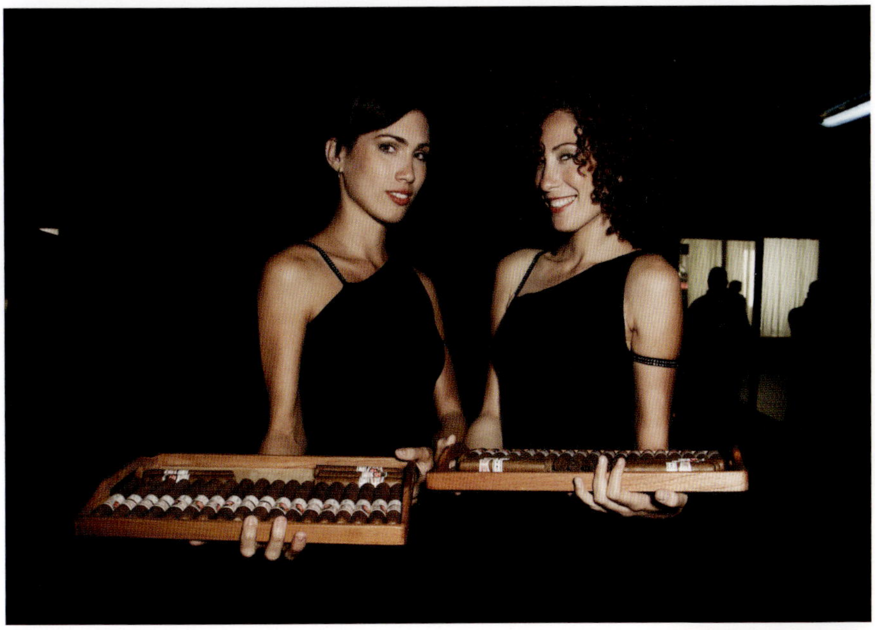

La Festival del Habano. The girls, glitz, gala—good times. (Below) Cigars and cocktails, Playboy–style.

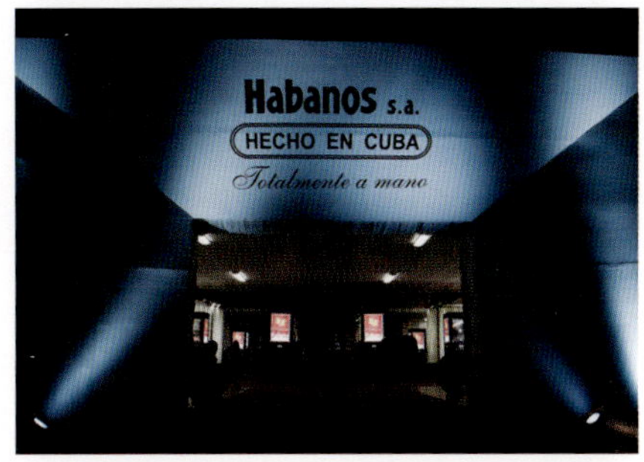

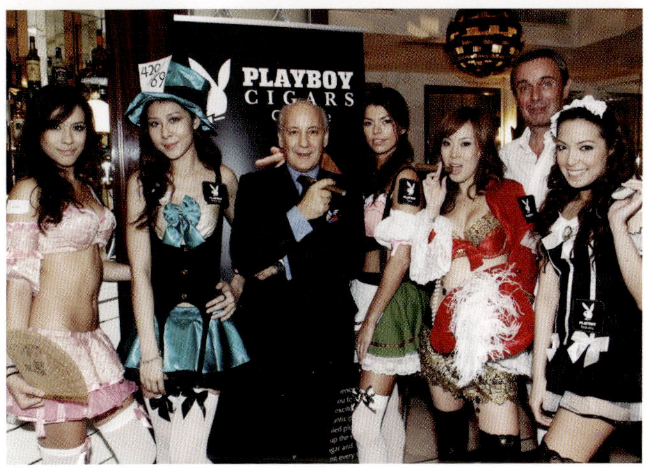

The Cohiba thirtieth anniversary dinner, though, was something to see—largely because of an appearance by El Lider Maximo himself. It had been rumored that Castro would make an appearance at the Partagas 150 dinner, too, and when he refused to materialize, it was a distinct disappointment. So, when the same sort of rumors began to swirl around the Cohiba event, they were greeted with a degree of skepticism. When Castro actually walked into the room that night, there was an audible gasp. Onstage, he (via his English translator) launched into an extemporaneous speech about cigars that lasted an hour and a half—the equivalent of a few brief remarks, considering the man's propensity for five-hour talks. Hearing Castro speak in person made it easier to understand how he kept the island nation under his control for almost forty years: sheer force of charisma. By the end of his speech, if he had asked us all to take a short walk on a long pier off the Malecón, we might have very well done so. *That* was a cigar dinner.

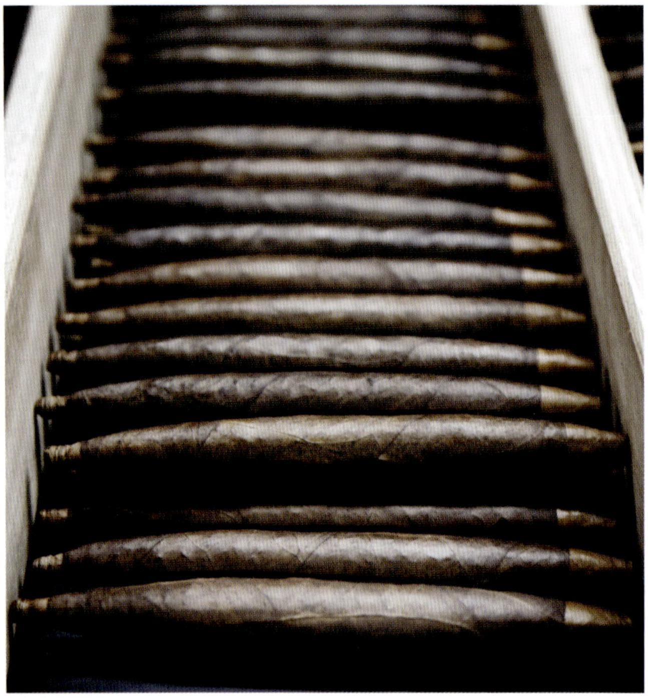

AGING > Just as wines "age" via the interaction between liquid and oxygen corked inside a bottle, so too do cigars mature as their leaves' oils and aromatic compounds interact. As "bottle aging" allows wines to smooth out and become rounder and more complex, cigars age in their humidor and their flavors achieve a kind of harmony.

But how long should a cigar be aged? This is a matter of contention and debate.

In my opinion, a cigar will start to lose its desired flavor somewhere after seven to ten years after it was rolled. Most cigars are best smoked either immediately after being rolled or between one and two years after being boxed.

Cigars are just not like premier cru Bordeaux; they will not be better twenty-five years later. Therefore I believe that when it comes to cigar aging, it's best to live and light up for today; the future may never come.

My friend and longtime collaborator, Dr. Adrian Bartoli, holds a contrary view. So does Min Ron Nee, author of *An Illustrated Encyclopedia of Post-Revolution Havana Cigars* (2003).

Bartoli once wrote: "Anyone who has tasted a pre-Revolution cigar will recall its seemingly limitless complexity, a certain musty élan, the sweet kiss of decay that the cigar left gently lingering on your lips. What it comes down to, of course, is aging."

Now that's a guy who likes an old stogie.

For the millennial new year, Bartoli was kind enough to share with me a box of 1961 Montecristo No.1, perfectly stored for thirty-nine years, and as vintage as vintage gets. To me, however, they were rendered nearly flavorless, with only the faintest nuance of the famed Cuban Monte blend. Bartoli loved them, of course, but I maintain that one shouldn't settle for a mere hint when they could have the peak of flavor in a five-year-old cigar.

Inevitably, discussions among the local cigar posse will drift into tall tales about pre-Revolution and other vintage smokes. The virtues of these cigars will be extolled from the rooftops, which is fine (even great), but it puts the unwary cigar pontificator at risk of becoming a (dreaded) 'Gar Geek.

At a Habanos Festival a few years back, a friend invited me to a tasting held at the El Laguito Cigar Factory. There, we would compare and contrast two Cohiba Lanceros rolled ten years apart. However, there was only one box of the 1996 Lanceros, which was empty before it had circulated around the conference table to me.

The tasting's host offered no apology, but out of respect for my buddy (even though the only available drink was tea served by a dude in a half-kimono) I stuck around.

Thirty minutes after the 2006 cigars were served, the panel discussion-cum-reviews commenced. The host went around the table soliciting each guest's take on the two smokes, and when he didn't get the desired response (something along the lines of, "This is the greatest cigar . . . ever. It's better than the best sex I've ever had!"), he would pepper the respective respondent with questions until they relented to his views.

Not being able to withstand this exercise at length, I exited the room and walked the grounds of the stately mansion-turned-fabrica even though it was pouring rain. The moral was—and is— simple: cigars are many things—fun, fraternal, etc.—but nothing beyond your family and career should be taken that seriously.

Cigars change as they age; anyone who has bought a box of cigars, smoked a few, and put the rest away for a few months has undoubtedly discovered this fact. Without question, this aging process is most pronounced in the first year.

Nee, in his book, breaks down cigar's existence along the following timeline:

Sick Period (first 1–2 years)
First Maturation (2–15 years)
Second Maturation (15–25 years)
Third Maturation (more than 25 years)

The sick period is marked by the presence of a pungent ammonia odor. Afterward, the cigar begins its true maturation—which in Nee's eyes can extend for quite some time. He has been known to remark upon the "smell of a fifty-year-old Don Candido" cigar with such glee that he can hardly contain himself.

My position is that a cigar suitable for aging goes through the following:

Fresh Rolled (first 1–4 weeks)
Sick Period (first 1–12 months)
The Mature Period (1–7 years)
The Plateau (7–10 years)
Decline (10+ years)

To me, the Mature Period represents the cigar at the pinnacle of the taste/blend envisioned by the cigar maker himself. The Plateau is simply that; the cigar will grow physically older, neither substantially improving nor diminishing in flavor and strength. It is a veritable purgatory in the cigar's existence, a nebulous period between perfection and passing.

Decline, the final stage, is where oils and aromatic compounds start to dissipate at a perceptible (often even pronounced) rate, irrespective of the storage conditions. During this period, a cigar will achieve a second plateau, one in which the cigar's flavor will no longer evoke the intended blend, but rather the box (the oil from the cigar box's wood having deeply penetrated and mingled with the tobacco leaf oils) and the environment in which it was stored.

A quick story to illustrate that last point; one day, while visiting a tobacconist in London, I was offered a 1926 Hoyo de Monterrey straight from the private collection of a peer of the realm. Although aged properly, the cigar tasted both like the wood box in which it had been housed and the minerals from the water vapor that kept it moist. In other words, it tasted like the basement that had been its home for decades, one that definitely didn't taste like a cigar.

Who is right? Tell me in fifty years and let me know how Nee's third maturation turns out.

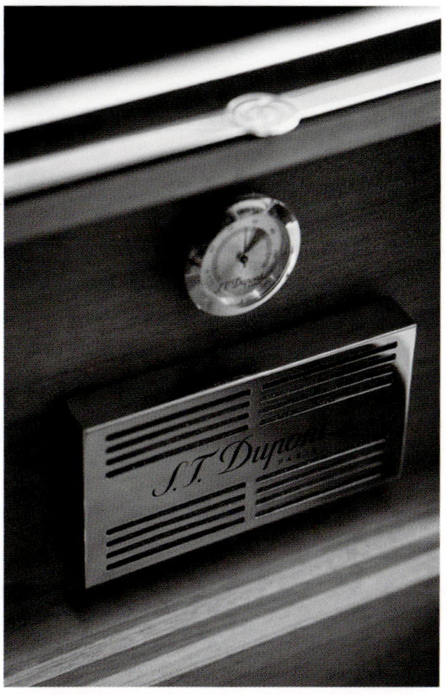

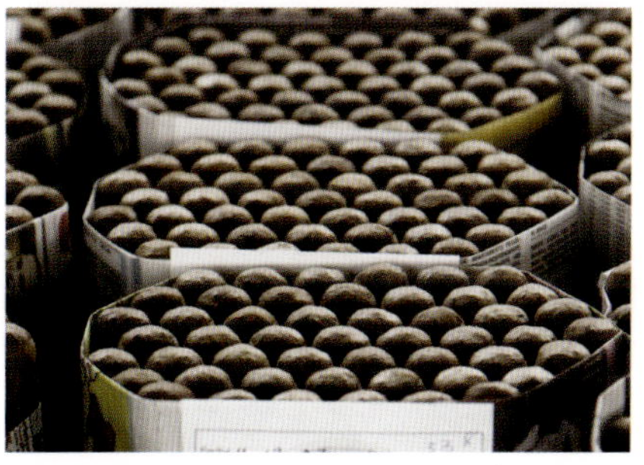

SICK PERIOD

The term for this uniquely-named stage of aging is borrowed from the wine term "bottle sick," in which newly bottled wines go into "shock" from contact with oxygen and sulfur in the bottling process. Author Min Ron Nee believes that continuing maturation of the cigar's tobacco will make the ammonia dissipate at the rate of "90 [percent] gone in a few months, [95 to 99 percent] gone by the end of the first year."

Some people prefer young (fresh) cigars, while others like an older stick—it's all a matter of taste. Either smoke a cigar within the first month of purchasing it, or age them at least a year; but if you suspect your cigar is in Nee's "sick period," do not even sample—just wait.

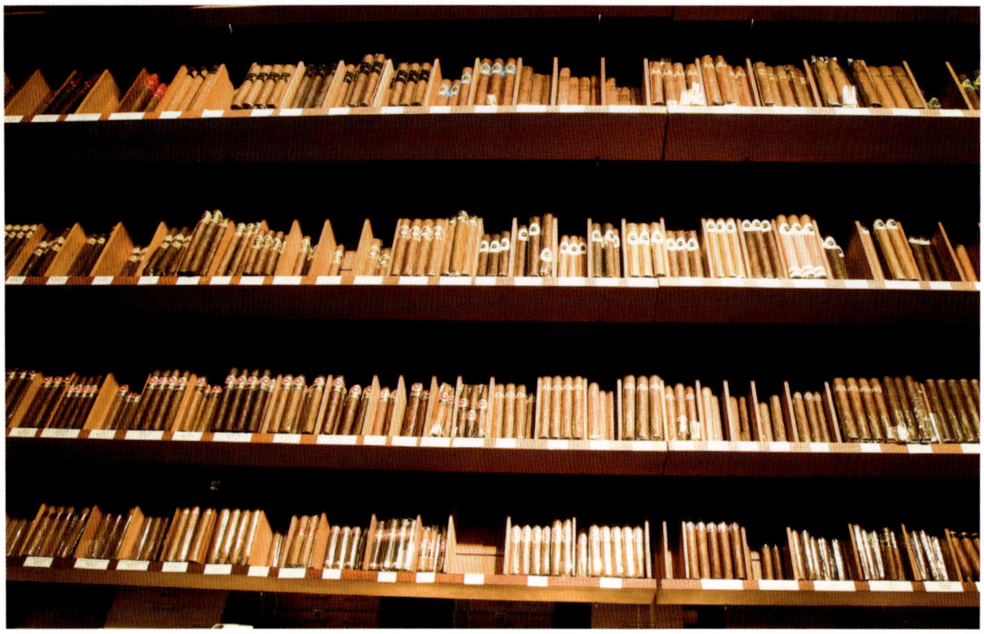

It is often easy to become overwhelmed by the bountiful selection; however, not all cigars are suitable for aging—ask your tobacconist if you are unsure.

SUITABLE CIGARS > The basic ingredients of cigar aging are:

Cigars
Storage
Time

The last thing you want happening after you age your cigars for a year or more is to find that they taste like dirt. This is where cigar type and your method of storage come into play.

First, think about the type of cigars you're going to age. Cuban cigars and select Nicaraguan and Dominicans seem to benefit most from aging. The rule of thumb in determining which cigars will withstand the rigor and challenge of sitting motionless in a box for a really long time is to choose full-flavored and full-bodied cigars, rolled from darker and richer tobacco. Keep in mind, though, that even though heavier cigars will have pleasantly rich flavors when aged; they may smell overwhelming when young, much in the same way that most fine wines are too tannic to drink when young. A corollary of this cigar rule states that if you start out with a really light, floral cigar, you will have a box that has been rendered flavorless in just a few years.

In addition to selecting prime tobacco, one must make sure the cigars are also well-crafted; obviously, if you're going to invest the time and energy in aging cigars, you want something smokable when the time comes. A too-loosely-rolled cigar may lose its entire flavor by the end of the aging process, while one too tightly rolled may crack its wrapper with changes in temperature and humidity.

The size of a cigar is also important. Those with ring gauges north of 50 tend to be better suited for aging, as they are somewhat shielded from the outside environment and less apt to be affected by fluctuations in humidity and temperature. The added stability that larger cigars provide makes them highly desirable for long-term aging.

As I mentioned in a previous chapter, the wrapper determines a large measure of a cigar's flavor, making this something you'll want to focus on when picking out your cigars. The oils and aromatic compounds are key elements in aging; the amount of natural oil in a cigar is revealed by the presence of small oil spots on the wrapper, the translucency of coloration, and the presence of variegation and mottling. None of these things is to be confused with bruising, (which occurs along the veins and indicates the leaf has been crushed) or the small, white, harmless sunspots that dot the occasional wrapper.

Aromatic compounds impart the wrapper with a yellow to reddish tint, turning what would otherwise be a pale brown to a deeper shade of reddish-brown. These naturally darker cigars—as mentioned before—may be more appropriate for aging.

Don't be confused by Maduro wrapper cigars, whose dark coloration and distinctively strong, sweet flavor is the result of forced aging. These cigars have found a place in many people's hearts, but while the binder and filler will age nicely, these cigars' wrappers have been "fixed" (essentially, undergone an extreme fermentation technique) as far as additional aging is concerned.

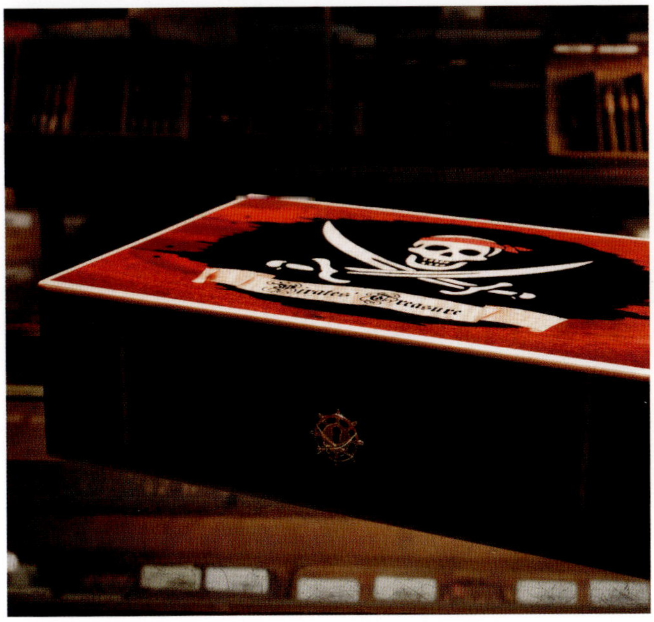

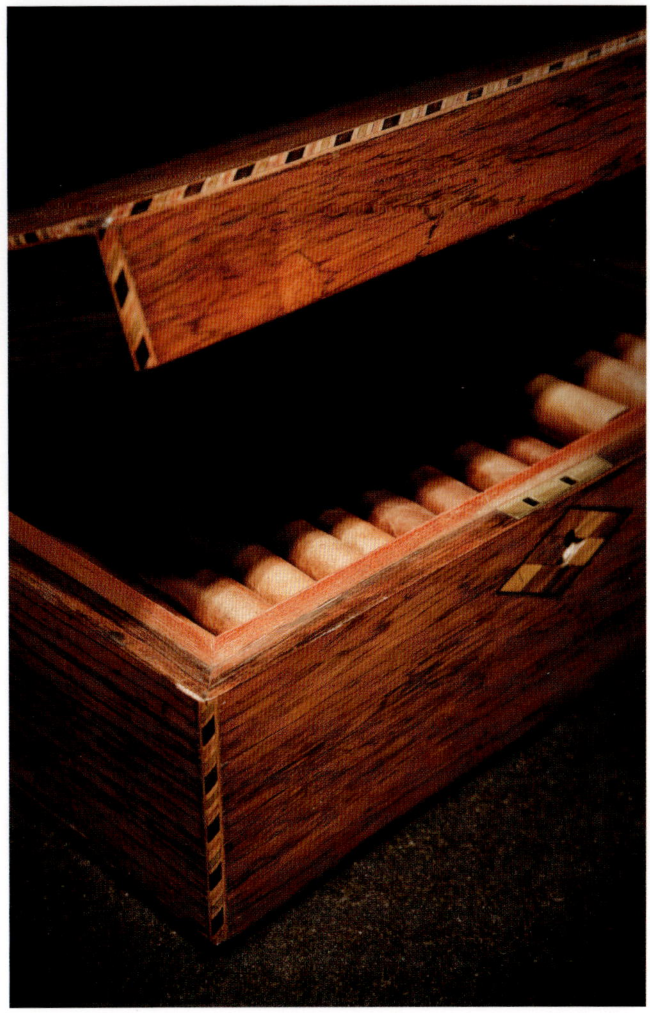

PROPER STORAGE > As previously touched upon, cigars should be kept at 70 degrees and 70 percent humidity. Any more humidity or heat and your cigars will rot, any less and the aging process begins to be impeded. The most crucial aspect of aging is maintaining a stable environment. Rapid changes in temperature and humidity cause cigars to expand and contract, cracking their wrappers.

Keep in mind that this is not just a matter of your humidor's interior, but also the surroundings in which your humidor rests. Avoid setting your humidor either in direct sunlight or in rooms that experience swings in ambient humidity. Stable and consistent is the key.

Cigar aging is an active process. You can't just shut your cigars in a sealed box at a specified temperature and humidity and be done with it. The chemical reactions of the aging process also produce many (at times noxious) gases that would become an impediment to further aging if allowed to build. However, providing an egress for those gases would also let water vapor escape, spoiling any attempts at constant, stable humidity.

Solving this problem resulted in the invention of the humidor, an open box with a constantly replenished humidity element. In ideal circumstances, the space in the humidor should be at least twice the volume of cigars you intend to keep. Let 'em breathe a little.

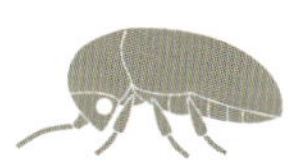

A BUG'S LIFE

Nothing breaks the heart of a smoker more than opening a box of beautiful cigars and finding them reduced to dust by beetles (Lasioderma serricorne). To prevent this from happening:

Proper storage: Make certain (as much as possible) that your cigars are stored in conditions that are both humidity-controlled and temperature-controlled. One way to ensure this, especially for larger cigar collections, is to purchase an active cigar cabinet (refer back to page 37).

Freeze: Place a box in a heavy-gauge Ziploc bag inside your freezer and leave it there for 72 hours. This will turn any beetles and larva into the six-legged equivalent of Jack Nicholson at the end of *The Shining* (that's popsicle-like, for you non–horror movie buffs). Let the cigar defrost (still in the bag) in your refrigerator's empty crisper for a few hours, then take the box out of the plastic bag before placing the box and/or cigars in your humidor.

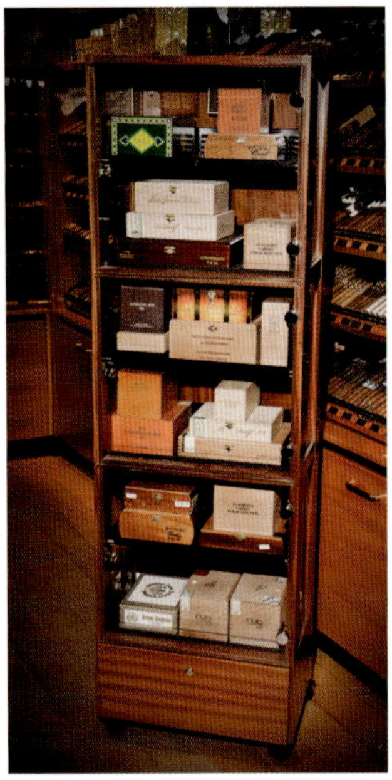

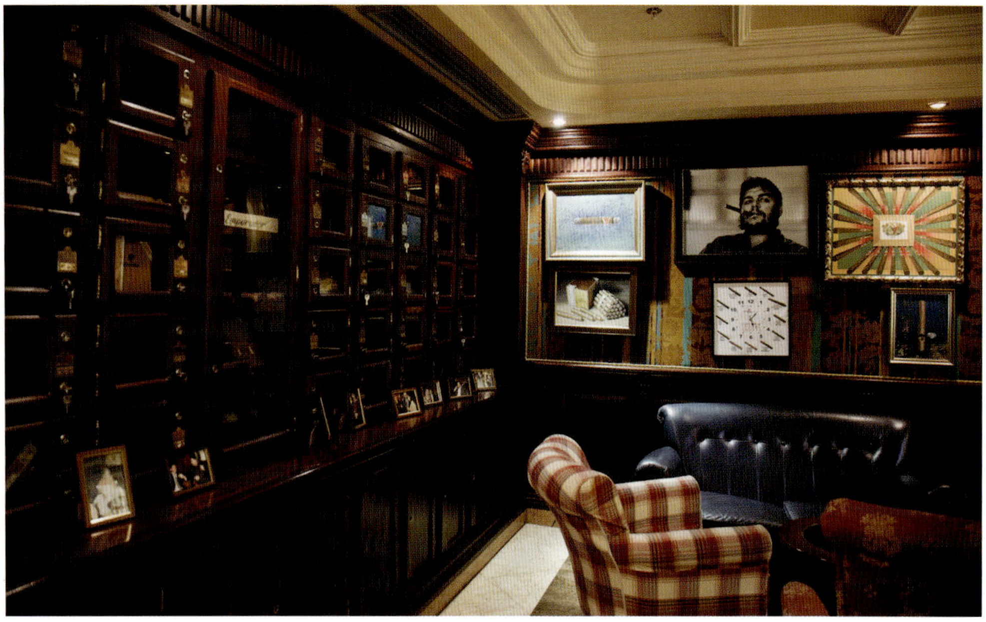

LOCKERS > Whether you're a spatially-challenged type like me who makes do with the tiny living area that a Manhattan apartment affords, or reside in a sprawling *casa de la* 'burbs, chances are your cigar collection could become too large for even a not-so-humble humidor. In such a case, a cigar locker might be a solid option. If you are keen on aging certain select cigars, then lockers become a great option, if only because you'll be less tempted to sneak a smoke—out of sight, out of mind.

Many a cigar store or bar offers lockers for rent, usually for a reasonable annual fee. Should you be that customer who annually drops the cash equivalent of an all-options supercar at their establishment, some tobacconists will even provide you one (hopefully) free of charge.

For space reasons, I have almost always had cigar lockers—often with mixed results. Some humidification systems work, others don't; some work and then stop, and then work again. On occasion, tobacco beetle infestations occur, with the critters jumping from locker to locker until they are destroyed. It's akin to a lice outbreak at a nursery school: one kid gets them, every kid gets them.

Hours of access can also be a point of contention (sometimes, you simply need to puff away at that Dunhill you've been saving—who cares if it's midnight?). Then there's location, location, location, location; often after buying Cubans outside of the U.S., I've had to resort to lockers or shelf space in Toronto, London and Paris in order to store them—which was great as long as my travels took me to those places on a regular basis. Once a project in one of those places ended, though, it could be years before I visited again—and in the case of Toronto, I arrived at the tobacconist where I'd been storing my smokes only to find that—in my long absence—the store (and my cigars) had vanished.

Food for thought, indeed.

CLUB MEMBERSHIPS > My father had a set of philosophies that centered around one of his favorite expressions: "If it floats, flies, or fucks, rent it." This attitude extended to vacation homes and beach houses. He would say, "Why would anyone buy a place and go back year after year when you could rent the best suite in a hotel someplace new and different for two weeks every year for less money than the mortgage, insurance, and maintenance of a second home?" And I have to agree: purchasing equals commitment.

Clubs and club memberships fall into the same category. If you want to smoke a cigar in the same place day after day (and perhaps year after year), then a club might be great for you. Since lockers and club memberships often go hand in hand, it might be worth it to join in order to obtain a prime locker—I won't stop you. While I loved my father, I didn't necessarily agree with all his adages; to that point I've often enjoyed being both a guest and a member at such clubs.

And if you truly do believe variety is the spice of life, you can be like my friend Adam, who has multiple cigar lockers in many different locations. Recently, he sent me an e-mail when we were trying to decide where to meet up to light up that in part read: "I'm like a dog with a big backyard burying bones . . . I plant cigars all over the city and then decide what kind of mood I'm in . . . This week it's been Cigar Inn all week . . . by next week I could be back @ Nat's, and within a few weeks when it gets warmer we'll be on the terrace of the Williams Club."

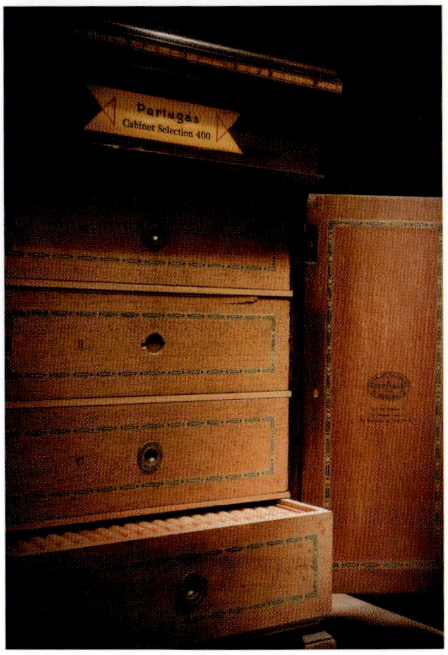

A highly collectible antique humidor filled with equally aged cigars worthy of a Christie's auction, Edición Limitada offerings from Cuba and the Dominican Republic.

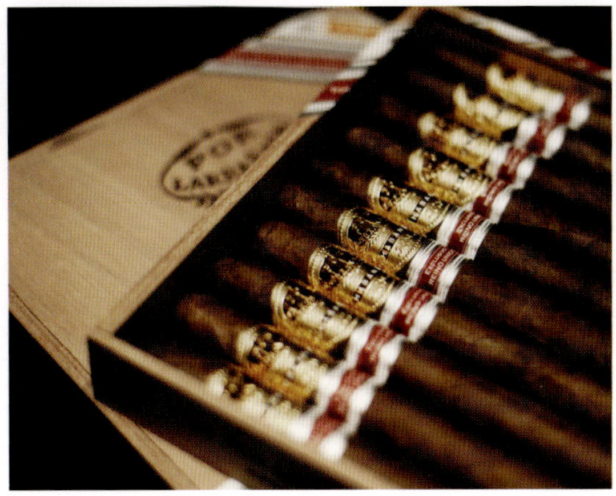

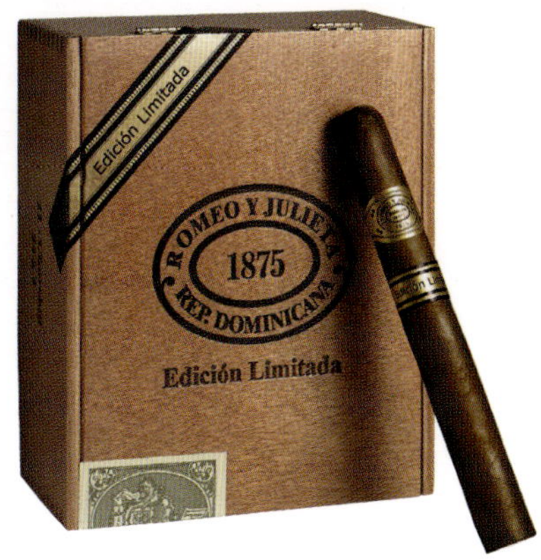

COLLECTING LIMITED PRODUCTION CIGARS, LIMITED EDITION CIGARS & SPECIAL OCCASION HUMIDORS > The natural extension of aging is, of course, collecting. If you were the kid with every *Star Wars* action figure in the original packaging (which you then sold on eBay to buy your first house), then you are probably predisposed to the collecting bug.

There are some incredibly impressive and encyclopedic cigar collections out there, often tended by some truly passionate but often eccentric cigar collectors. I have happened across a variety of people in that genre, including a dethroned porn king, a rather fastidious TV producer, and a tax-dodging fish expert—though I will only go into detail about one of them.

I visited Al Goldstein on any number of occasions at his Pompano Beach, Florida, estate. I marveled at the fact that this onetime publisher of *Screw* magazine had converted an entire bedroom into a giant walk-in humidor, filled with the most eclectic collection I had ever seen. Everything was there, from vintage Cubans to well-aged La Platas.

Al loved cigars so much that he launched a newsletter, titled *Cigar,* in 1980, complete with cigar reviews written by Bill Cosby, his neighbor on Manhattan's Upper East Side. Sadly, *Cigar* folded after only four issues. I always had a great affection for Al, even as and after he lost his mind and company, followed soon by his fortune.

The eclectic nature of his collection was unrivaled compared to anything I had ever seen. He would age a selection of Te-Amos —the cabdriver's cigar—for fifteen years. Yet beside that he would have a splendid box of Cuban Davidoff Chateau Latour that had been maturing splendidly for at least a decade. There was no rhyme or reason, just a lack of organization and aesthetics, with cigars jammed into a wide mix of small and large humidors—but whether the cigar in question was a throwaway or one of the most valuable ever, he treated them all with equal care. That was the important part.

You too can collect cigars of suitable quality. However, those who consider themselves to be true connoisseurs have a propensity to gravitate toward the rare and obscure. These are divided into three broad categories:

Limited Production: A recurring range of cigars—either produced year after year or for a limited number of years—which has a rigidly set limited annual production run, irrespective of demand. While limited, the quantities are far greater than limited editions—comparable to a winemaker's estate or private reserve. The Dominican Edición Limitada by Altadis U.S.A., Fuente Fuente OpusX, La Aurora Cien Anos (initially 300,000 made over three years between 2003–06, the Preferido was released in 2009, however, with only 800 boxes made available, going from limited production to a very limited edition—see below), and the Padron 1926 Series are all examples of limited production cigars.

Limited Edition: The name says it all. Like any other limited edition collectible, these cigars are numbered (either on the individual bands, the boxes, or both) and in some cases signed on production tags either inside the box or on the box itself.

Limited Edition undertakings have no set rules on what makes them limited (shape, size, tobacco, blend) or the quantity in which they are produced. Often, the cigars contain vintage or select tobacco that had an incredibly low yield . . . only enough to produce a small batch of sticks. Cigar makers Peter Johnson and Litto Gomez often develop very limited edition and much coveted products, with the Cuban Edición Limitadas being perhaps the best example.

Special Occasion Humidors with Cigars: Often the most limited offering (in some cases true one-offs), these custom cabinets or desktop humidors come with a few dozen to a couple hundred cigars inside, and are usually for the serious collector. Prices for these often go into five (and occasionally six) figures—not surprising, considering that only a few dozen to a few hundred are typically made.

PART II

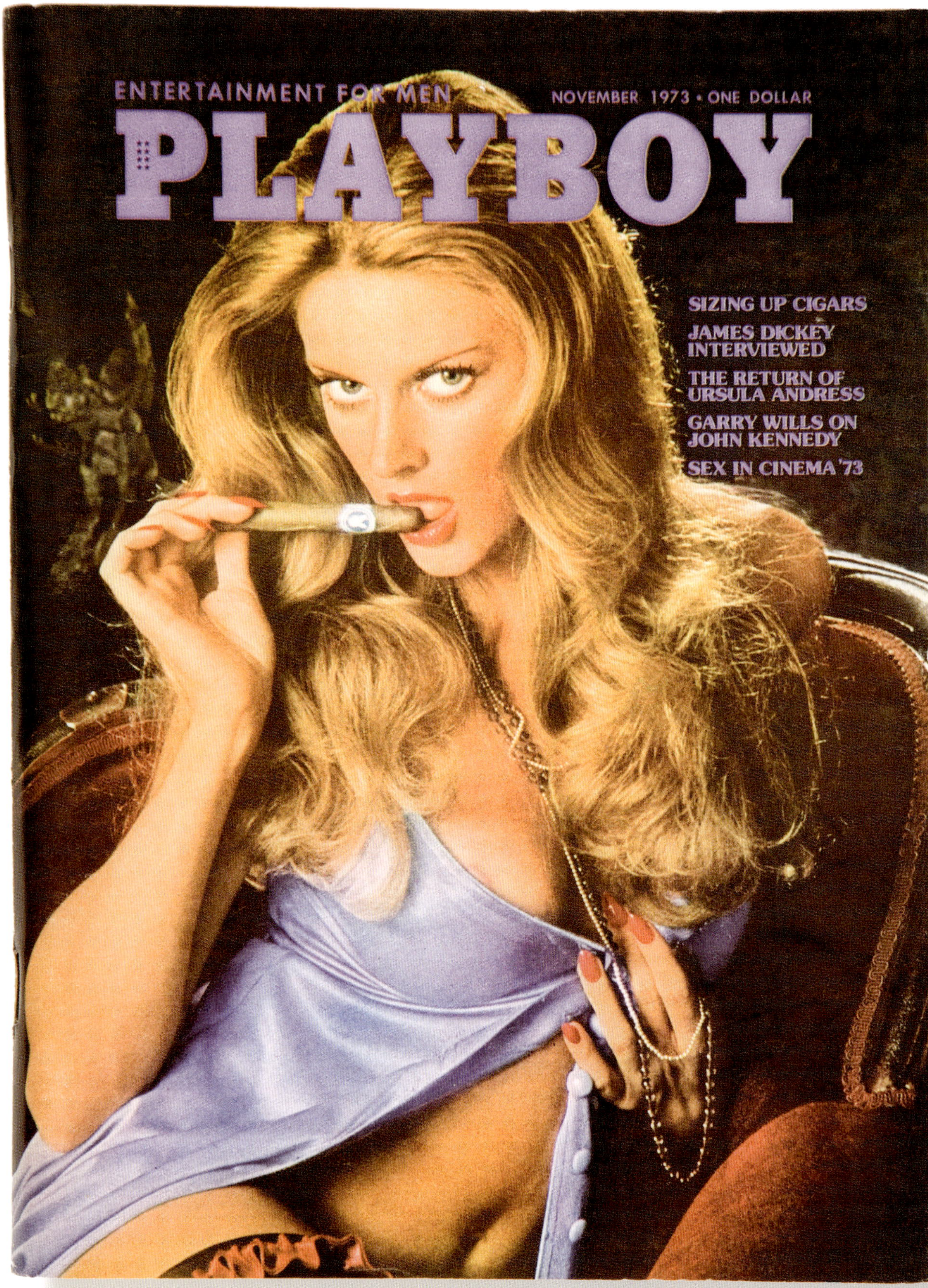
ENTERTAINMENT FOR MEN
NOVEMBER 1973 • ONE DOLLAR
PLAYBOY
SIZING UP CIGARS
JAMES DICKEY INTERVIEWED
THE RETURN OF URSULA ANDRESS
GARRY WILLS ON JOHN KENNEDY
SEX IN CINEMA '73

1973

THE PLAYBOY archives

To underscore *Playboy*'s contributions, perpetuation, and quite possibly preservation of cigar culture, the following section offers up articles, illustrations, cartoons, and ephemera all related to the subject. In every case, the cigar is the ultimate accoutrement of the good life, emphasizing—in ways both overt and subtextual—the elegance and beauty of the subject at hand (remove the smoke from any of the images on the following pages and suddenly they seem a bit emptier). With the cigar comes the allure, the *je ne sais quoi* that *Playboy* was first to bring to audiences everywhere.

1973

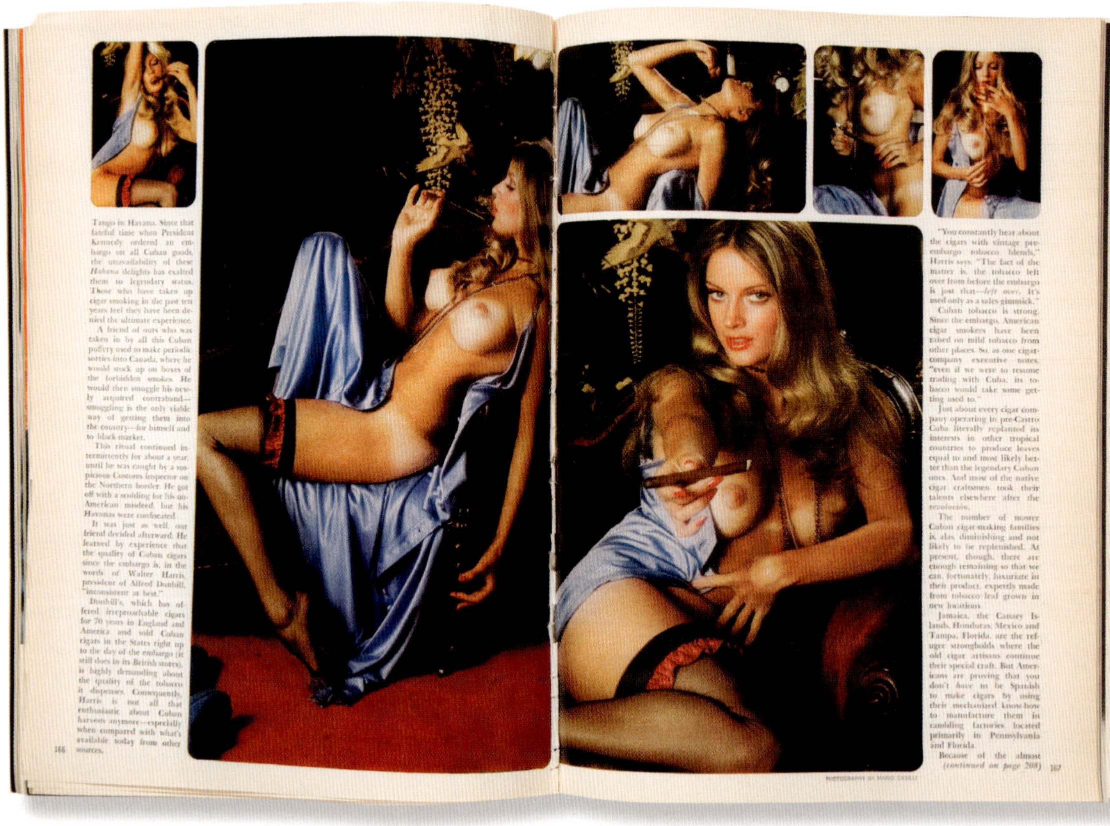

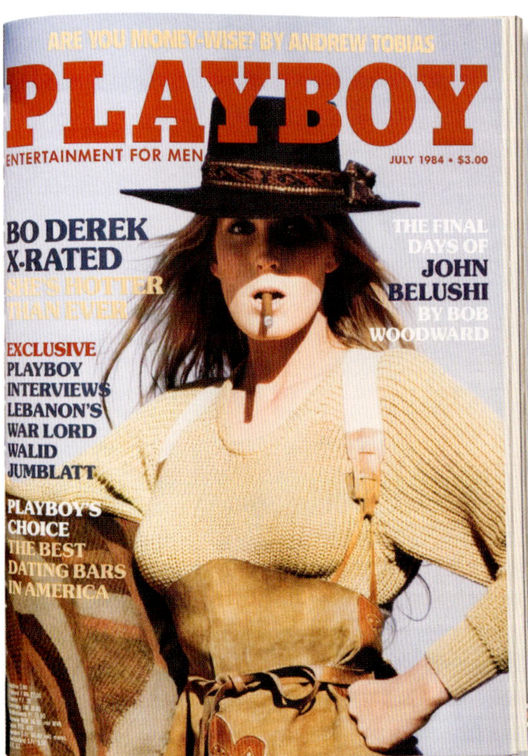

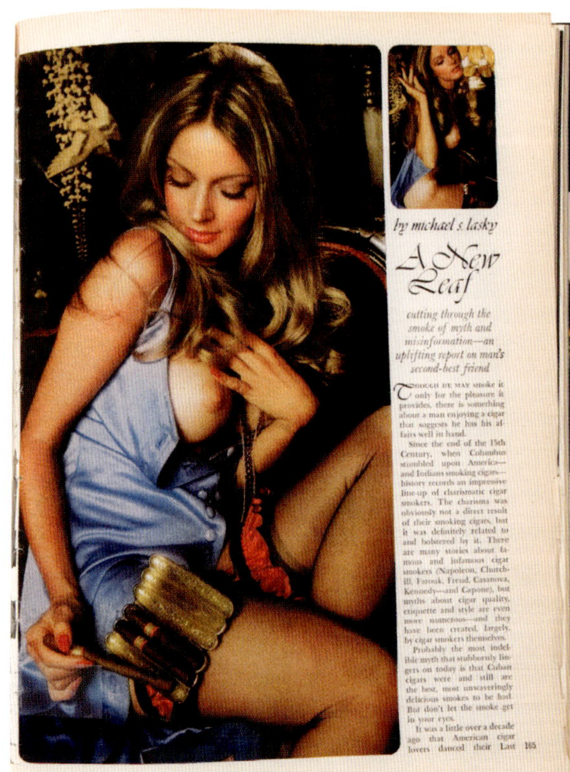

1984

1973

1996

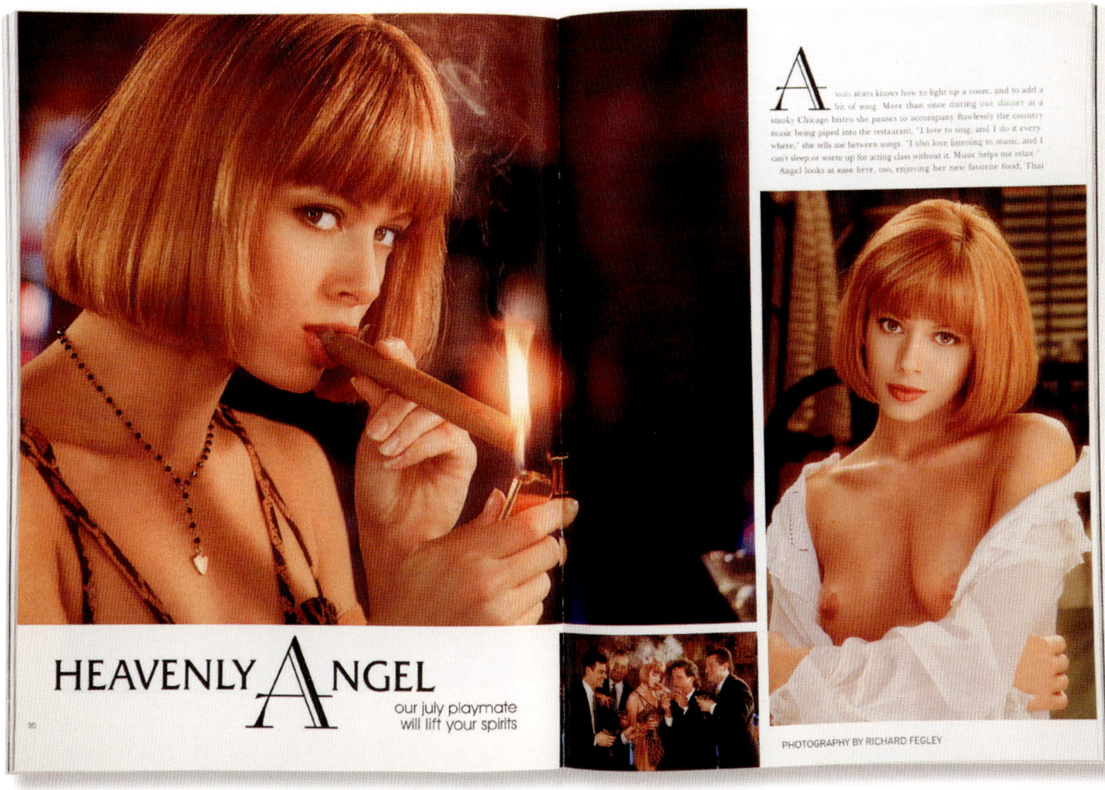

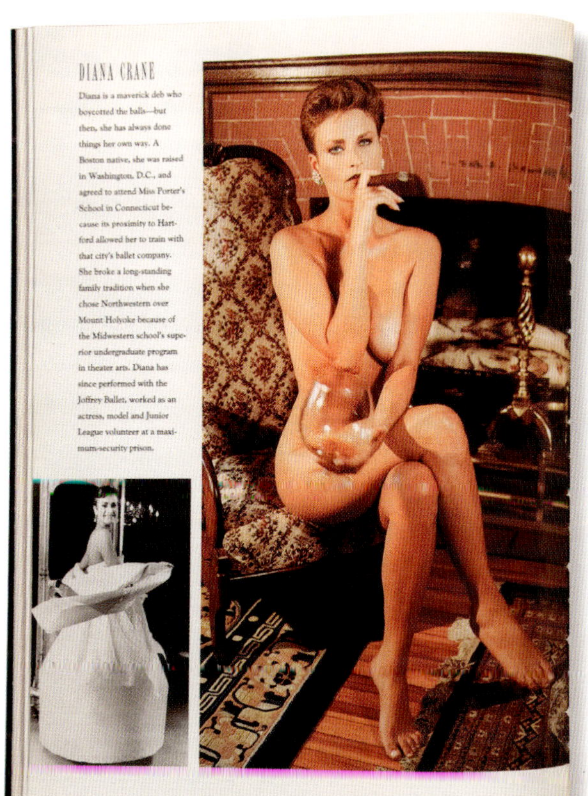

1992

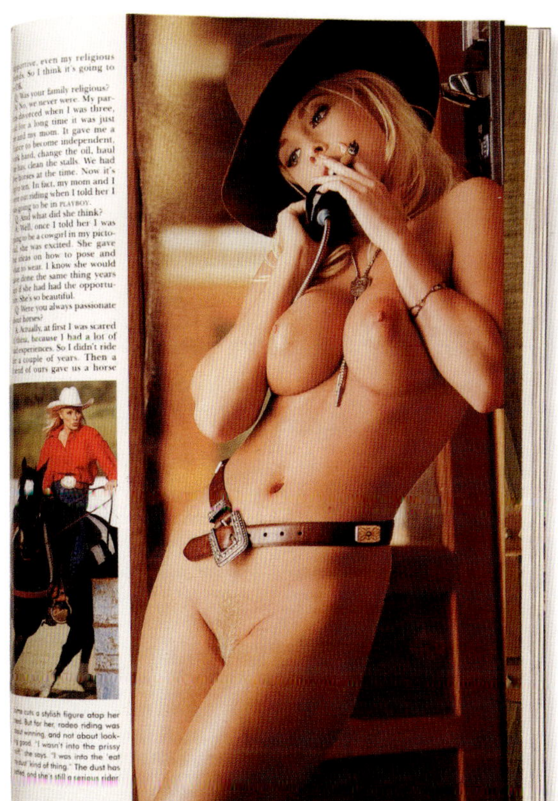

1999

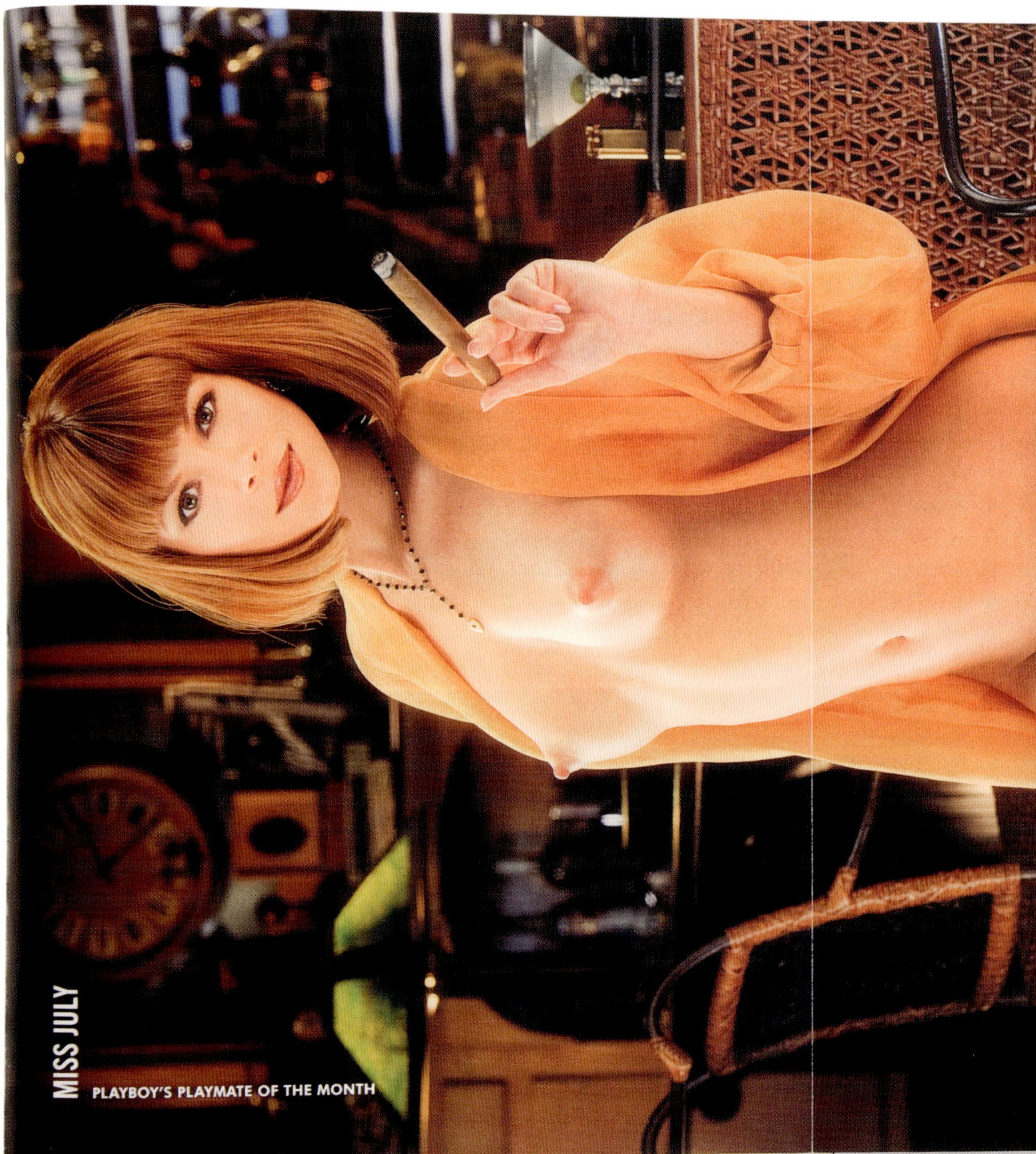

1996

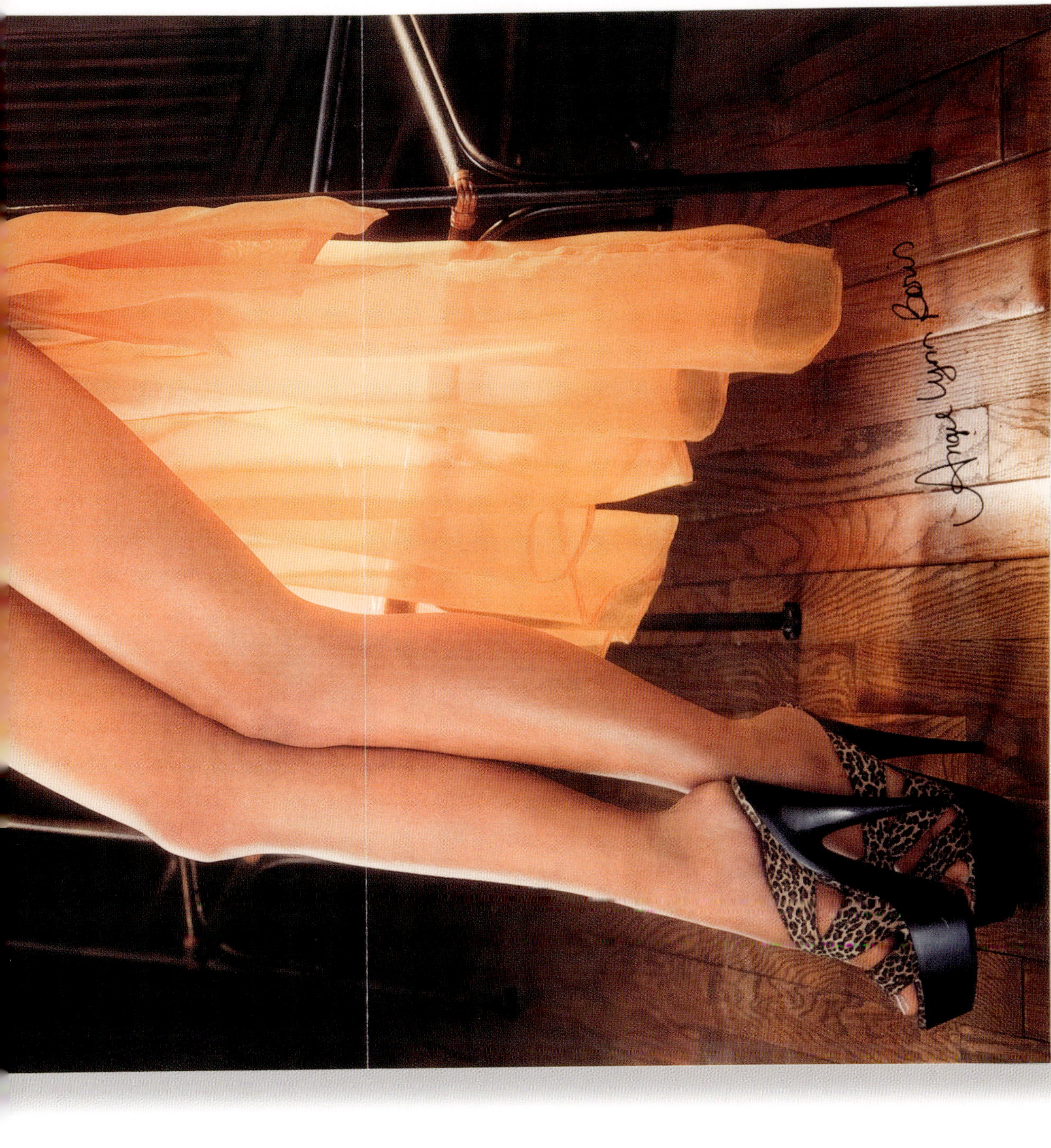

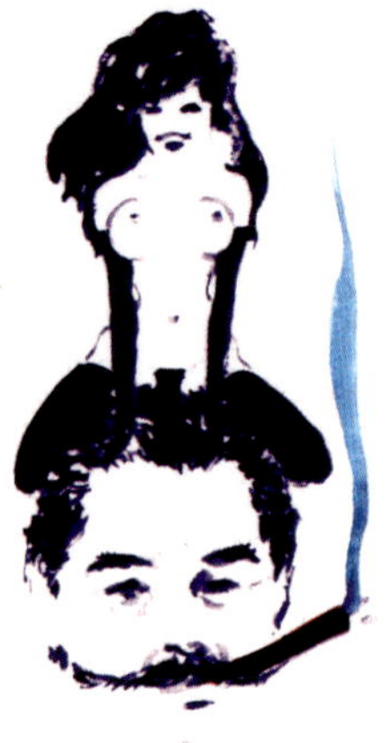

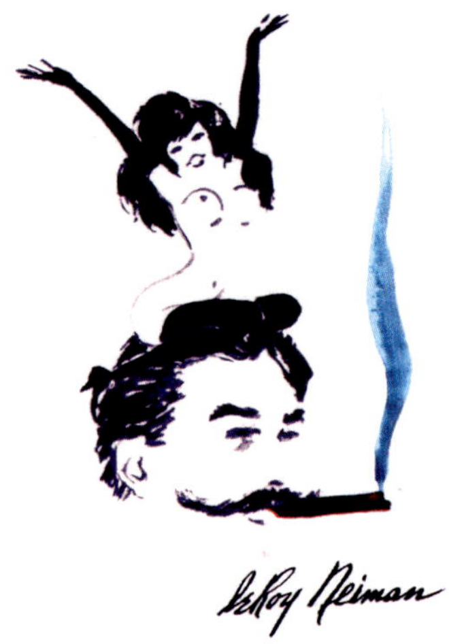

1985

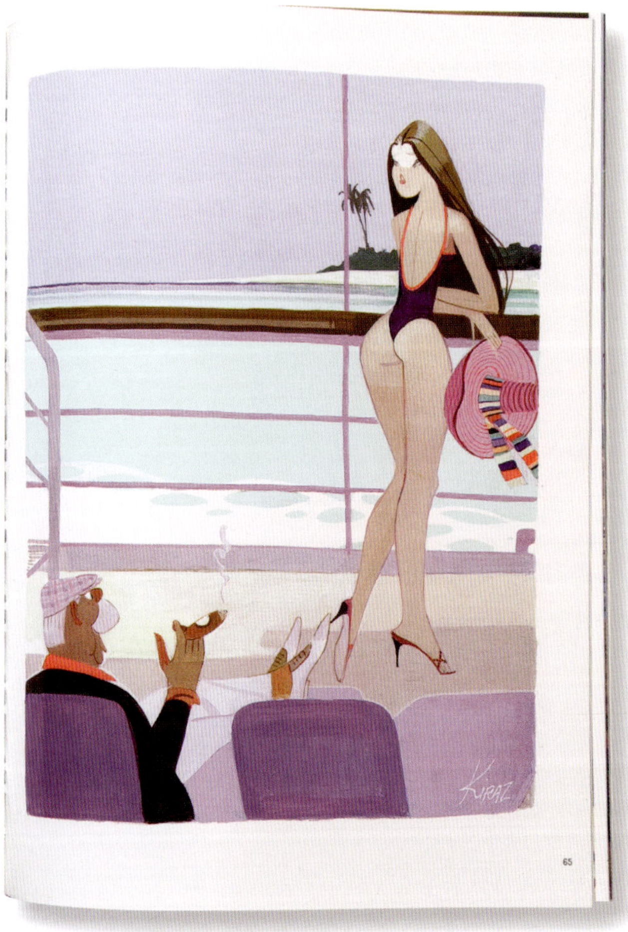

1996

"Oh, no—you're not hiding the view... quite the contrary...!"

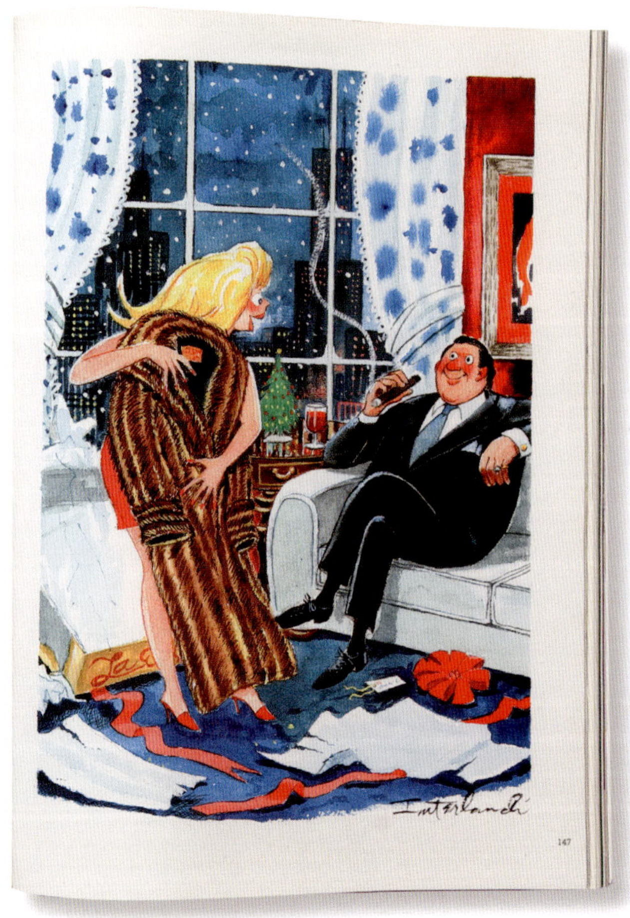

1973

"I'm delighted you're not one of those who thinks it's the thought that counts!"

2008

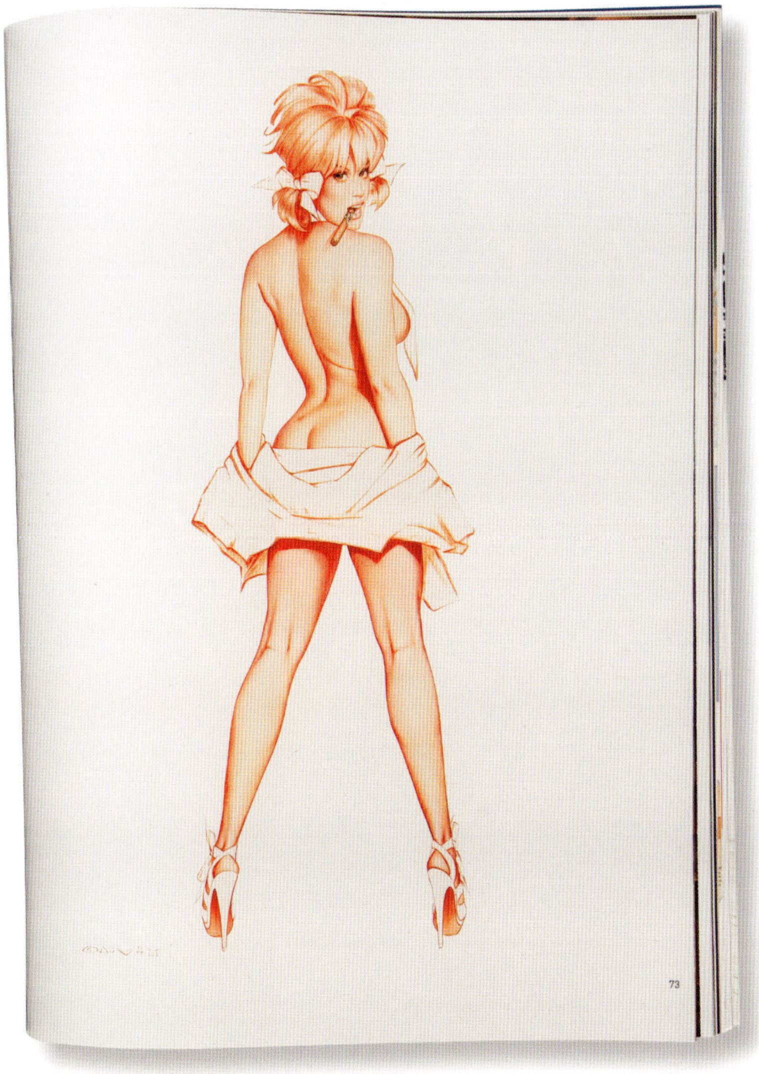

"Got a light?"

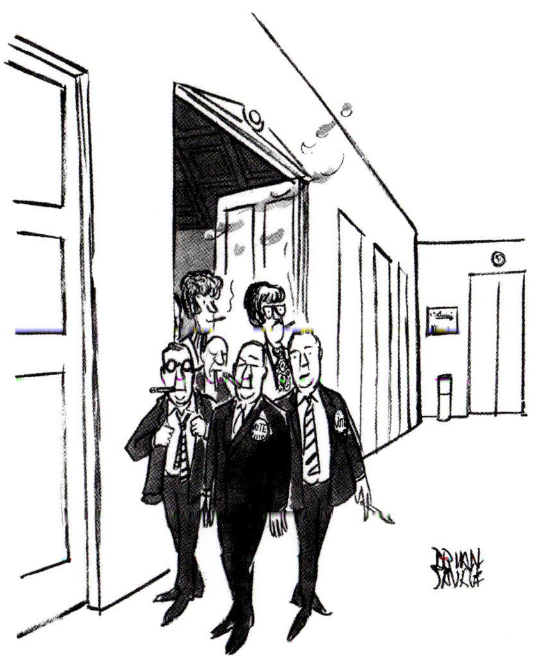

1972

"One thing about youngsters participating in politics—the smoke-filled rooms sure smell different."

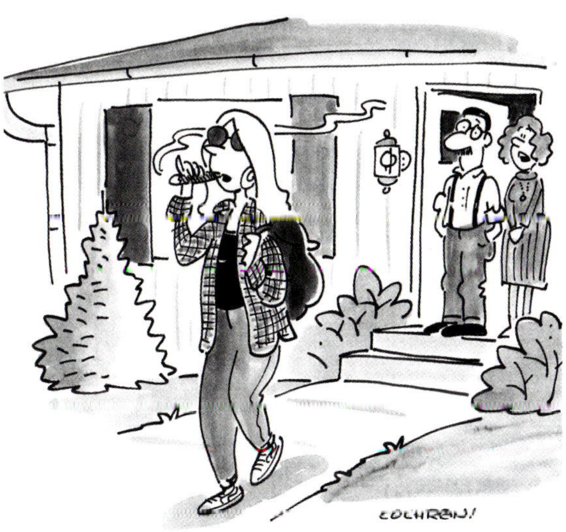

1999

"She makes good grades and she practices safe sex, so I suppose we should overlook the stogies."

1997

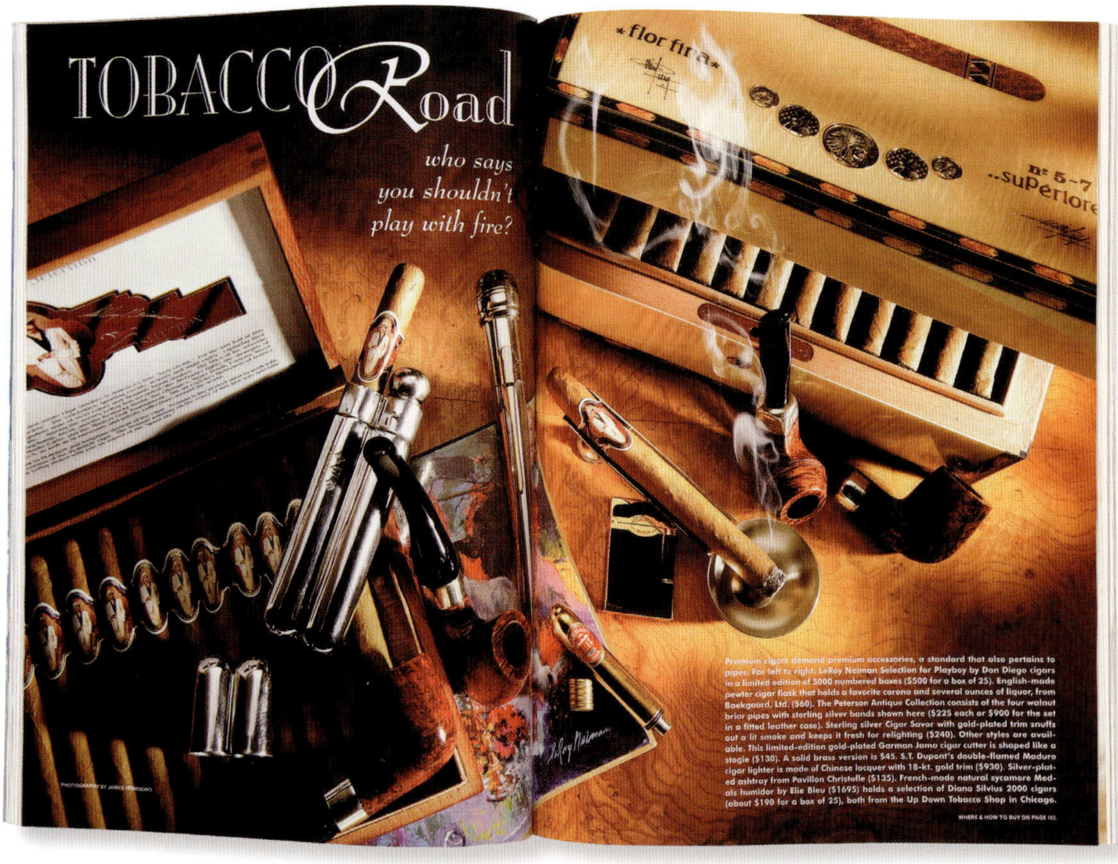

TOBACCO Road

who says you shouldn't play with fire?

Premium cigars demand premium accessories, a standard that also pertains to pipes. Far left to right: LeRoy Neiman Selection for Playboy by Don Diego cigars in a limited edition of 5000 numbered boxes ($500 for a box of 25). English-made pewter cigar flask that holds a favorite corona and several ounces of liquor, from Baekgaard, Ltd. ($60). The Peterson Antique Collection consists of the four walnut briar pipes with sterling silver bands shown here ($225 each or $900 for the set in a fitted leather case). Sterling silver Cigar Savor with gold-plated trim snuffs out a lit smoke and keeps it fresh for relighting ($240). Other styles are available. This limited-edition gold-plated Garman Jamo cigar cutter is shaped like a stogie ($130). A solid brass version is $45. S.T. Dupont's double-flamed Maduro cigar lighter is made of Chinese lacquer with 18-kt. gold trim ($930). Silver-plated ashtray from Pavillon Christofle ($135). French-made natural sycamore Medals humidor by Elie Bleu ($1695) holds a selection of Diana Silvius 2000 cigars (about $190 for a box of 25), both from the Up Down Tobacco Shop in Chicago.

WHERE & HOW TO BUY ON PAGE 155.

2008

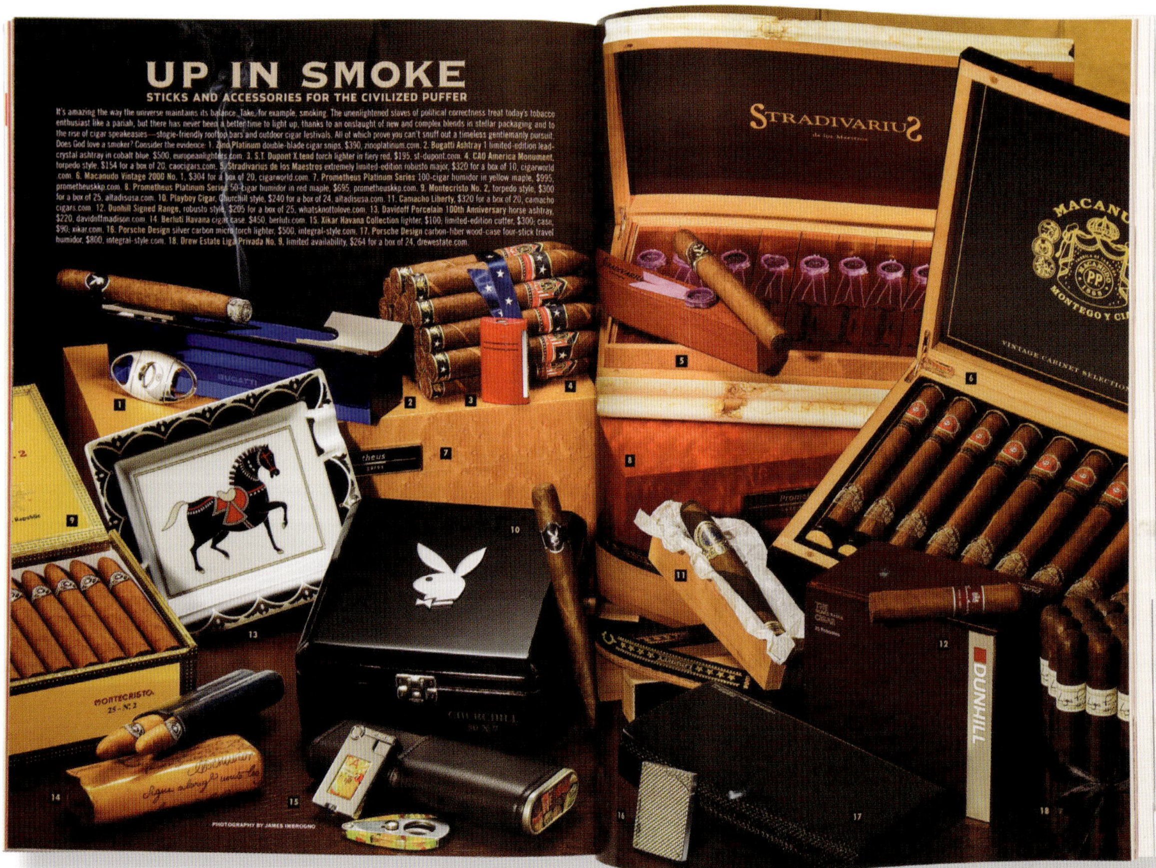

UP IN SMOKE

STICKS AND ACCESSORIES FOR THE CIVILIZED PUFFER

It's amazing the way the universe maintains its balance. Take, for example, smoking. The unenlightened slaves of political correctness treat today's tobacco enthusiast like a pariah, but there has never been a better time to light up, thanks to an onslaught of new and complex blends in stellar packaging and to the rise of cigar speakeasies—stogie-friendly rooftop bars and outdoor cigar festivals. All of which prove you can't snuff out a timeless gentlemanly pursuit. Does God love a smoker? Consider the evidence: 1. Zino Platinum double-blade cigar snips, $390, zinoplatinum.com. 2. Bugatti Ashtray 1 limited-edition lead-crystal ashtray in cobalt blue, $500, europeanlighters.com. 3. S.T. Dupont X.tend torch lighter in fiery red, $195, st-dupont.com. 4. CAO America Monument, torpedo style, $154 for a box of 20, caocigars.com. 5. Stradivarius de los Maestros extremely limited-edition robusto major, $320 for a box of 10, cigarworld.com. 6. Macanudo Vintage 2000 No. 1, $304 for a box of 20, cigarworld.com. 7. Prometheus Platinum Series 100-cigar humidor in yellow maple, $995, prometheuskkp.com. 8. Prometheus Platinum Series 50-cigar humidor in red maple, $695, prometheuskkp.com. 9. Montecristo No. 2, torpedo style, $300 for a box of 25, altadisusa.com. 10. Playboy Cigar, Churchill style, $240 for a box of 24, altadisusa.com. 11. Camacho Liberty, $320 for a box of 20, camachocigars.com. 12. Dunhill Signed Range, robusto style, $205 for a box of 25, whatsknottolove.com. 13. Davidoff Porcelain 100th Anniversary horse ashtray, $220, davidoffmadison.com. 14. Berluti Havana cigar case, $450, berluti.com. 15. Xikar Havana Collection lighter, $100; limited-edition cutter, $300; case, $90; xikar.com. 16. Porsche Design silver carbon micro torch lighter, $500, integral-style.com. 17. Porsche Design carbon-fiber wood-case four-stick travel humidor, $800, integral-style.com. 18. Drew Estate Liga Privada No. 9, limited availability, $264 for a box of 24, drewestate.com.

1992

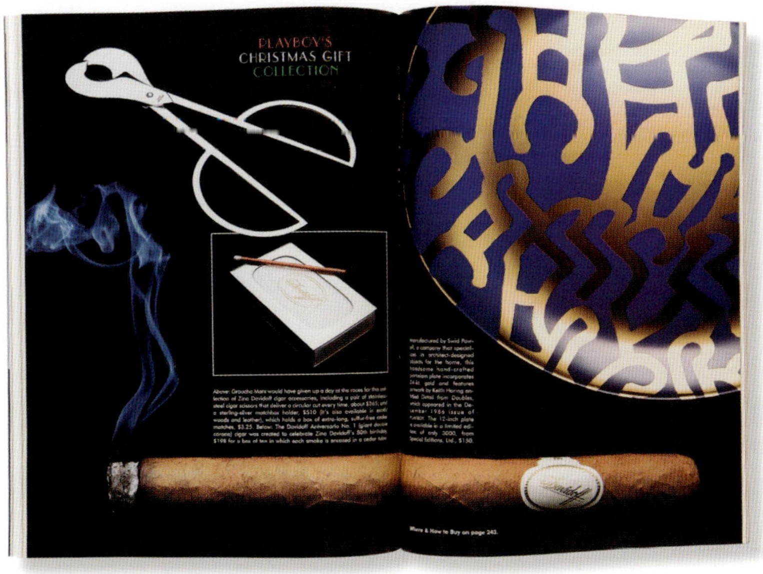

1996

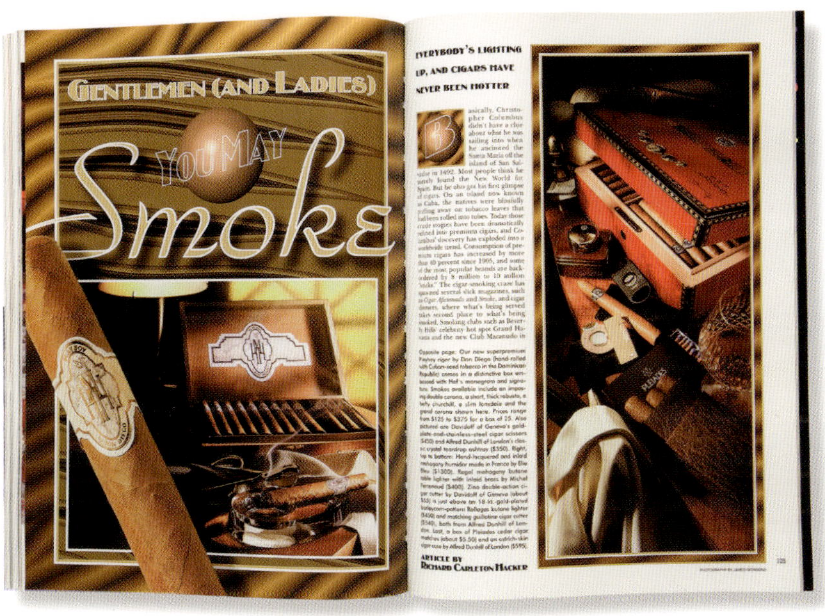

1984

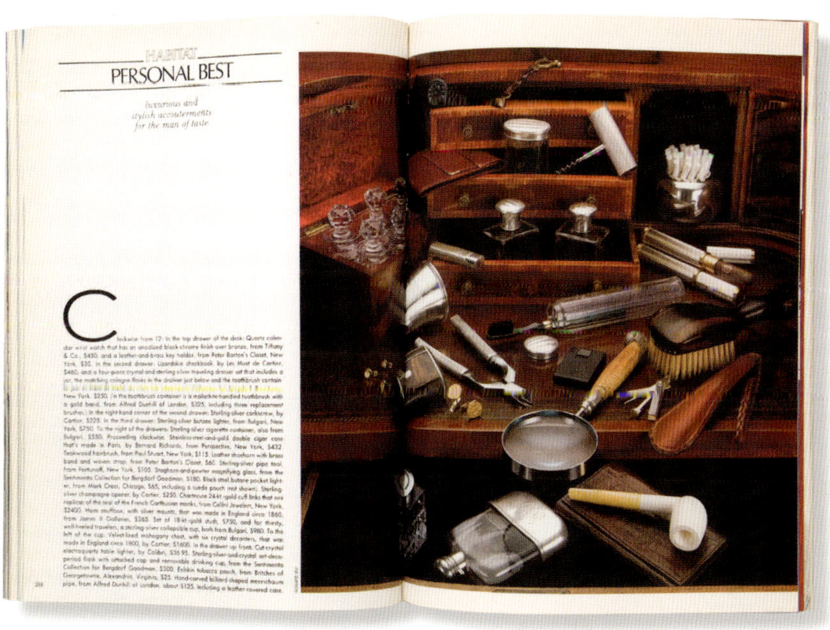

1969

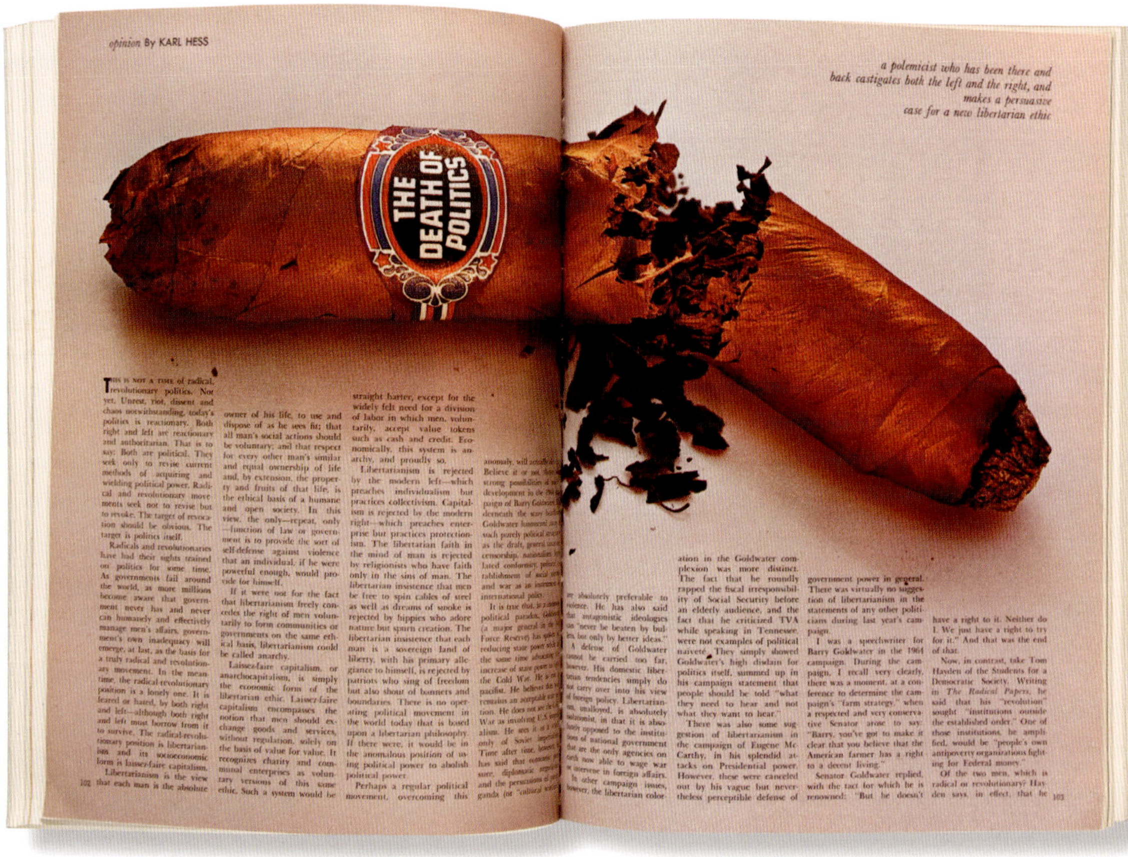
opinion By KARL HESS
THE DEATH OF POLITICS
a polemicist who has been there and back castigates both the left and the right, and makes a persuasive case for a new libertarian ethic

1972

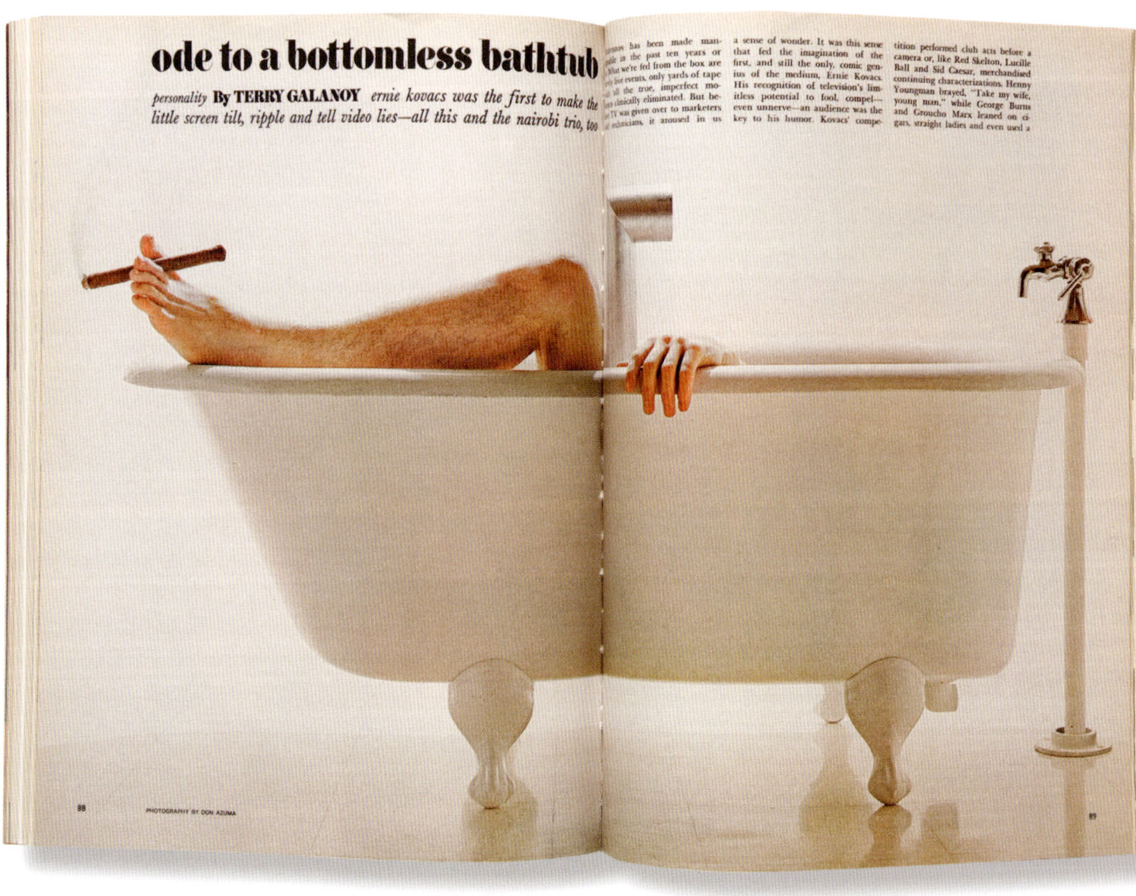
ode to a bottomless bathtub
personality By TERRY GALANOY ernie kovacs was the first to make the little screen tilt, ripple and tell video lies—all this and the nairobi trio, too
PHOTOGRAPHY BY DON AZUMA

1999

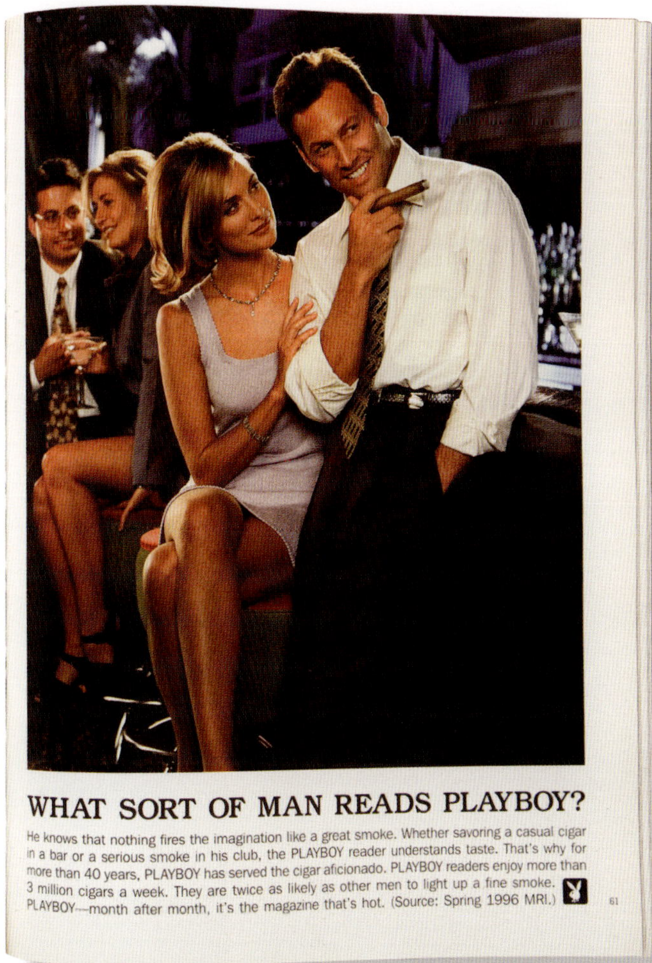
WHAT SORT OF MAN READS PLAYBOY?
He knows that nothing fires the imagination like a great smoke. Whether savoring a casual cigar in a bar or a serious smoke in his club, the PLAYBOY reader understands taste. That's why for more than 40 years, PLAYBOY has served the cigar aficionado. PLAYBOY readers enjoy more than 3 million cigars a week. They are twice as likely as other men to light up a fine smoke. PLAYBOY—month after month, it's the magazine that's hot. (Source: Spring 1996 MRI.)
61

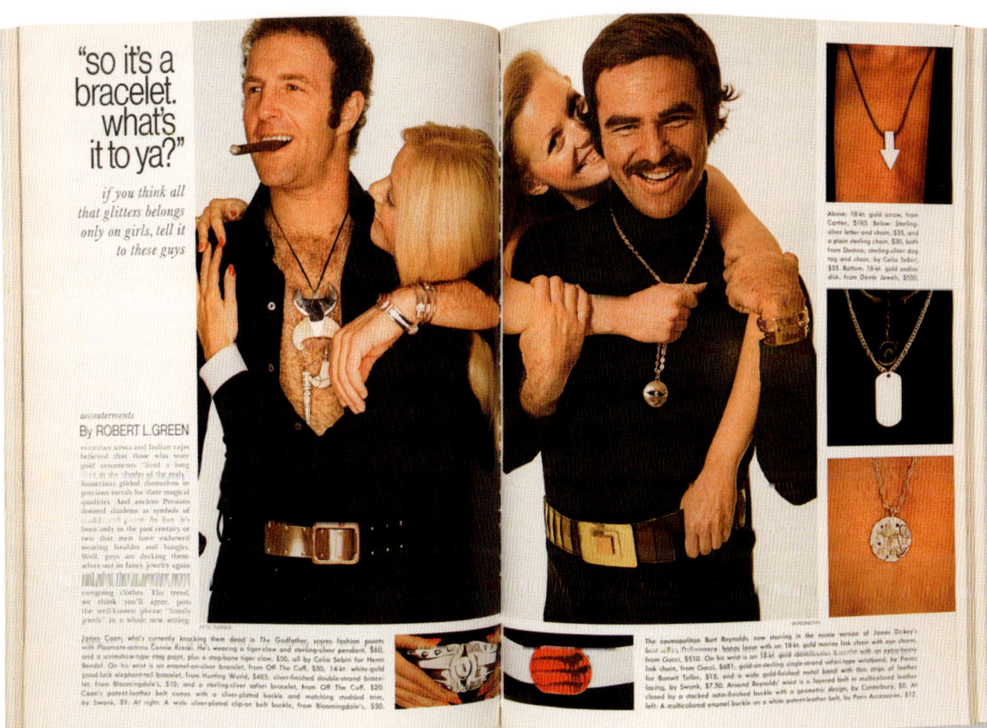
"so it's a bracelet. what's it to ya?"
if you think all that glitters belongs only on girls, tell it to these guys
accouterments
By ROBERT L. GREEN

1972

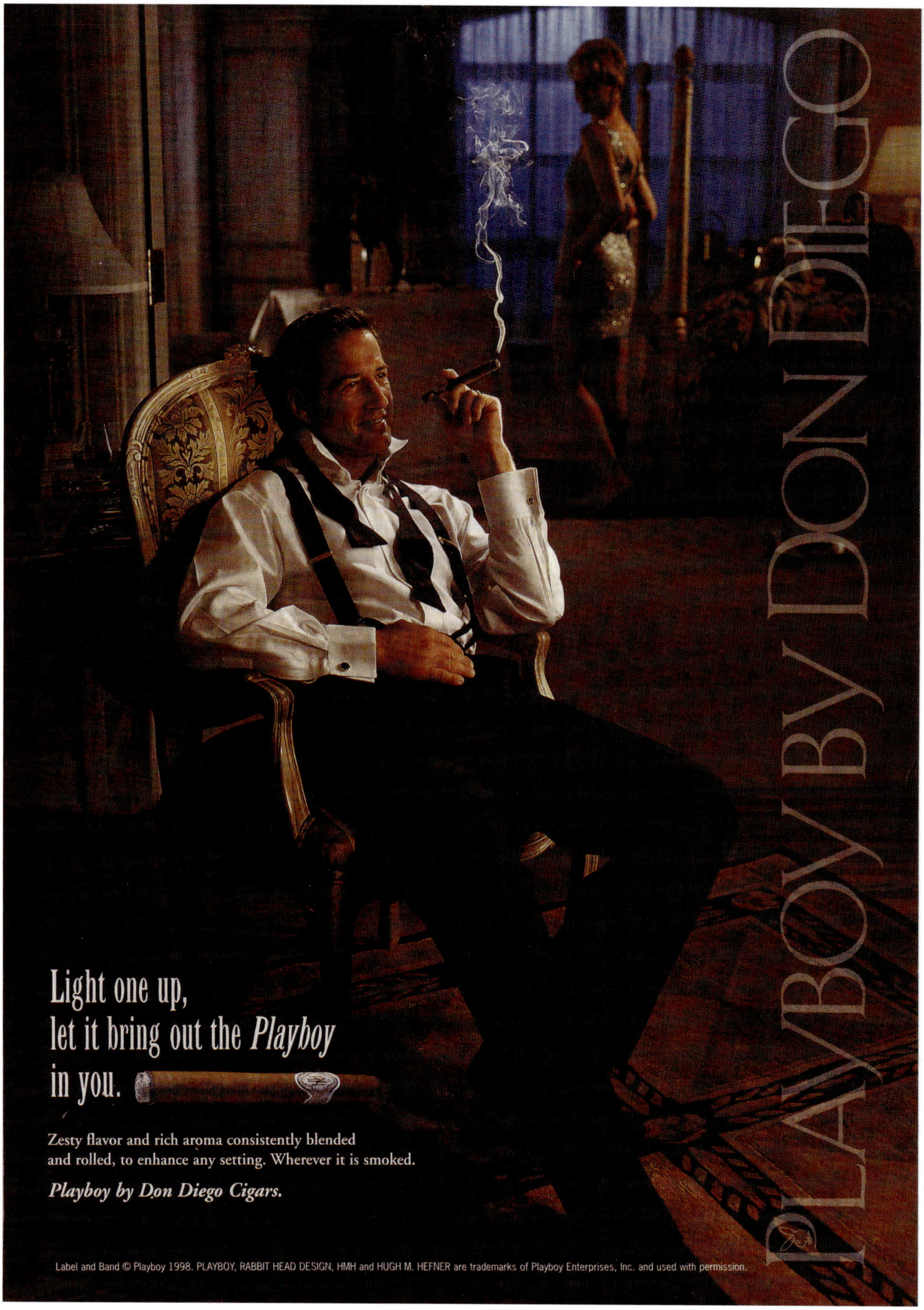

PLAYBOY BY DON DIEGO
Light one up,
let it bring out the *Playboy*
in you.
Zesty flavor and rich aroma consistently blended
and rolled, to enhance any setting. Wherever it is smoked.
Playboy by Don Diego Cigars.
Label and Band © Playboy 1998. PLAYBOY, RABBIT HEAD DESIGN, HMH and HUGH M. HEFNER are trademarks of Playboy Enterprises, Inc. and used with permission.

Ads 1950s to today

Back in the 1950s, when men were men and unafraid of the three-martini business lunch, some of Madison Avenue's most creative minds (and, in the case of El Producto, that mind belonged to iconic American art director Paul Rand) made cigar print advertising into an art form all its own. Interspersed among a *Playboy* issue's interviews, pictorials, party jokes, and cartoons, these ads told a unique, captivating story.

That creative drive didn't end in the Mad Men era. During the cigar boom of the 90s, a second wave of adventurous ad minds, such as Manhattan-based Bill and Sheila McCaffrey, and West Coaster Chad Farmer, left their distinctive (and smoky) mark on audiences and clients.

Not surprisingly, mass-market cigars, as well as catalogs, were the primary ad offerings all the way through the mid-1980s. Premium print cigar advertising found during prior decades was primarily consigned to Havanas, and select upscale retailers such as Alfred Dunhill in London and Nat Sherman in New York. Consequently, it should come as no surprise that the veritable bonanza of premium cigar advertising that we know today commenced with the onset of the cigar boom of the 90s.

The following pages show how some advertising, as with the editorial images displayed earlier (page 50), seems incomplete without a touch of smoke.

1950's

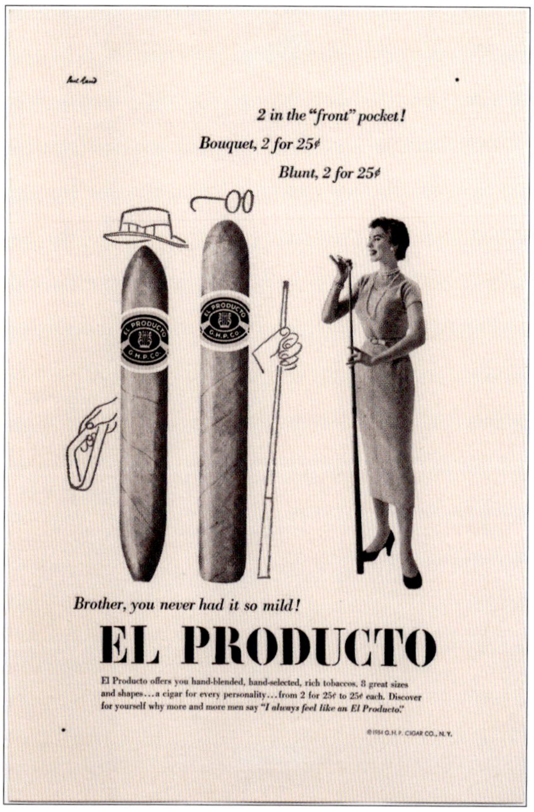

2 in the "front" pocket!
Bouquet, 2 for 25¢
Blunt, 2 for 25¢
Brother, you never had it so mild!
EL PRODUCTO
El Producto offers you hand-blended, hand-selected, rich tobaccos. 8 great sizes and shapes...a cigar for every personality...from 2 for 25¢ to 25¢ each. Discover for yourself why more and more men say "I always feel like an El Producto."
©1954 G.H.P. CIGAR CO., N.Y.

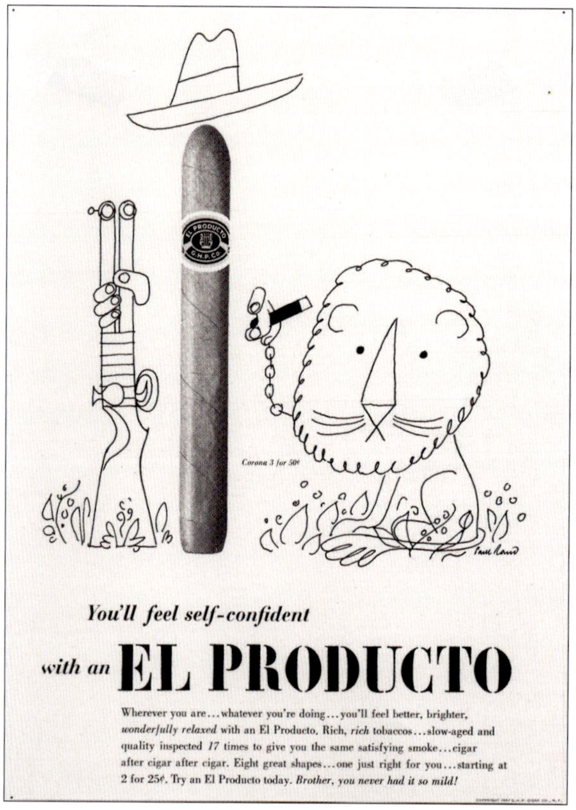

Corona 3 for 50¢
You'll feel self-confident
with an EL PRODUCTO
Wherever you are...whatever you're doing...you'll feel better, brighter, wonderfully relaxed with an El Producto. Rich, rich tobaccos...slow-aged and quality inspected 17 times to give you the same satisfying smoke...cigar after cigar after cigar. Eight great shapes...one just right for you...starting at 2 for 25¢. Try an El Producto today. Brother, you never had it so mild!

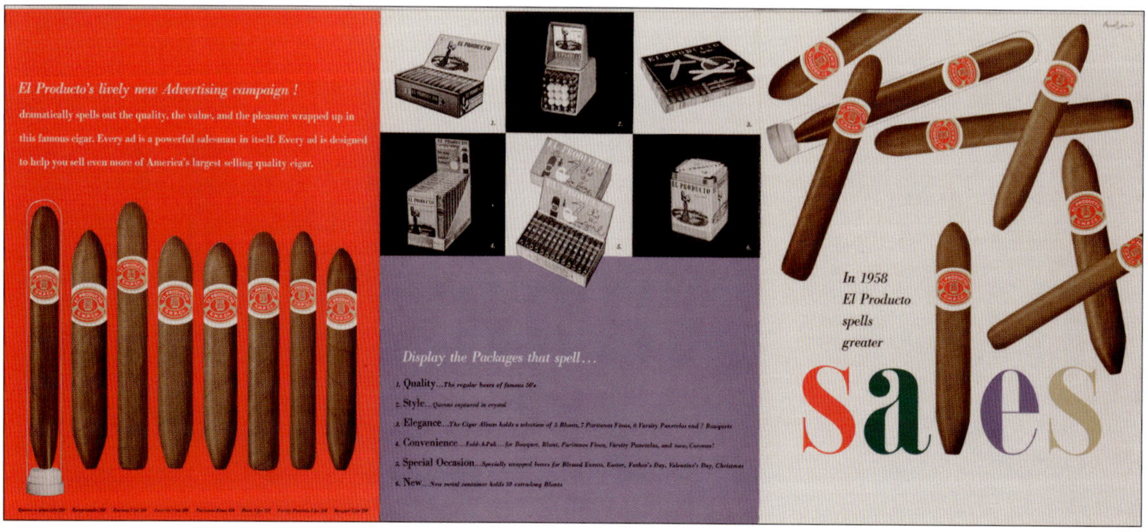

El Producto's lively new Advertising campaign !
dramatically spells out the quality, the value, and the pleasure wrapped up in this famous cigar. Every ad is a powerful salesman in itself. Every ad is designed to help you sell even more of America's largest selling quality cigar.
Display the Packages that spell...
1. Quality...The regular boxes of famous 50's
2. Style...Queens captured in crystal
3. Elegance...The Cigar Album holds a selection of 5 Blunts, 7 Puritanos Finos, 6 Varsity Panetelas and 7 Bouquets
4. Convenience...Fold-A-Pak...for Bouquet, Blunt, Puritanos Finos, Varsity Panetelas, and now, Coronas!
5. Special Occasion...Specially wrapped boxes for Blessed Events, Easter, Father's Day, Valentine's Day, Christmas
6. New...New metal container holds 50 extra-long Blunts
In 1958
El Producto
spells
greater
sales

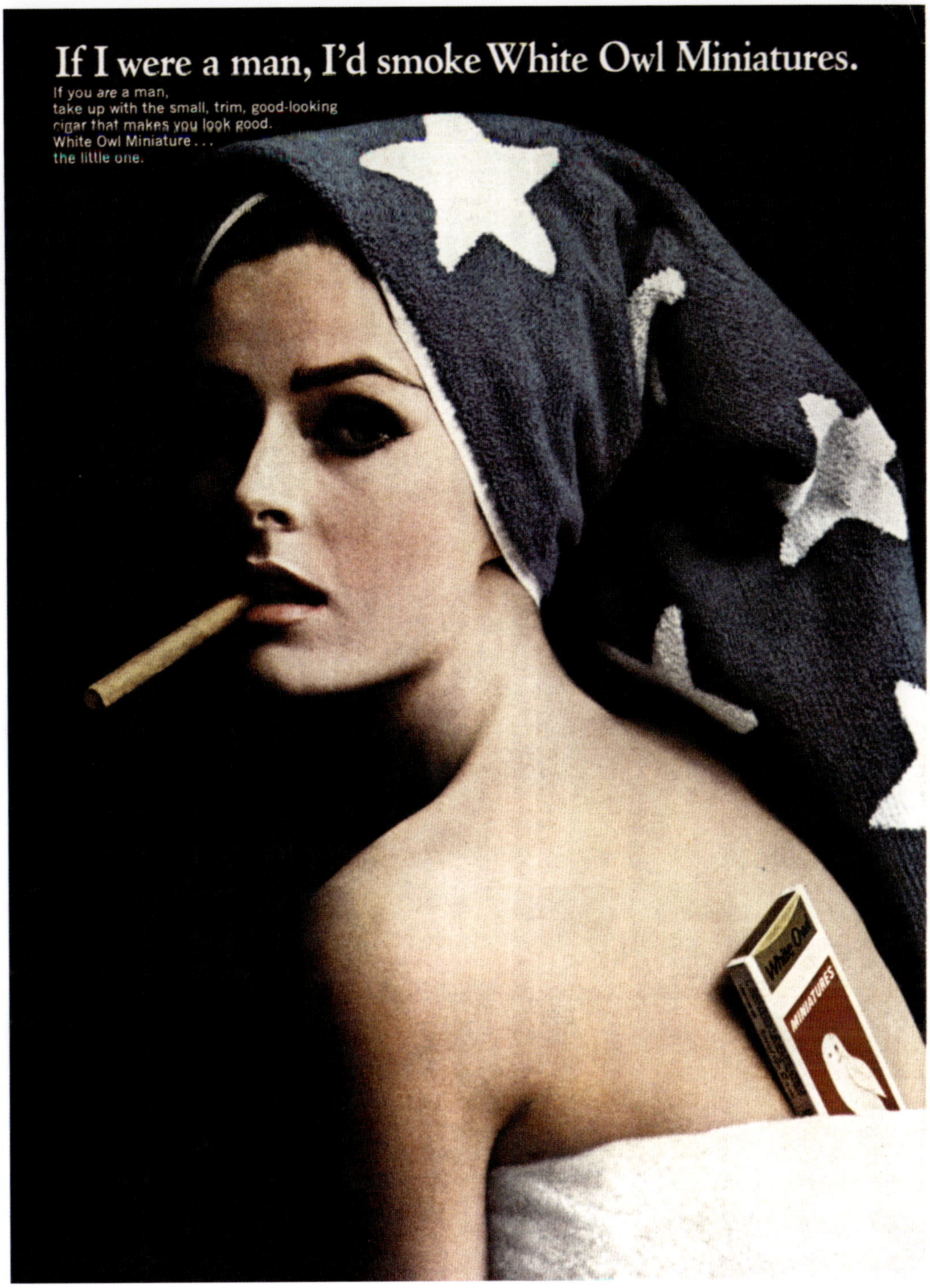
If I were a man, I'd smoke White Owl Miniatures.
If you *are* a man,
take up with the small, trim, good-looking
cigar that makes you look good.
White Owl Miniature . . .
the little one.

1960s

1970s >

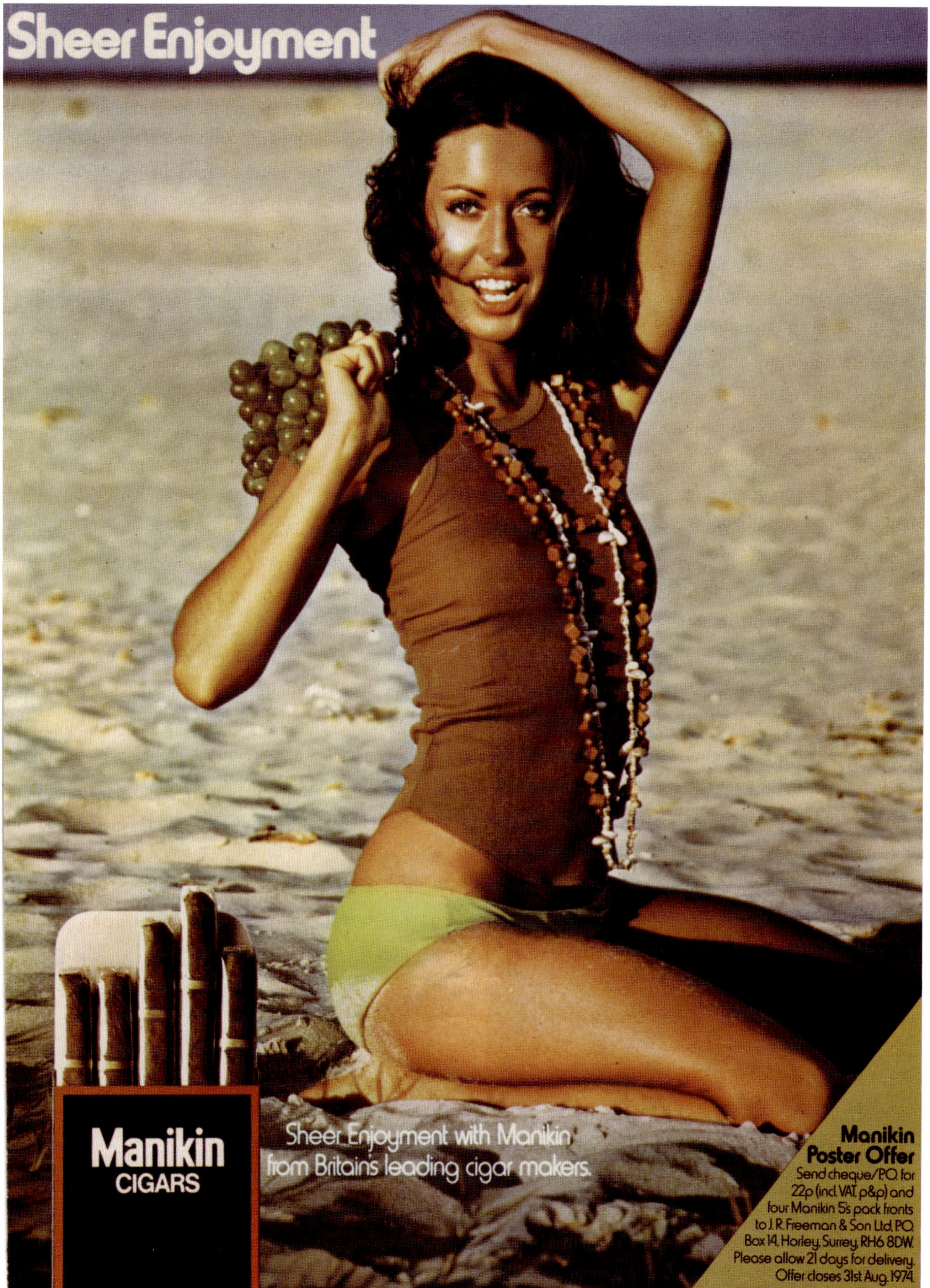
Sheer Enjoyment
Manikin
CIGARS
Sheer Enjoyment with Manikin
from Britain's leading cigar makers.
Manikin
Poster Offer
Send cheque/P.O. for 22p (incl. VAT, p&p) and four Manikin 5's pack fronts to J. R. Freeman & Son Ltd, P.O. Box 14, Horley, Surrey, RH6 8DW. Please allow 21 days for delivery. Offer closes 31st Aug. 1974.
Regd. Office: 65 Kingsway, London, W.C.2

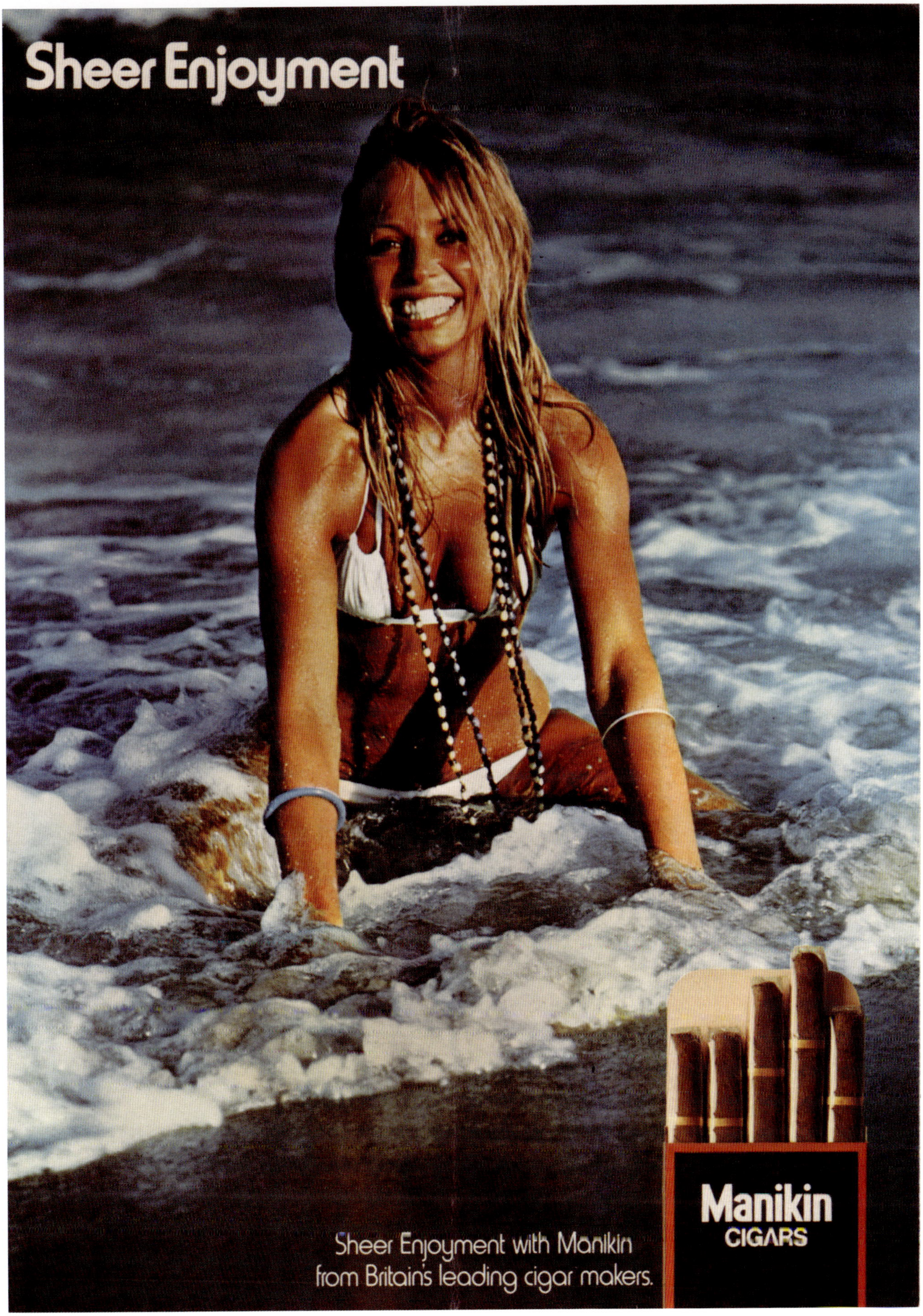
Sheer Enjoyment
Manikin
CIGARS
Sheer Enjoyment with Manikin
from Britain's leading cigar makers.

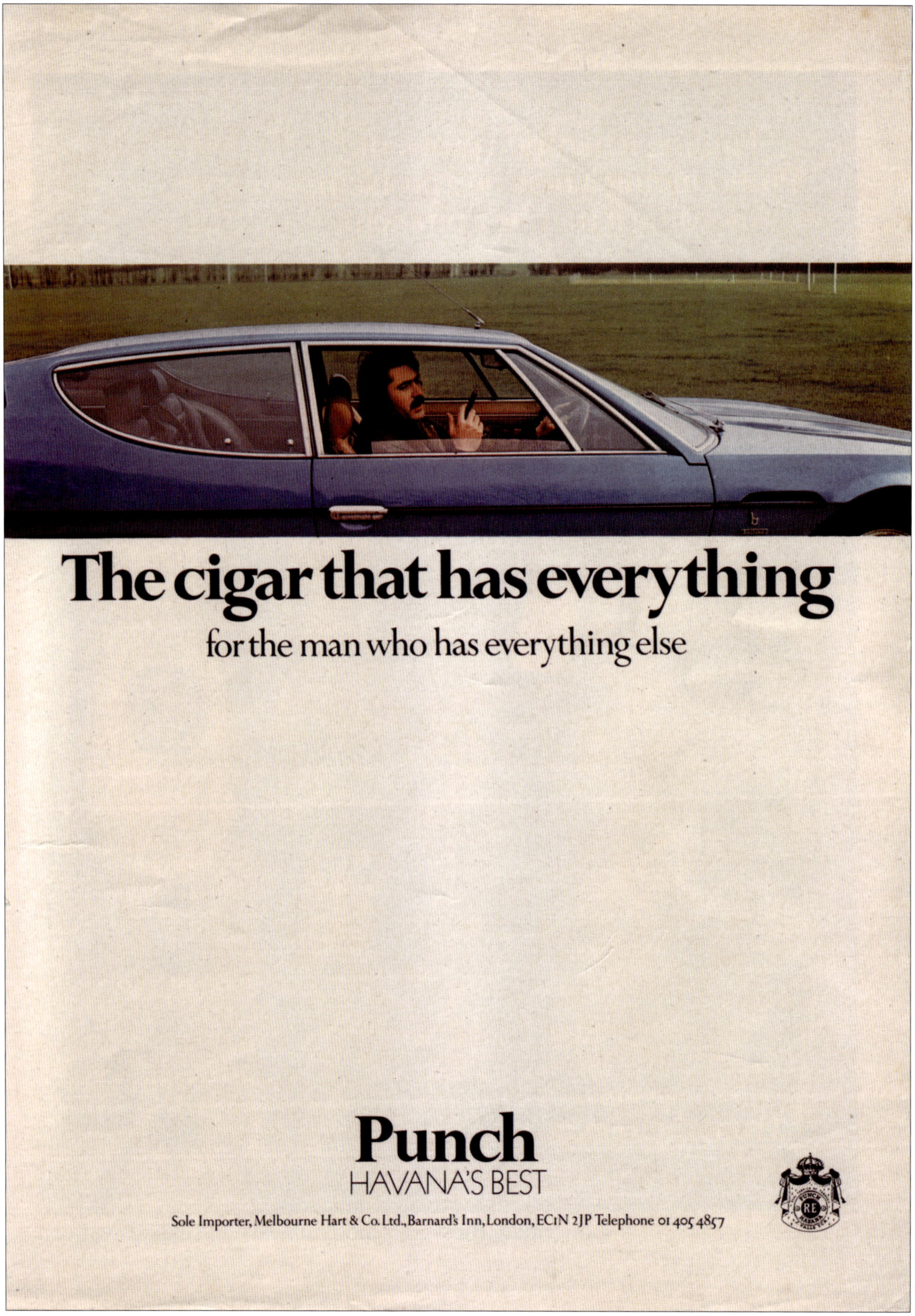
The cigar that has everything
for the man who has everything else
Punch
HAVANA'S BEST
Sole Importer, Melbourne Hart & Co. Ltd., Barnard's Inn, London, EC1N 2JP Telephone 01 405 4857

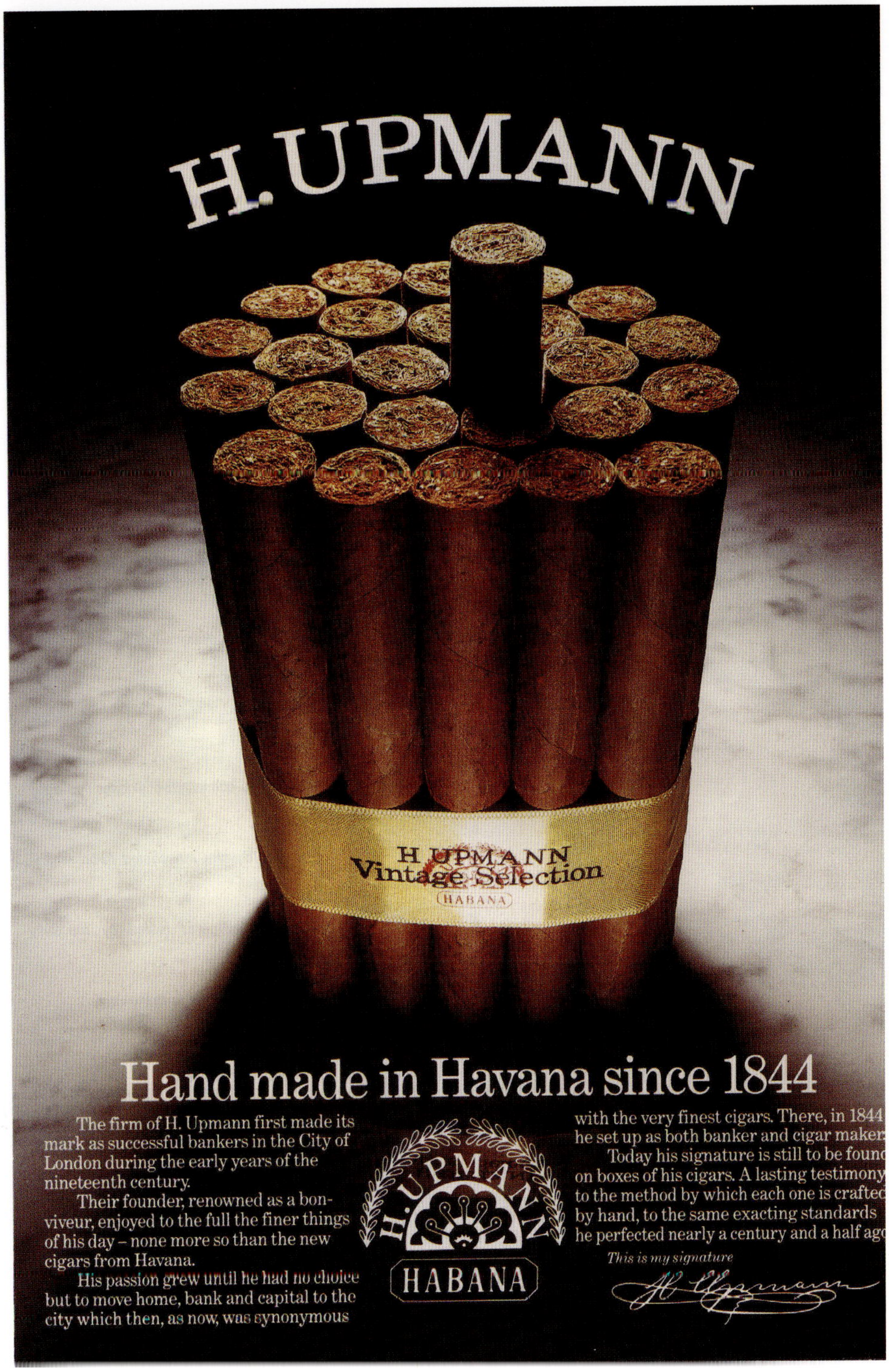

< 1970s **1980s** 1990s >

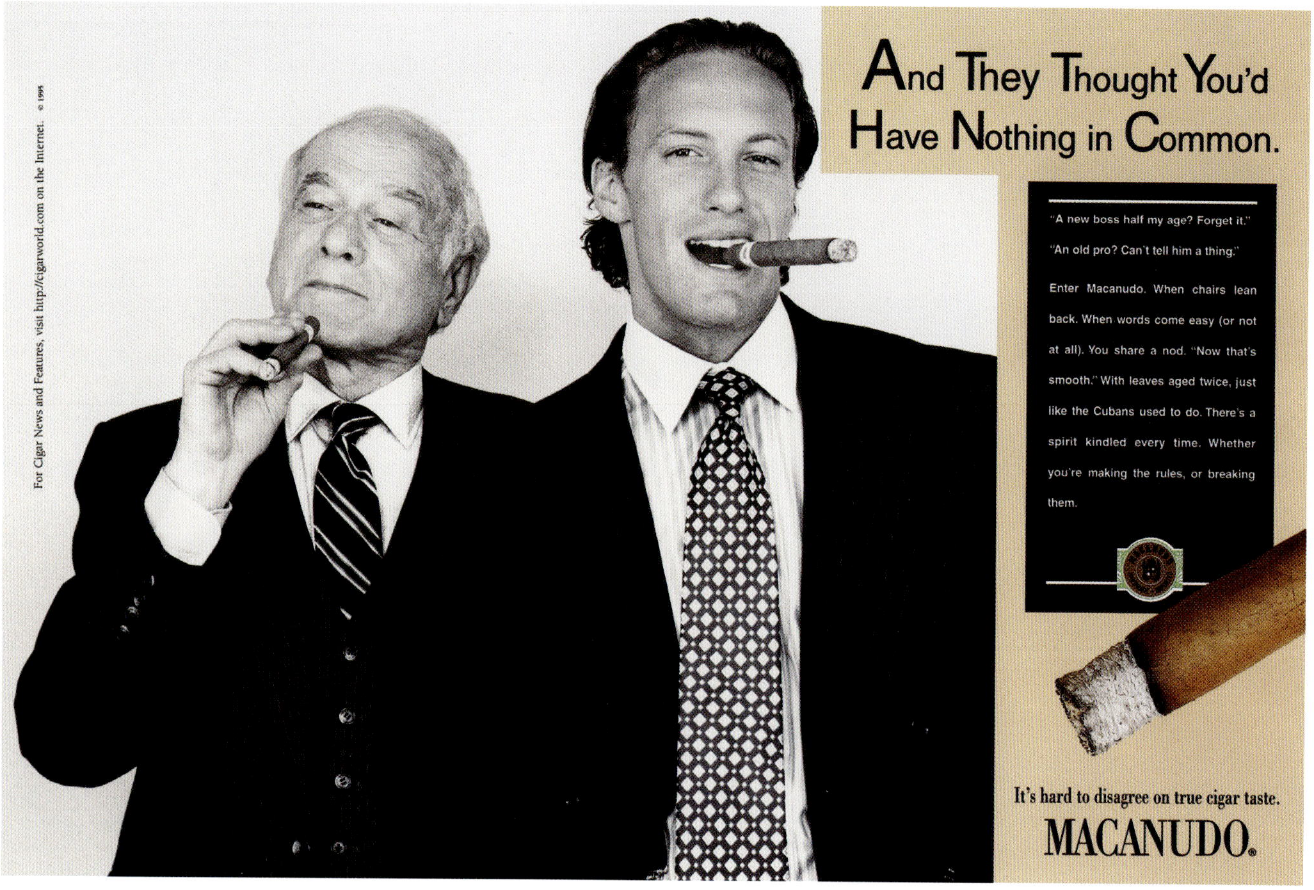
For Cigar News and Features, visit http://cigarworld.com on the Internet. © 1995
And They Thought You'd Have Nothing in Common.
"A new boss half my age? Forget it."
"An old pro? Can't tell him a thing."
Enter Macanudo. When chairs lean back. When words come easy (or not at all). You share a nod. "Now that's smooth." With leaves aged twice, just like the Cubans used to do. There's a spirit kindled every time. Whether you're making the rules, or breaking them.
It's hard to disagree on true cigar taste.
MACANUDO.

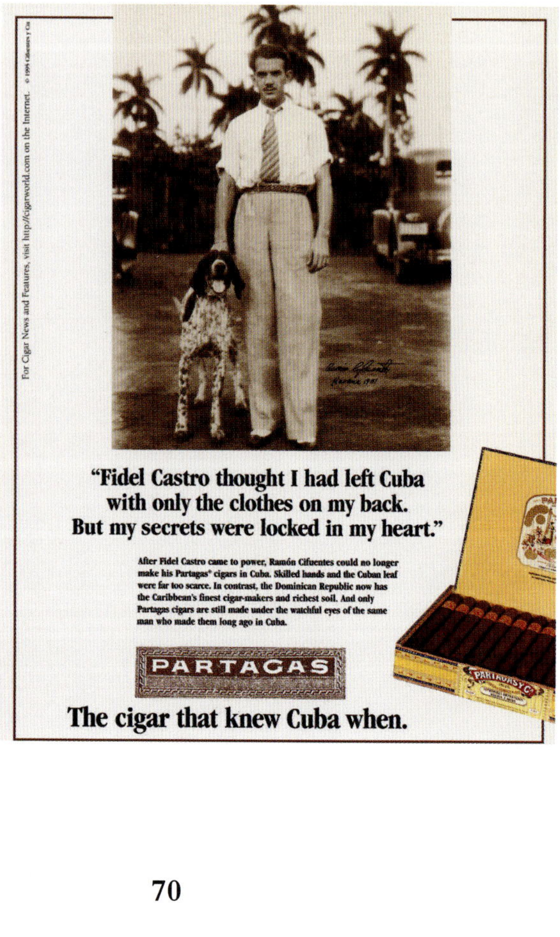
For Cigar News and Features, visit http://cigarworld.com on the Internet.
"Fidel Castro thought I had left Cuba with only the clothes on my back. But my secrets were locked in my heart."
After Fidel Castro came to power, Ramón Cifuentes could no longer make his Partagas® cigars in Cuba. Skilled hands and the Cuban leaf were far too scarce. In contrast, the Dominican Republic now has the Caribbean's finest cigar-makers and richest soil. And only Partagas cigars are still made under the watchful eyes of the same man who made them long ago in Cuba.
PARTAGAS
The cigar that knew Cuba when.

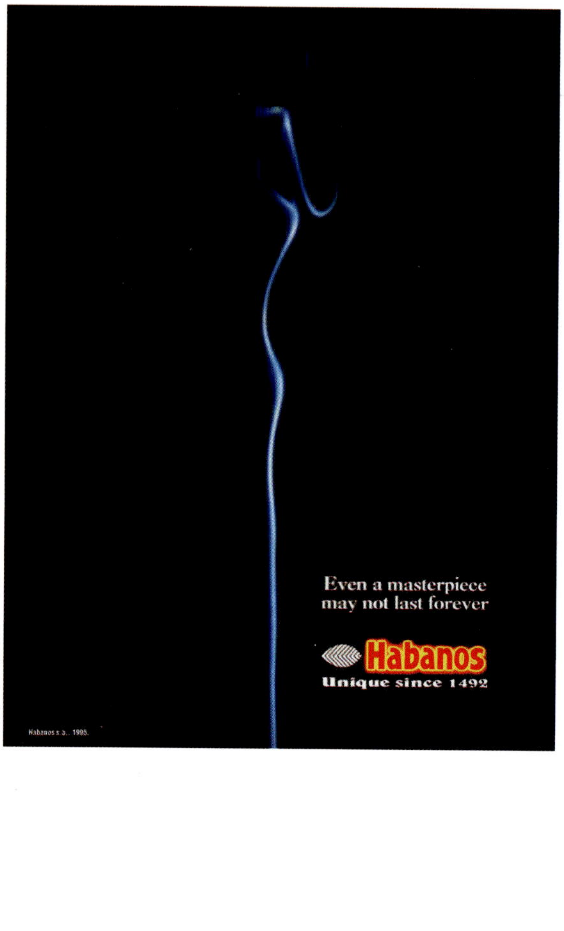
Even a masterpiece may not last forever
Habanos
Unique since 1492

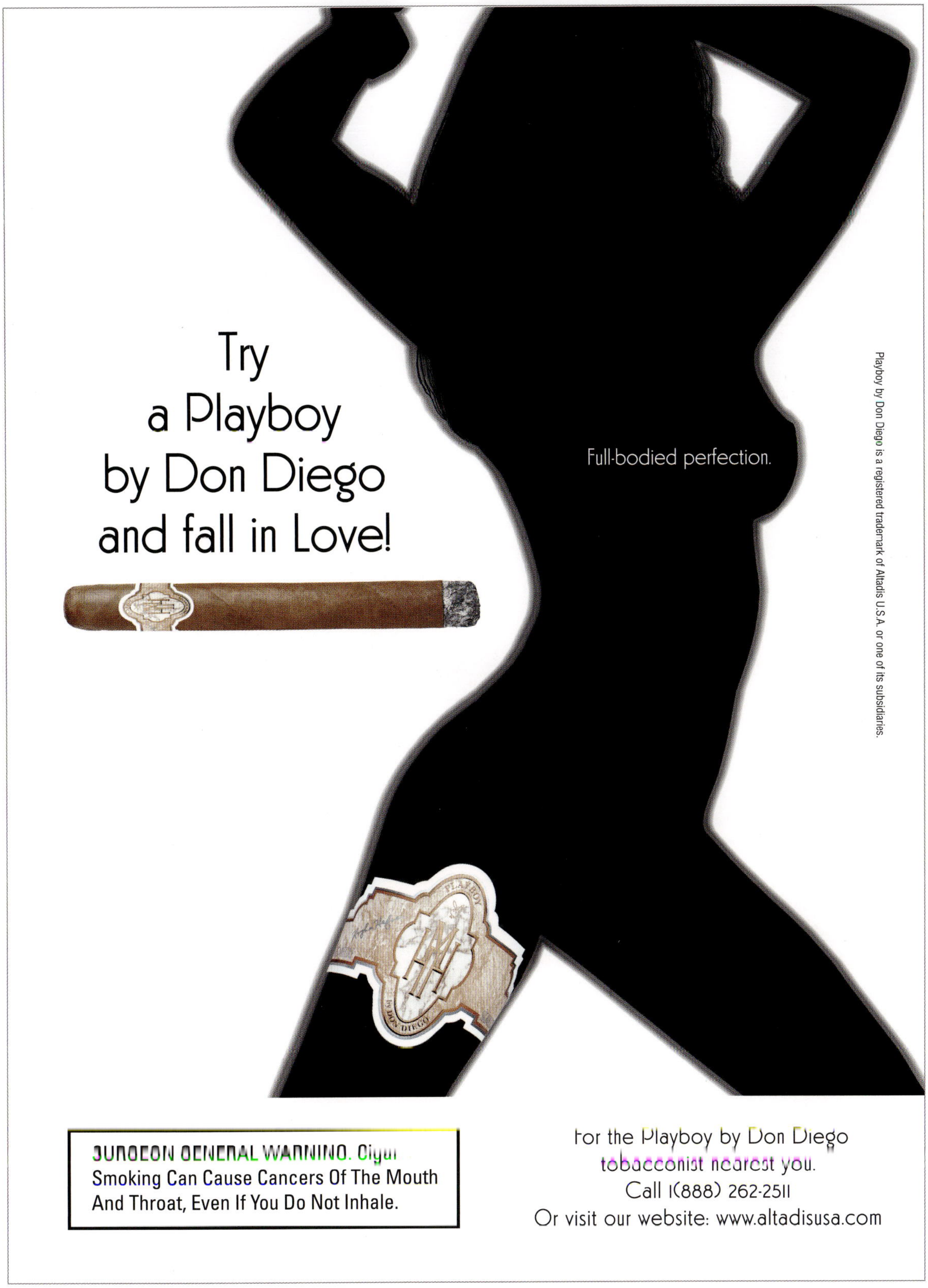

Try
a Playboy
by Don Diego
and fall in Love!
Full-bodied perfection.
Playboy by Don Diego is a registered trademark of Altadis U.S.A. or one of its subsidiaries.
SURGEON GENERAL WARNING: Cigar
Smoking Can Cause Cancers Of The Mouth
And Throat, Even If You Do Not Inhale.
For the Playboy by Don Diego
tobacconist nearest you.
Call 1(888) 262-2511
Or visit our website: www.altadisusa.com

1990s

2000s

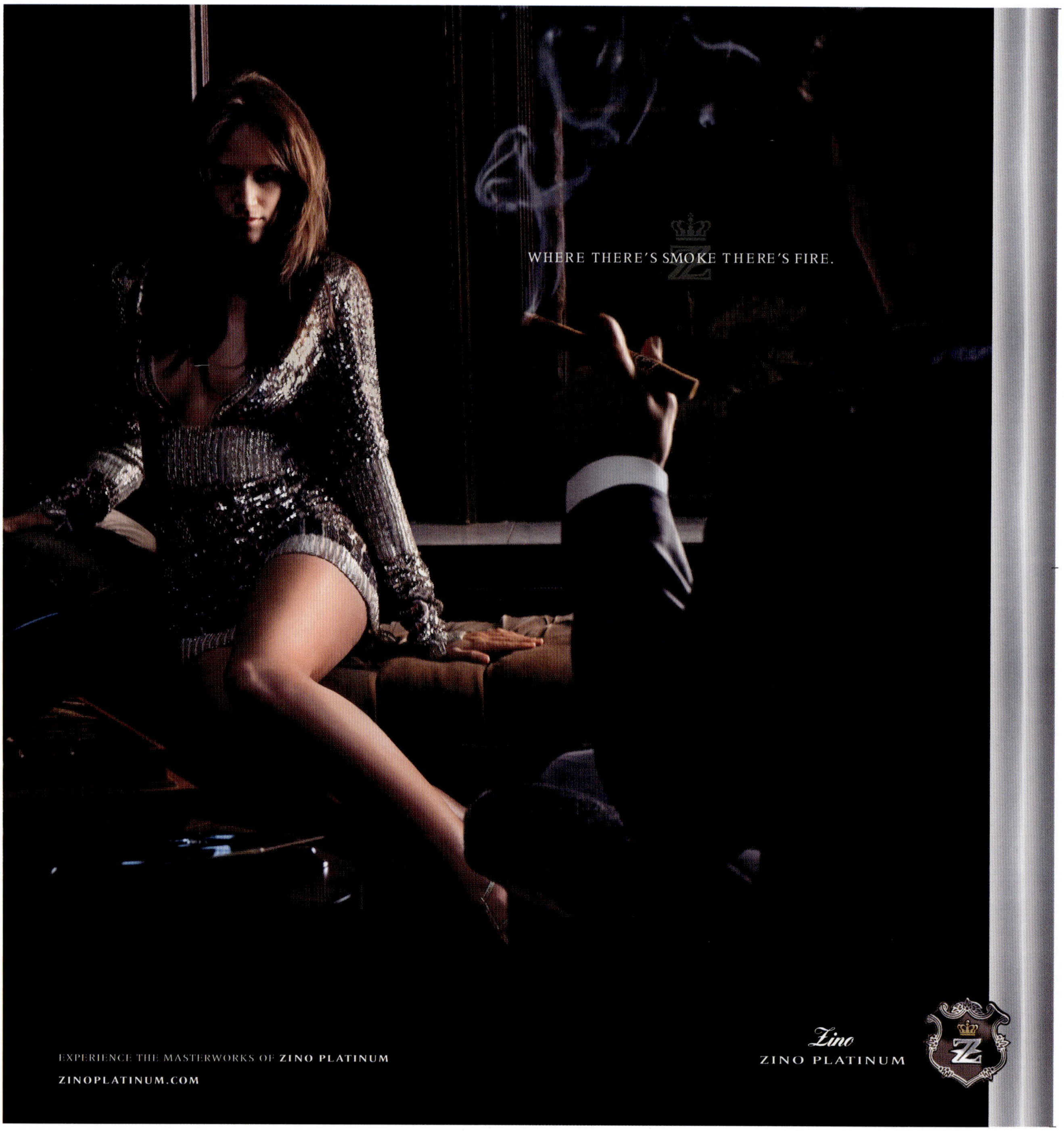

WHERE THERE'S SMOKE THERE'S FIRE.
EXPERIENCE THE MASTERWORKS OF ZINO PLATINUM
ZINOPLATINUM.COM
Zino
ZINO PLATINUM

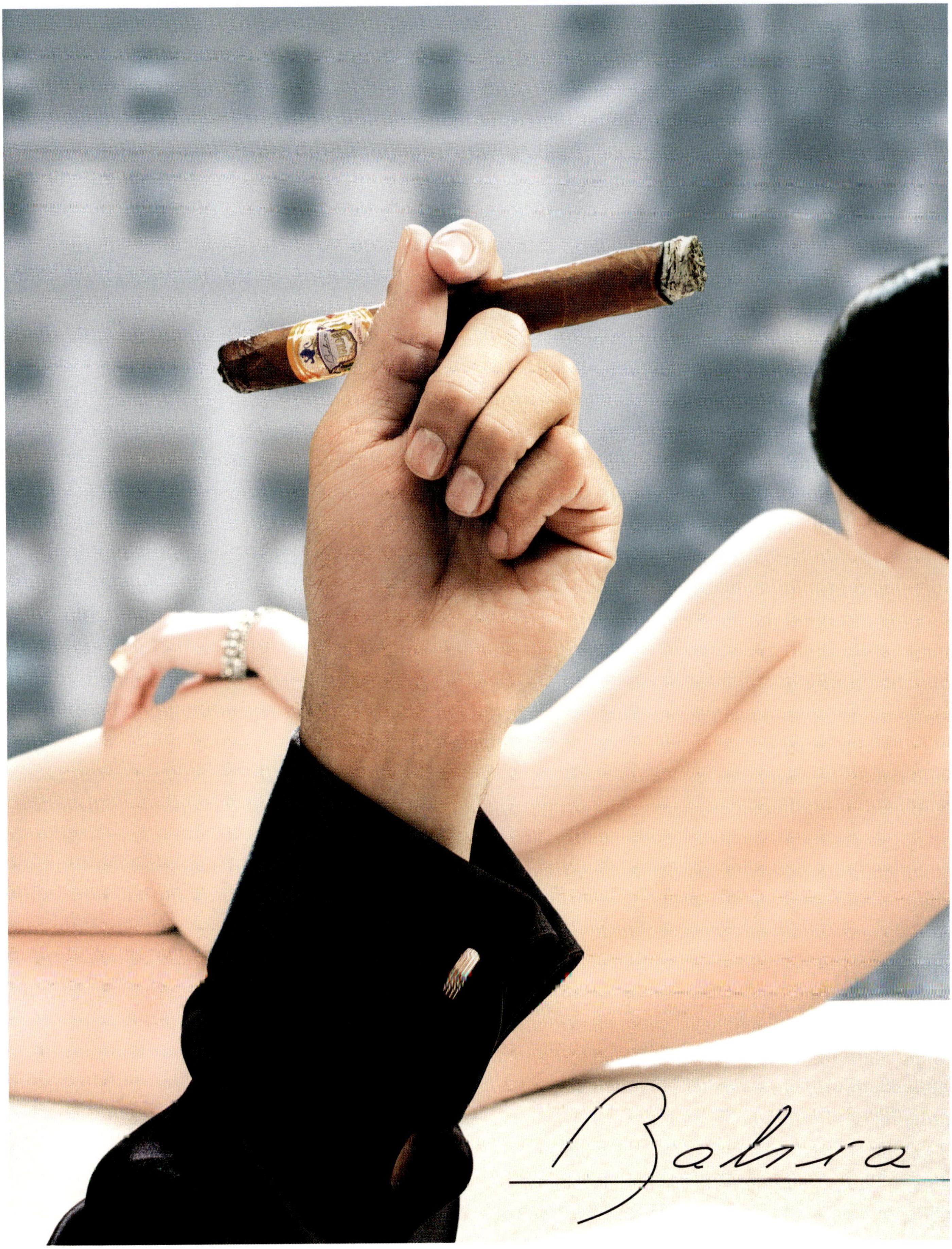
Bahia

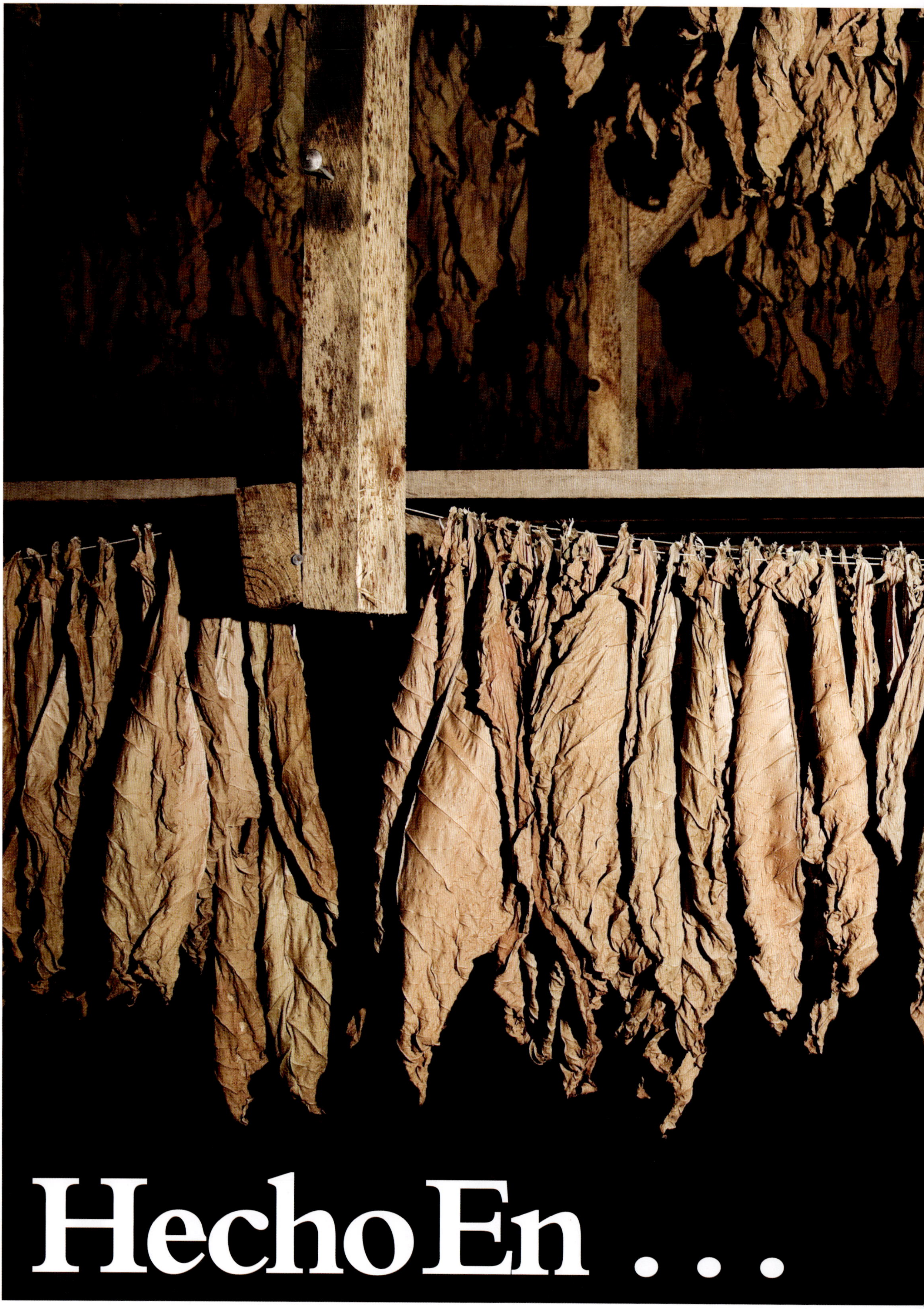

Hecho En . . .

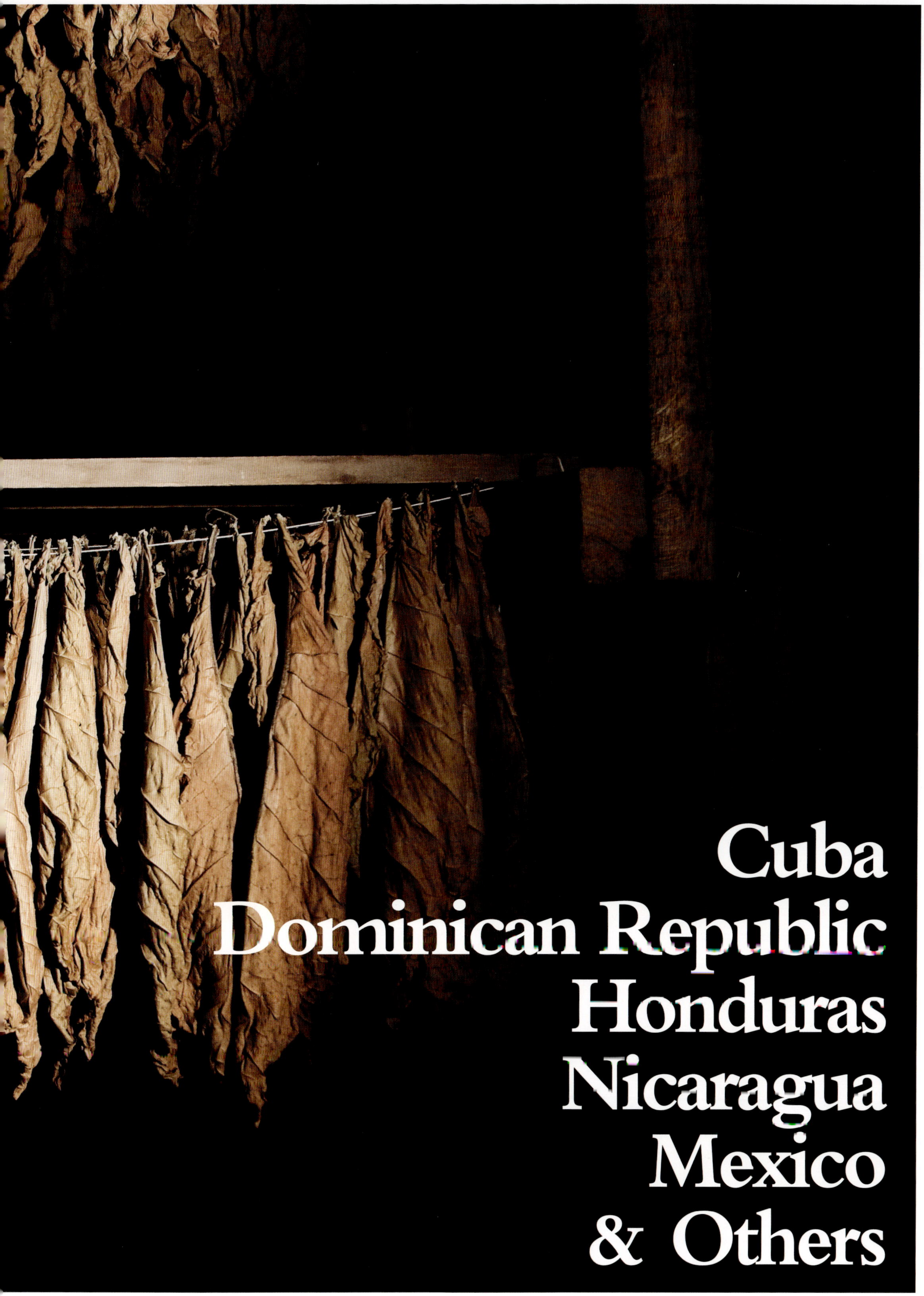

Cuba
Dominican Republic
Honduras
Nicaragua
Mexico
& Others

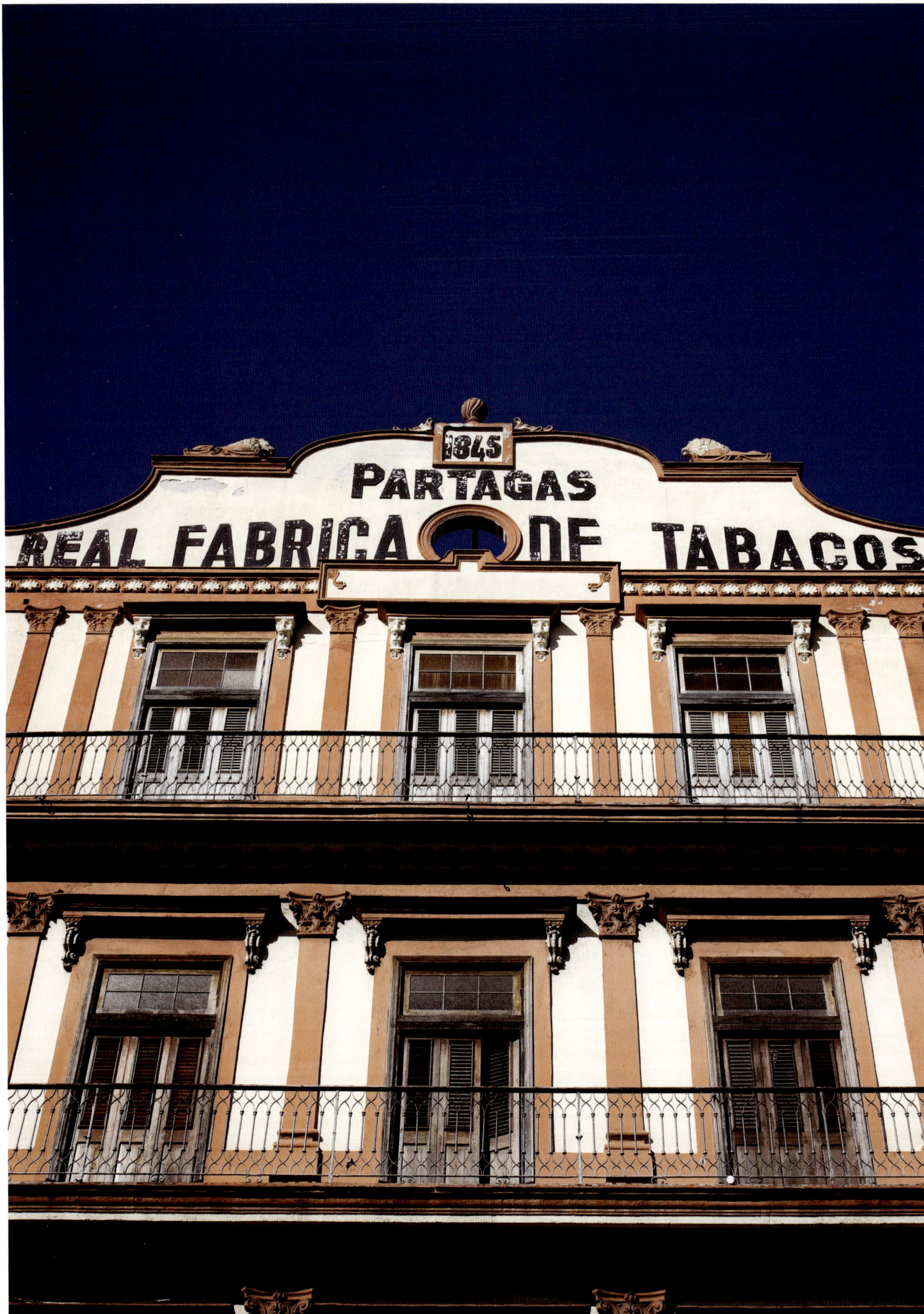
1845
PARTAGAS
REAL FABRICA DE TABACOS

Cuba

The 1956 Chevy-turned-taxi cruises away from Jose Martí International Airport, and in the wide backseat you've already clipped the first Montecristo. You're in Cuba, after all, the country where it seems sacrilegious not to have a stogie smoking at all times.

A millisecond before your flame begins to toast the tip of the cigar, and irrespective of having visited "La Isla" time and occasion prior, a thought hits you with the force of panic: I can't light this indoors! They shoot people for that back in the States!

Your eyes flicker up and meet the driver's in the rearview mirror. He scans lighter, cutter, and cigar in your hands and asks—without so much as a batted eyelid—in supremely passable English: "What is that you're smoking?" You show him the cigar's band, and he nods approval. *I could get used to this*, you think as you torch up.

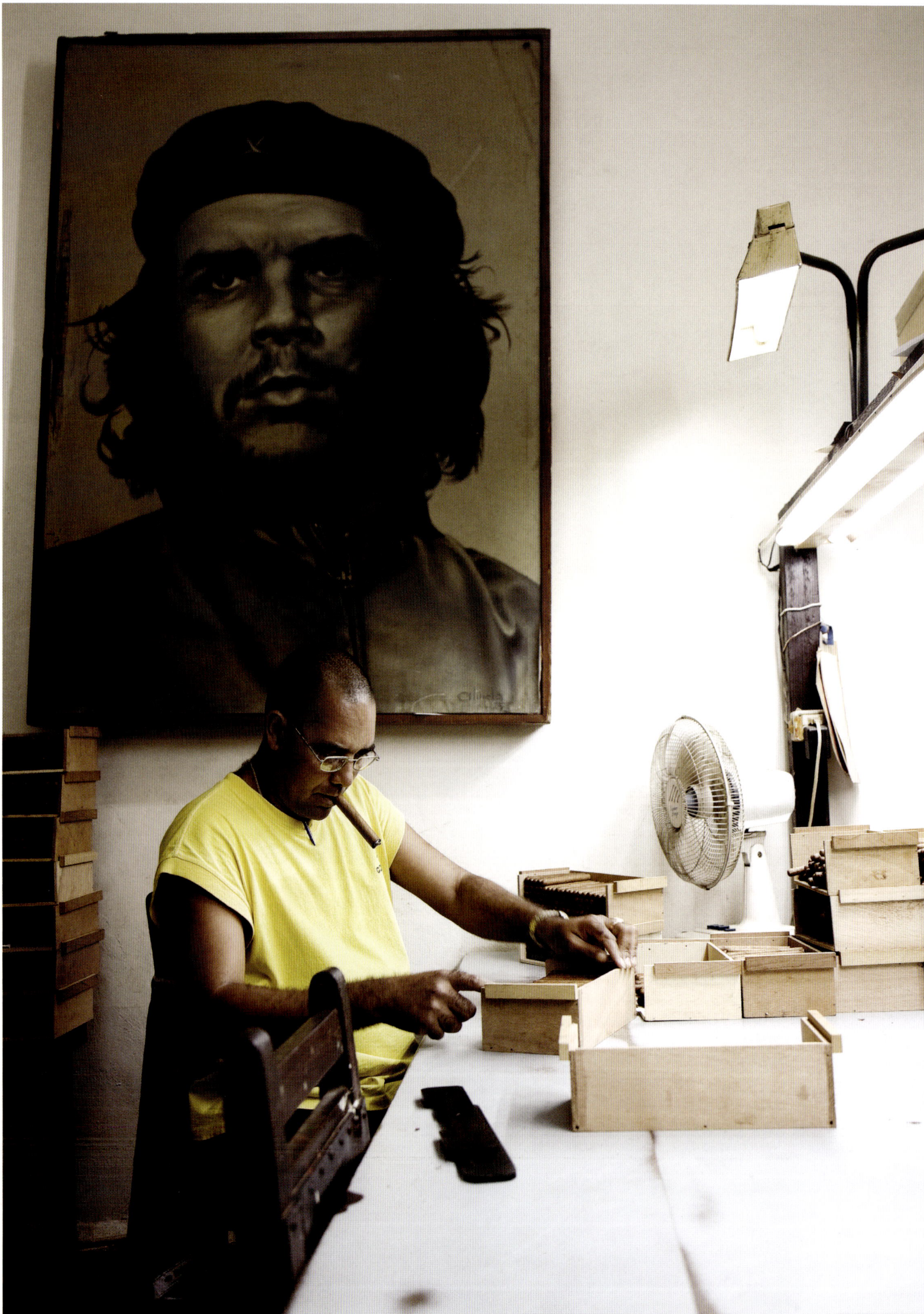

Despite five decades of U.S. embargo having left much of it in ruins, Cuba remains a defiantly totalitarian nation—and perhaps the last free smoking zone on the planet. Here, in what was once known as the Pearl of the Antilles, your cigar is welcome anywhere from restaurants to hotel elevators, as if it were still the glorious Technicolor days of sixty years ago, when the island was a playground for gangsters and the vacationing rich and powerful.

The cab swoops along the Malecón, the coast road, into Havana. If you hit "pause" on Paris in 1959, magically transported it to the Caribbean, sandblasted its pillared archways and exquisitely rendered fronts, seeded its wide boulevards with a dizzying array of 1950's Detroit iron and 1970's Russian automobiles, and then hit "play," you would have something very close to this city at the turn of the new century. Nearly everything here in the metropolis is peeling and crumbling, held together with bits of scavenged metal and layers of paint. The ghosts of the past endure even by light of day, along with the country's cigar legacy.

HECHO A MANO > Hemingway's presence looms large over Cuba. He lived here for a time, and local legend says the central character of his Pulitzer Prize–winning novella *The Old Man and the Sea* was based on a local fisherman. A greening statue of him stands in Cojimar, a small village east of Havana, and sometimes it seems as if no tourist trap is complete without some sign saying that the writer imbibed here, majestically, before shuffling home to whittle at his prose.

The man really did drink at El Floridita, an establishment whose constant hum of conversation is set to the rhythmic *click-click-click* of daiquiris being shaken by red-vested bartenders. At the massive dark-wood bar sits a bronze statue of Papa himself, smiling gamely for any tourist who wants a photo-op.

History aside, El Floridita remains a tourist spot. Tasting the real Havana—particularly its cigar culture—requires lighting a stick and heading back out into the tropical bustle of the city at midday. (A word of caution when crossing streets: Cubans tend to drive with suicidal sangfroid, slaloming around pedestrians at occasionally ludicrous speeds.) Curious Cubans in your path will inquire as to the brand smoking in your hand, others will whisper in your wake: "[illegible] good price [illegible] . . ."

Nestled within Havana's humid street life are the cigar *fábricas*. Some stand as architectural landmarks, true temples to the mystique of cigars, and accordingly, feature tourism-friendly amenities, such as the lounge and bar tucked away at the La Corona factory (which produces Punch and Hoyo de Monterey). Some factories come imbued with history, notably the mansion in Havana's Miramar neighborhood that was converted into El Laguito, ground zero for Cohiba and other top brands. Others run with a stripped-down utilitarianism that suggests a tropical variation on an Eastern Bloc factory.

A prime example of the latter is the José Martí (formerly H. Upmann) factory, located a few blocks from the landmark Cementerio de Cristóbal Colón in Havana's Vedado neighborhood. The stark exterior here may lack the Old World charm you find at the Partagas *fábrica* a few miles away, but, as with all the factories, the focus here is completely on production. At José Martí, over six hundred workers roll and ship some 22,000 cigars every day, slicing away with their sharp chavetas to the rhythm of the day's newspaper read into a microphone. Posters on the walls shout Revolutionary slogans, and Ché Guevara glowers from a large red poster nailed to a storeroom wall.

Workers at their fastest can roll filler, binder, and wrapper leaves into a new cigar every four or five minutes. Their training takes months, and mastery takes years. Only a small percentage are allowed to roll the truly flagship products.

Certain Cuban factories subject their cigars to the Drawmaster, a desktop device with a metal tube that takes a fireless pull on each cigar to test whether the draw is within acceptable limits. This seems an attempt to counter one gripe about Cuban cigars: that they are inconsistent in their manufacture (the Cubans themselves argue strenuously that their quality control is sound). Not that you'd ever say anything negative about quality to one of the rollers, at least not when he has one of those curved *chavetas* close at hand.

Across the square from the domed El Capitolio (modeled—perhaps ironically in retrospect—after the U.S. Capitol) and behind a classic façade, the Partagas factory produces some eight million sticks per year. Like every other *fábrica* on the island, it's part of Habanos S.A.; this corporation—jointly owned by the government and Britain's Imperial Tobacco—produces roughly 125 million cigars for export, with worldwide sales of over $400 million. Habanos S.A. accounts for three-quarters of the worldwide premium cigar market outside of the United States.

COUNTERFEITS

If cigars remain a source of pride and fascination for many here, they also represent a source of under-the-table income for others, who push counterfeits and factory rejects on the unsuspecting. The connoisseur should avoid these at all costs, and only purchase their sticks at one of the city's authorized stores.

HAVANA HABITATS

Since its opening in 1930, hordes of international visitors have chosen to stay at the classically luxurious Hotel Nacional de Cuba, architecturally modeled after the Breakers hotel in Palm Beach, Florida. Perched on a hill overlooking Havana Bay, the eight-story Spanish Colonial–style structure features 457 rooms, fifteen suites, and a presidential suite, and its veranda and wide lush lawn are perfect for a smoke break. Famous faces ranging from Winston Churchill to Ernest Hemingway have smoked here at one point or another.

For those who prefer more modern-style accommodations, the 462-room Meliá Cohiba (located five minutes down the Malecón from the Nacional) and the 409-room Meliá Habana in the swank neighborhood of Miramar stand as Cuba's answer to the standard-issue glass/marble/steel luxury hotels found all over the world.

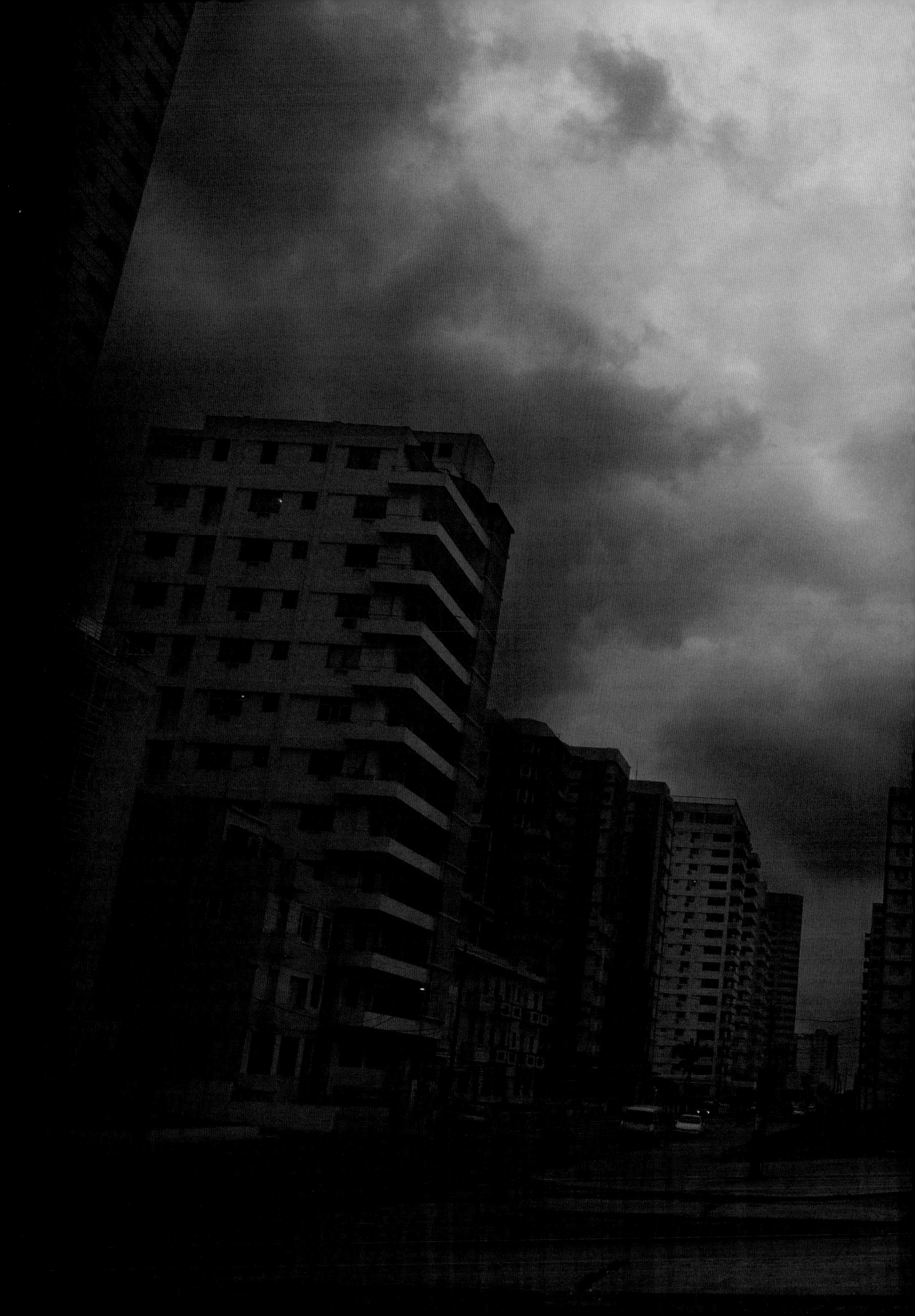

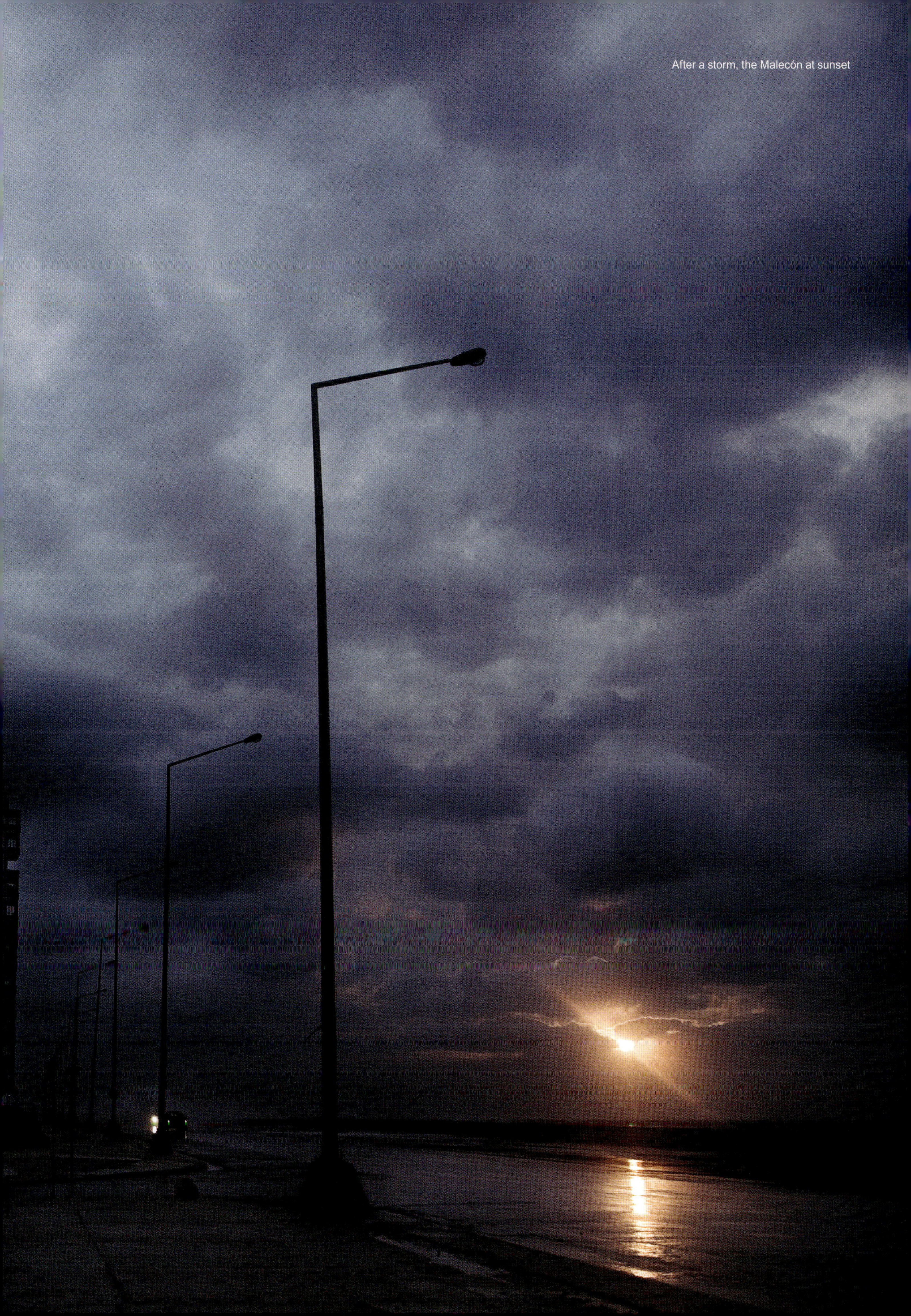

After a storm, the Malecón at sunset

A BRIEF HISTORY OF HABANOS S.A. > On the night of February 6, 1962, Cuban cigars were freely available for sale at any fine U.S. tobacconist, including those visited by Pierre Salinger, press secretary of John F. Kennedy in Washington, DC. The president had ordered his aide (and fellow cigar devotee) to round up every H. Upmann Petit Corona he could find. Much to Salinger's credit, he managed to purchase roughly 1,200 by the next morning.

Upon being told of the stash, Kennedy supposedly smiled, then removed a long piece of paper from his desk drawer and signed the executive order establishing the trade embargo with Cuba.

"Cuban cigars were now illegal in our country," Salinger later wrote. "The only time I could get a few . . . was when I traveled abroad with the President to countries like France, Austria, and Great Britain." With his own humidor nicely loaded, though, Kennedy wasn't about to cut any members of the presidential party any slack; later that year, Khrushchev offered Salinger a box of 250 Cubans during a Moscow trip, elating the latter beyond belief, at least until a scandal-concerned Kennedy ordered him to turn them over to U.S. Customs for destruction.

The embargo, meant to starve Cuba into regime change, sent it even more firmly into the welcoming arms of the Soviet Union. Later that year, the Cuban Missile Crisis froze U.S.–Cuba relations to near-absolute zero. But even the embargo had a hard time stopping a Cuban cigar industry already well on its way to recovery after the shocks of the 1959 Revolution. After Castro swept across the island from East to West, routing the increasingly demoralized army of dictator Fulgencio Batista and securing Havana, Cuba's cigar families fled, leaving their property behind to be nationalized and a local cigar industry in temporary disarray.

Even as those exiled families registered their cigars' names as international trademarks, the Cuban authorities created Cubatabaco, a state-run tobacco monopoly that later changed its name to Habanos S.A., and under its authority started producing the old brands again. Although the U.S. embargo deprived the revived industry of its then-largest customer, the Europeans continued their lifelong obsession with the cigar. Within a few decades, European cigar companies such as Tabacalera S.A. (later folded into Altadis S.A.) began pumping tens of millions of dollars into Habanos S.A., helping keep its product quality high and its business functional. Other entities such as British cigar distributor Hunters & Frankau likewise infused cash into the corporation.

RED SOIL > The collapse of the Soviet Union marked the beginning of what Cubans refer to as "The Special Period," and ushered in a rough time for cigar production. Suddenly deprived of everything from pesticide to fuel—and not helped in the least by a series of hurricanes that tore across the island—the industry's output was cut nearly in half by the early 1990s, and only careful attention and much work brought it back from the brink.

If nothing else, however, the centuries have proven the Cuban people to be exceptionally resilient. A few hours west of Havana lies the vaunted Pinar del Río area, where some of the world's best tobacco is grown. When you arrive in Vuelta Abajo—its most renowned growing region—you'll notice the soil is reddish. Cigar experts rave about how the mix of nutrient-rich earth here, sunlight, and weather produces superior-quality tobacco in the same way that the local conditions in Provence produce unmatched wine grapes. It seems that, regardless of the terroir product being grown, it truly all comes down to location, location, location.

To reach the fields from the highway, you turn onto cracked asphalt roads lined with shanties and then steer from those onto deeply rutted dirt roads that wind their way to the island's small farms.

For a socialist country, the farmers here were granted a startling degree of autonomy in the wake of the Revolution; in addition to keeping their land, they sell their

THE LECTOR

The tradition of having a lector read to the assembled workers started in 1850, when the employees of Cuba's Calle de la Industria demanded they hear the classics while they rolled. As the practice spread, rollers took their literary education one step further by taking their newest creations' names from literature—hence, Romeo y Julieta, Montecristo, and the like.

INTERNATIONAL BESTSELLER

Although it's one of those brands that everyone seems to gravitate toward, Cohiba is a relatively new addition to the Cuban cigar canon. First developed as Castro's personal cigar in the 1960s, it gained legendary status as a gift given to diplomats and visiting luminaries before finally being made available for commercial consumption in the early 1980s.

Today, the cigar represents some 25 percent of Habanos S.A. sales. Montecristo and Romeo y Julieta (Winston Churchill's personal favorite) follow up at second and third, respectively. Cuba's cigars are distributed worldwide through a network of Casa del Habano stores, currently open in 133 locations.

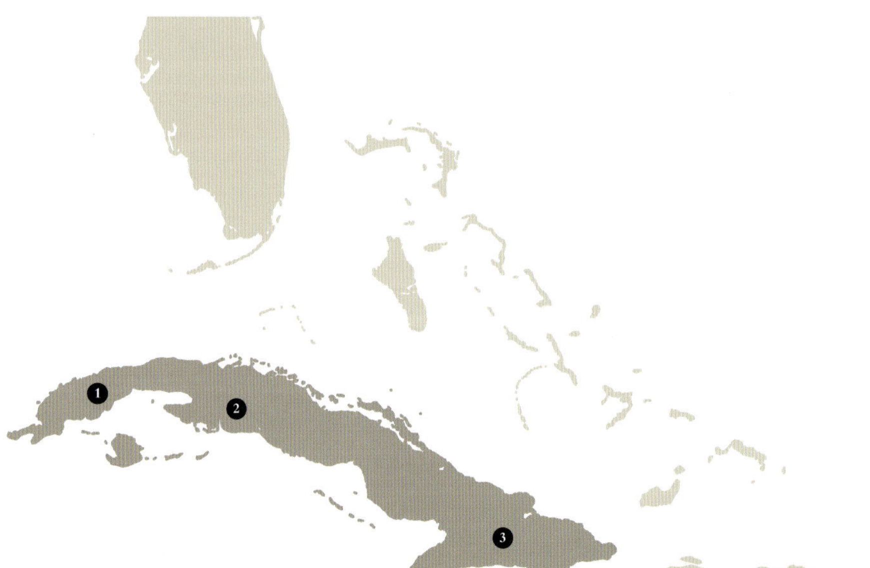

WHERE IT ALL BEGINS

Today, Cuba has prime tobacco-growing regions, located in the west (1. Pinar del Rio), center (2. Partido, known for its wrapper and filler), and east (3. Remedios and Oriente).

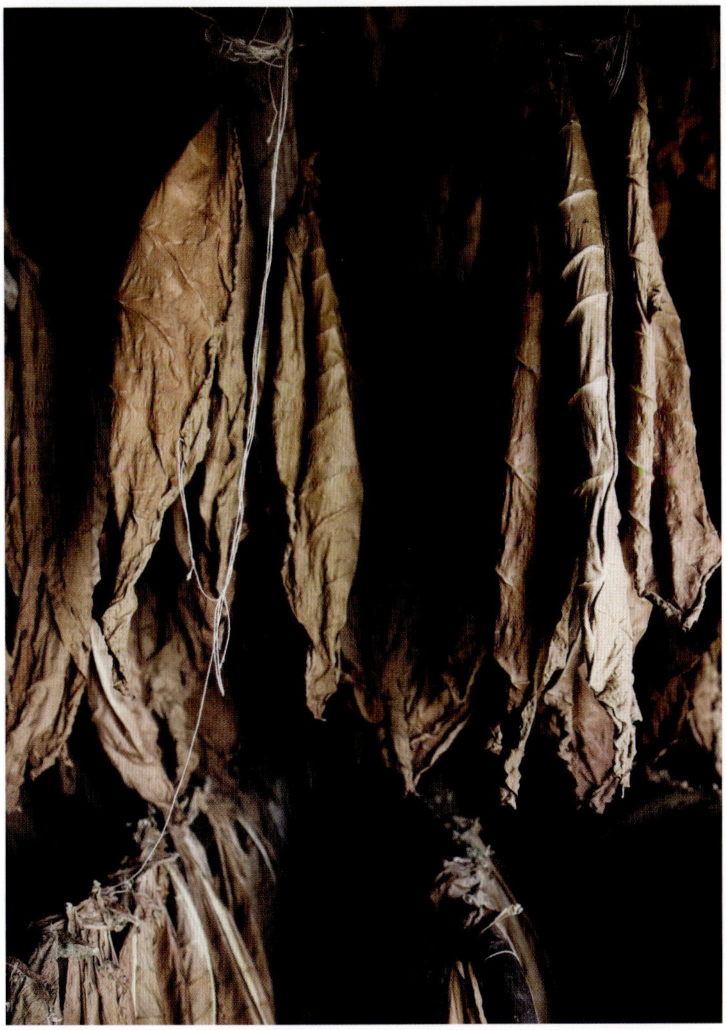

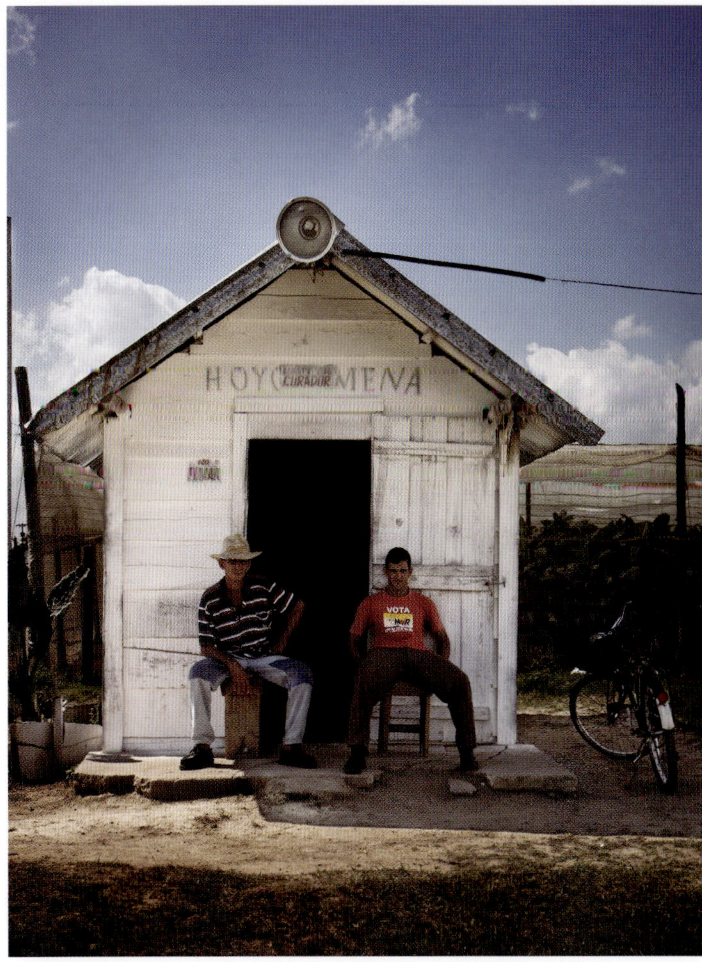
CURADOR
VOTA

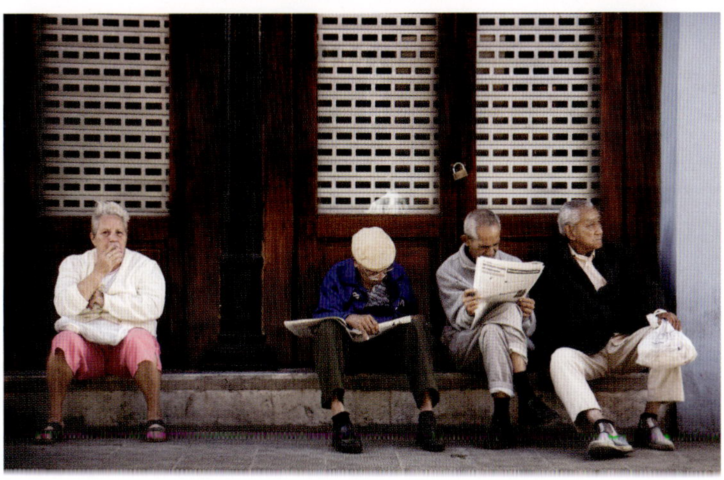

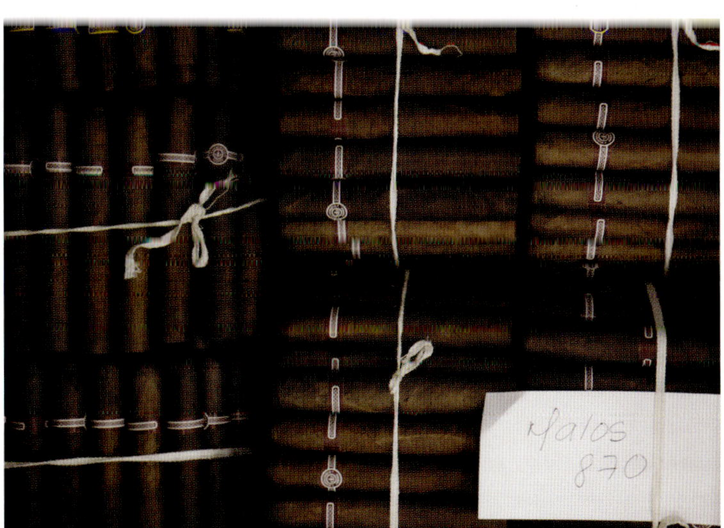
Malos
870

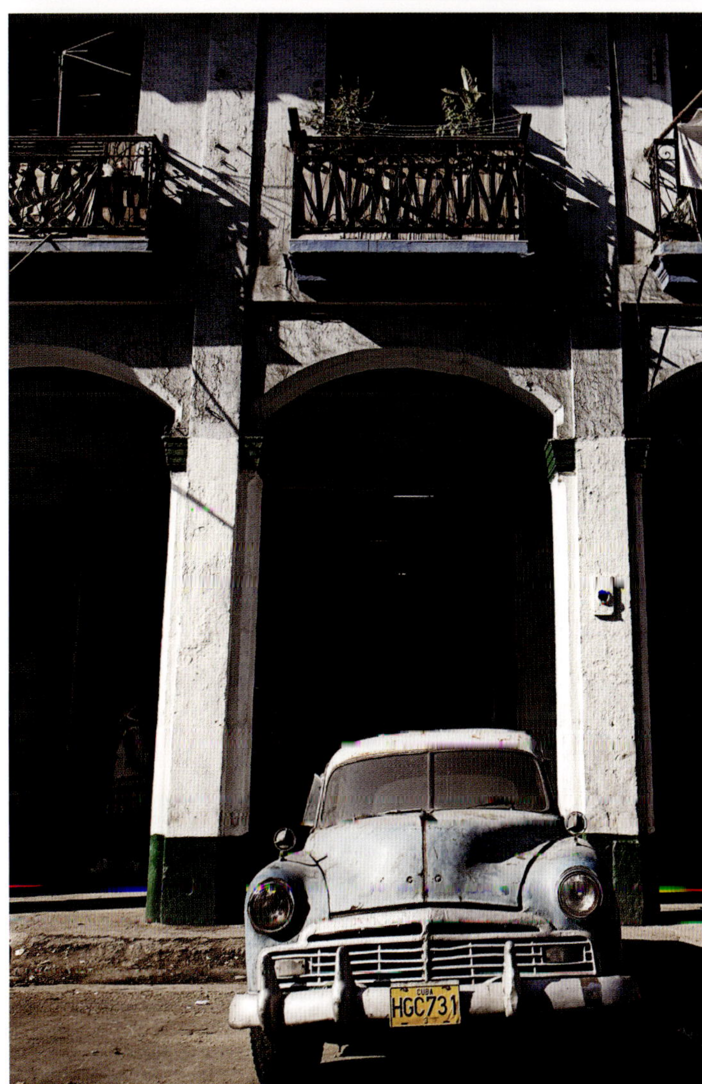
HGC731

tobacco to the state at a price decided by the leaves' variety, size, and shape. On a cool and sunny winter day, their seemingly endless fields may be covered by untold yards of billowing white fabric, as the tobacco underneath begins its life in the shade. Walk through their curing barns and stare up into the darkness at the tiers of tobacco hanging from poles, fermenting through the months.

Not least because of their abilities and peerless instincts, the tobacco farmers here are revered; one in particular, Alejandro Robaina, is a genuine star in a country where much of the cigar industry is kept faceless. A small and timeworn man, Robaina has spent decades growing some of the world's finest wrappers on his family plantation in Pinar del Río. Cigar-lovers make pilgrimages to sit on his rustic porch, and very nearly boost him onto their shoulders at festivals.

The Robaina clan, along with the rest of the island's farmers, carries on a tobacco-growing tradition that extends back centuries to Cuba's colonization. By the early nineteenth century, state-run plantations had spread across the island and the Spanish crown granted Cubans the right to roll their own cigars—effectively putting the *fábricas* in Seville and other Spanish towns out of business. Ships left Havana's port heavy with cigars bound for the wider world, and with the bountiful cash from those sales, Cuban families began assuming prestige and power.

That period saw the rise of the iconic cigar brands: Partagas, H. Upmann, El Rey del Mundo, Romeo y Julieta and others rolled out during a prolific multi-decade period stretching from the 1820s through the 1850s. Their reputation quickly increased throughout the world, as they won accolades at exhibitions and competitions from Moscow to Chicago. Barons such as José Gener and J.F. Rocha operated as vertically integrated entrepreneurs, controlling every step of the process—from growing the tobacco to shipping the finished product—and cigars largely remained a family business until the Revolution.

THE END IS THE BEGINNING OF THE END OF THE BEGINNING > But by the time the Revolution had done its work, the cigar families had fled, leaving their compatriots to ride out the swells of history and make do with what they had. If Cuba's cigars are still prized around the world, it all comes down to the tenacity and pride of those thousands who still stream into the factories, day in and day out, to roll smokes under trying circumstances.

On a rainy winter Monday in Havana, as an offshore storm sends waves bursting over the concrete wall separating the Malecón from the Caribbean, a navy blue Soviet-era sedan coughs to a halt on a flooded side street beside the five-star Meliá Cohiba. As the driver leapt out, preparing to revive the engine with an improvised squiggle of metal, his passenger walked over to an American journalist to chat.

Zino Davidoff, the Ukrainian-born founder of the eponymous firm, used Cuban tobacco for his cigars until he shifted operations to the Dominican Republic in 1990. He once called Cuba's confluence of soil and weather "irreplaceable virtues" that made the island "magic" for tobacco growers.

The man inquired, in Spanish, as to the brand of cigar smoking in the journalist's hand; and upon being told it was a Bolivar, nodded approval. The nod became a full-on smile when the journalist offered one over, but not before the man took a quick glance around to see if la policia were lurking about. Fraternization with the "enemy" is something actively discouraged among ordinary Cubans, even as the government has relaxed its policies on ownership of cellphones and other (nearly unobtainable) electronic devices such as microwaves.

Smoking the local pride-and-joy in the light rain, and staring beyond the concrete wall and frothing breakers toward the gray sea once sailed upon by conquistadors, the Cuban sighed and said, "New York, Miami, I would like to go." His head tilted for the pavement, and he spat. "Can't."

Not for the moment, at least. That will change; at times you can almost feel the modern world trembling to enter in full force, to fast-forward Havana into a city of shiny new fuel-efficient Fords and a bright fast-food joint on every corner. When that day comes, ships will again leave Havana's harbor loaded with Cuban cigars, to feed the inevitable spike in U.S. demand.

On that day Cuba will change—and though they may even ban smoking in cabs and El Floridita—its cigar legacy will be forever assured.

CLOSE CALL

Legend tells that, soon after he assumed power in the Revolution, Castro advocated consolidating all the island's cigar brands into a single "people's cigar" called the Siboney. His compatriots were quick to dissuade him; legend holds that even Ché—that Marxist revolutionary par excellence—thought it too radical a decision (perhaps he was also thinking that his time spent tromping through the bush would be that much more monotonous if there was only one variety of Cuban to smoke).

Fortunately, Castro backed down, clearing the way for future generations of smokers to torch up a Romeo y Julieta, Montecristo, or any other of Habanos S.A.'s twenty-seven current premium brands.

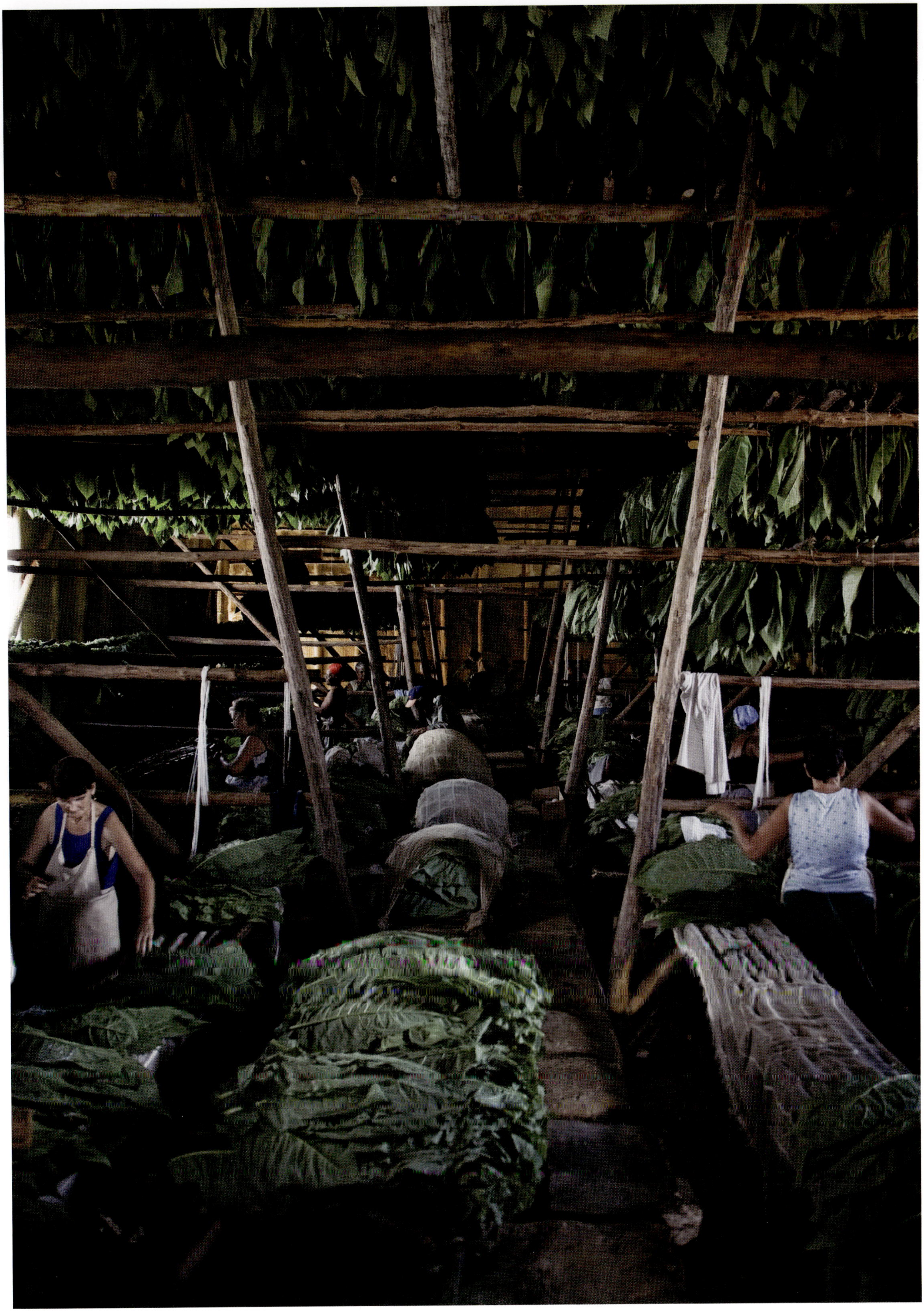

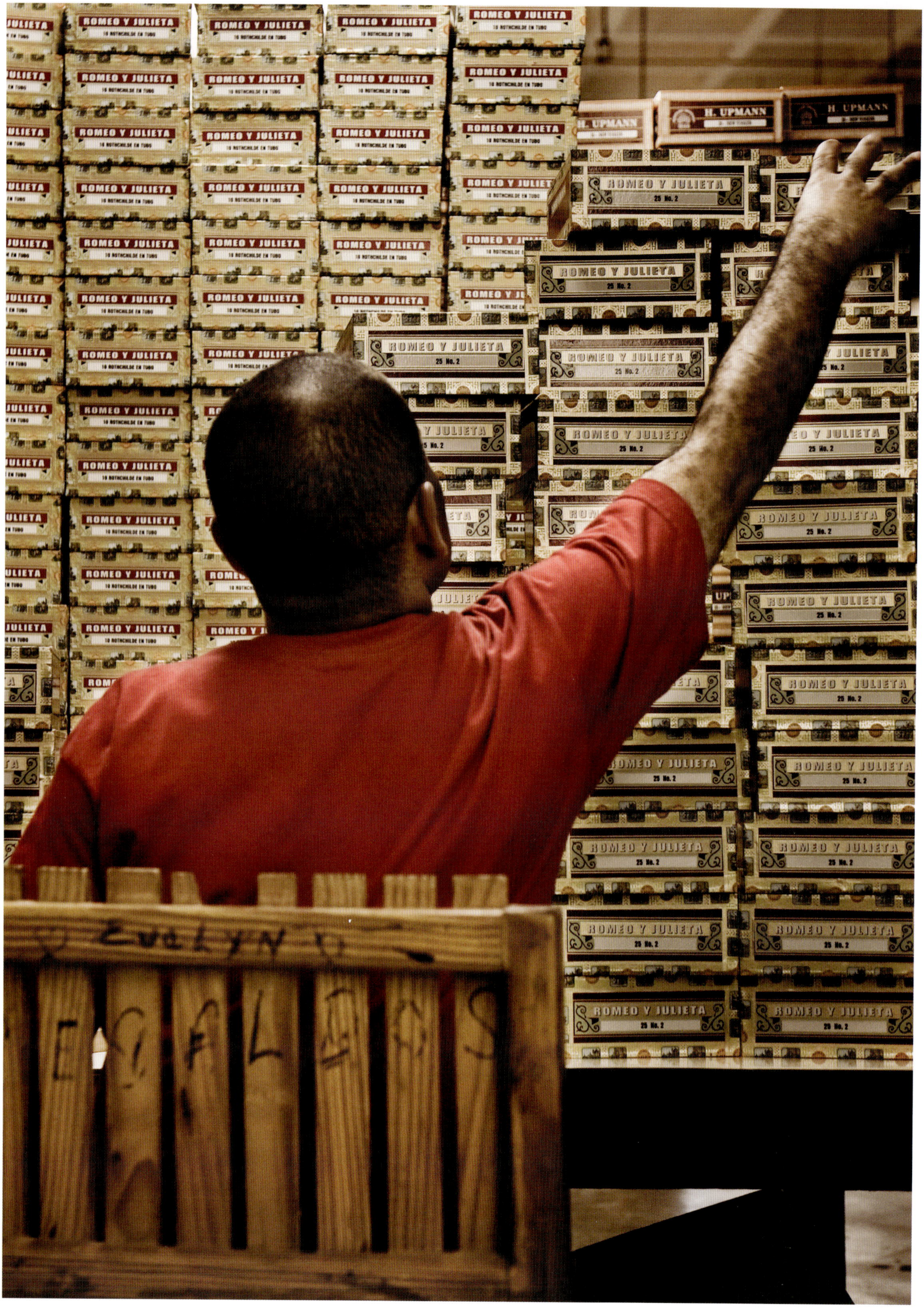
ROMEO Y JULIETA
H. UPMANN
25 No. 2

Dominican Republic

You could call the town of La Romana the best of both worlds. It's home to the golfing resort of Casa de Campo, whose ocean-side Pete Dye course is considered one of the finest in the Caribbean; it is also the address of Tabacalera de García S.A.S., which at 270,000 square feet is the world's largest premium cigar factory. Under the watchful eye of master cigar maker José Seijas (who's been here since 1974, except for a brief stint spent in the Canary Islands), the *fábrica* produces tens of millions of the Dominican Montecristo, H. Upmann, Romeo y Julieta, and other brands. This means that you can smoke one while teeing off and watching your "perfectly aimed" ball disappear into the sea.

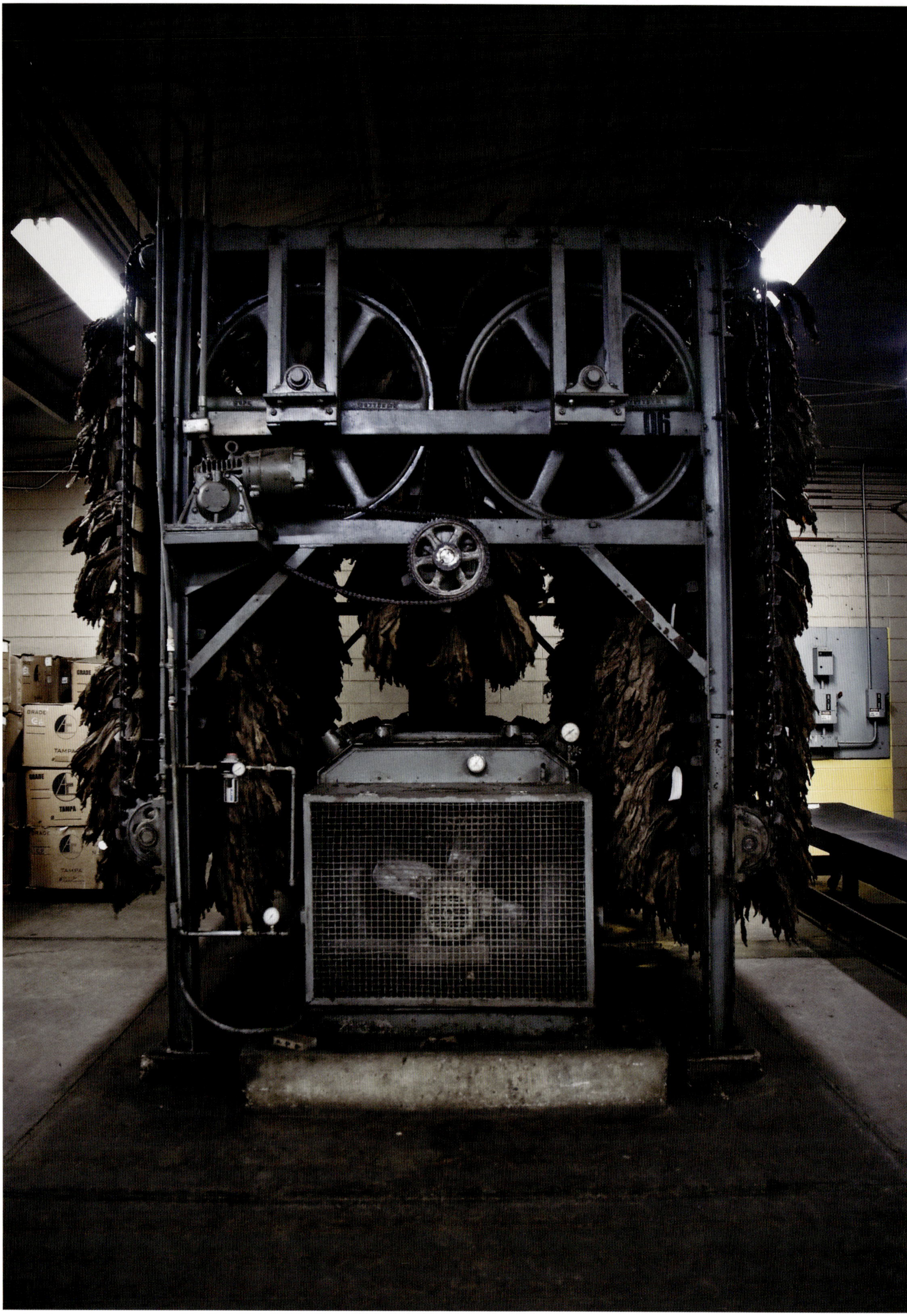
06
GRADE
TAMPA

Ownership of Tabacalera de García has shifted over the years, from multiple incarnations and owners, from Consolidated Cigar Corporation to Altadis U.S.A., as the business side of the cigar world underwent some substantial mergers-and-acquisitions action. During that time, different brands have rolled out of its loading docks (including the Playboy cigar). But despite these shifts around and inside, the factory is as much a fixture of the landscape as La Romana, the golf course or even the ocean. In its infinite wisdom, the Dominican government made Tabacalera de García the country's first tax-advantaged free zone in the early 1970s, demonstrating the island's commitment to its cigar culture (not to mention commerce in general).

For more proof that cigars have a prominent place in the heart and soul of this Caribbean nation, you need to drive far west, into the industrial town of Santiago. There, on a warm spring night (one of those rare ones where the smog has cleared away and left the air as fresh and clean as the day Spanish explorers first saw this wide valley), the local cigar industry's best and brightest have assembled on a stage near a replica of the Dominican's first, humble cigar factory where Eduardo León Jimenes's rollers crafted the first Dominican cigars a century ago.

One of the men onstage is Seijas; he and the other master cigar makers with him represent ProCigar, the cigar world's equivalent of OPEC—a group bound together for the good of all. Tonight is the first night of the first annual ProCigar Festival—their upstart-yet-elegant answer to Cuba's famous Habanos Festival—and the juxtaposition between the small and "antique" *fábrica* behind them and the glamorous crowd at their feet couldn't be more distinct: From modest beginnings, the industry here has expanded to the point where it sees itself as capable of challenging Cuba for its tobacco crown. Indeed, the cigar makers start taking the microphone to hammer that point home:

"We export the finest premium handmade cigars in the world . . ."

"This is cigar country!"

Some 516 years after Columbus and his merry band sighted the coast of the island they named La Española, or "The Spanish Island" (later mutated into Hispaniola), the Dominican Republic stands poised at a historical turning point. "We're not really Third World," one cigar titan says as he eases his SUV through the bright chaos of Santiago's major thoroughfares. "At this point, we're more like Second World."

A number of duty-free "free zones"—the first of which was Tabacalera de García—dot the country, hosting factories that produce millions of sticks per year. From dawn to dusk, the factories bustle with activity. Seated at wooden desks, rollers move with a precision that seems deceptively free and easy. Workers at long tables strip and bundle leaves and check the quality of finished cigars, under the watchful eye of both supervisors and cutouts of the Virgin Mary taped to the concrete walls. In some rolling rooms, the radio blares tinny pop; in others, the only music is the rhythmic thump of blades slicing tobacco leaf into shape, underscored by the thrum of wheeled carts shuttling through the mazelike corridors. Here is where the artistry of cigar-making—a craft that's existed here for centuries— firmly intersects with the pure commerce part of the business.

Much of the country's rising fortunes are due to its up-and-coming tourism industry and recent resort real estate boom, but cigars have been playing an increasing part as well. In 2007, the country exported 177.7 million cigars to the United States, a 3.8 percent increase from the year before, and part of a steady increase from a low period after the crash of the mid-1990s cigar boom. The quality of Dominican cigars has much to do with that rise–and so, too, does its situation with Cuba.

THE TIDES OF HISTORY > The fates of Cuba and the Dominican Republic have been entangled ever since Europeans first set foot on both islands; at alternating points, both served as the Spanish capital in the Americas. And like Cuba, the Dominican Republic has been in the tobacco-growing business for centuries, but for much of its history, the majority of the crop was exported to Europe for actual production.

However, in the nineteenth century, as Cuba took the reins of indigenous production, its neighbor remained mired in a seemingly endless pattern of revolutions, dictatorships, and invasions (principally by neighboring Haiti). In 1805, the Haitians conquered Santiago and effectively ended the city's tobacco production for years. In 1821, the Dominican Republic declared its independence, only to have Haiti invade it again. It would take four more decades before Juan Pablo Duarte and his band of rebels managed to finally evict the invaders, and even then, the country was too bled-out to support thoughts of cigar production.

The Dominican Republic was still something of a mess in 1903, when Eduardo León Jimenes came up with the idea of starting a small cigar concern near Santiago. He called his company La Aurora, and soon his profits allowed an initial handful of rollers to increase to a few dozen. Others, realizing that making cigars was a viable enterprise, started their own factories.

These now-legendary figures and their families spent the next few decades building their brands. They dealt with the country's lack of infrastructure, and endured the brutal thirty-one-year reign of dictator Rafael Trujillo (who was assassinated in 1961). Even before that, though, events were underway that would have a profound effect on the Dominican cigar industry.

In 1959, Castro came to power in Cuba. His socialist agenda and close ties to the Soviets led to the retaliatory U.S. trade embargo in 1962. Cuban cigar families' stories from the period are rife with tales of militia arriving at their offices to seal safes and seize property. With their businesses nationalized and their bank accounts frozen, many Cuban cigar makers had no choice but to flee the country. After

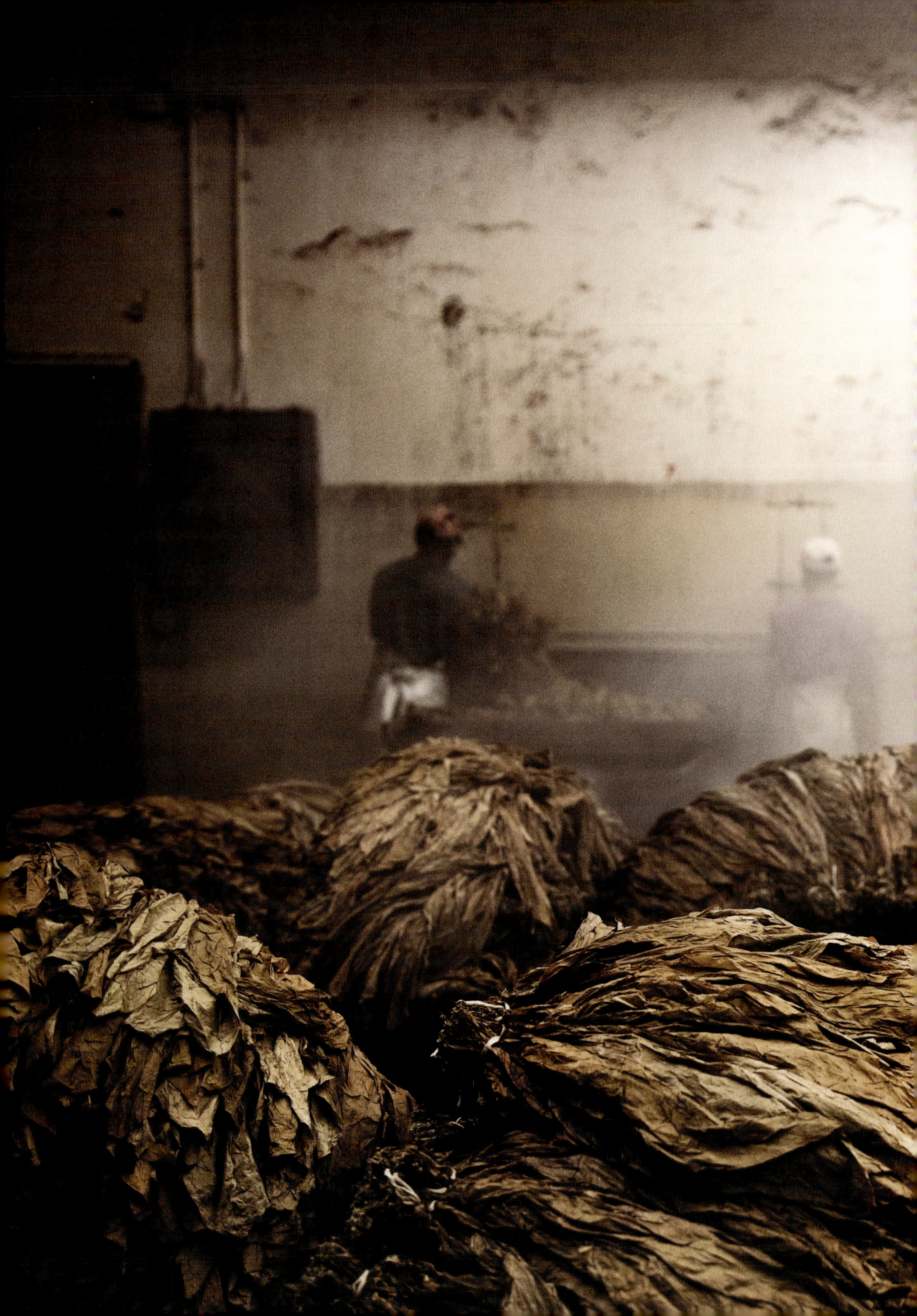

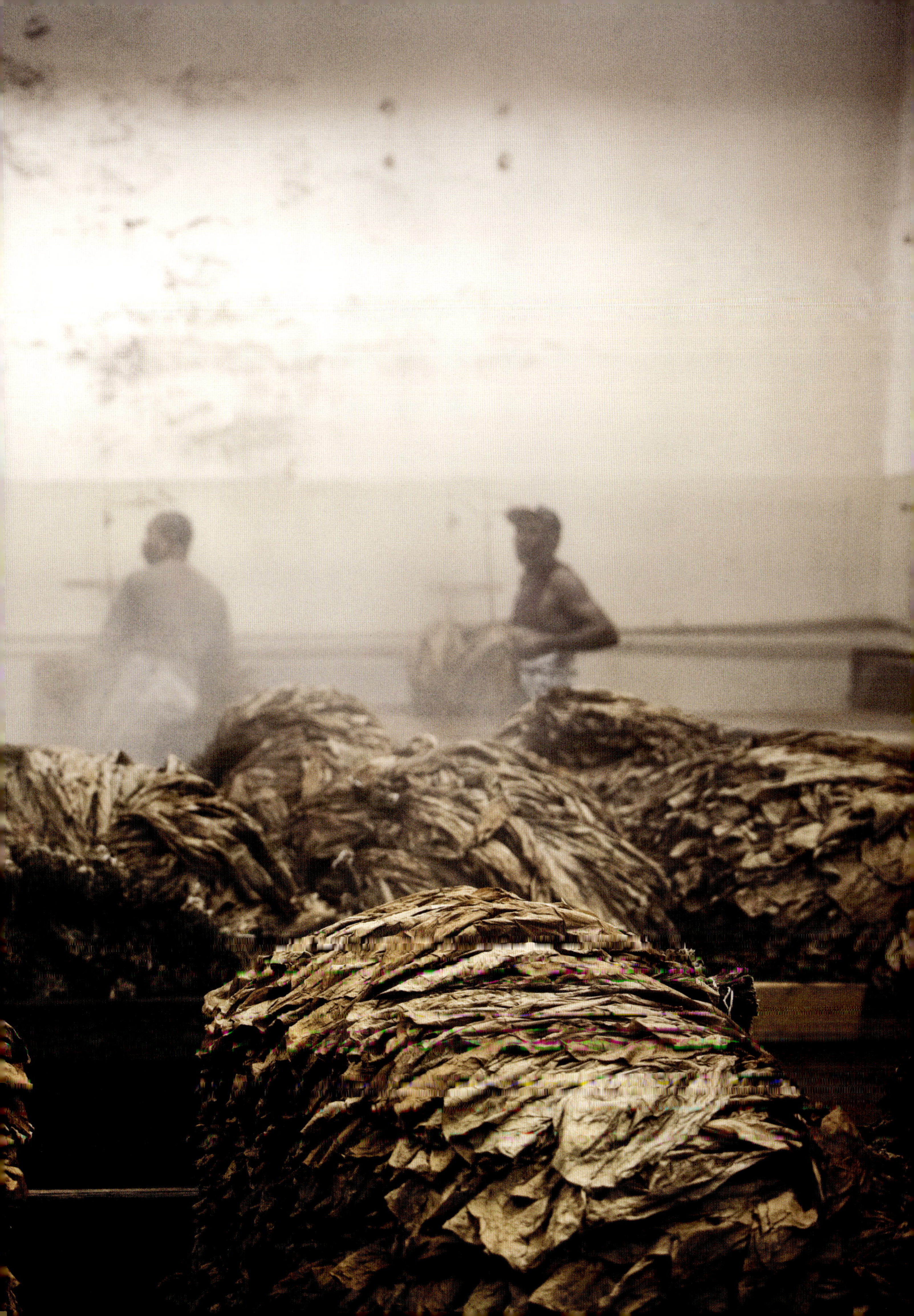

they left, the embargo came down like an iron curtain, cutting off Americans from their beloved Cuban cigars. They would need another source for their quality smokes.

In the end, irrespective of their sometimes convoluted route, many of them found their way to the Dominican Republic.

With the death of Trujillo, the country had developed a certain political stability; that, combined with its long tradition of growing tobacco, attracted a variety of formerly Cuba-based players to set up shop. And there they prospered.

BOOM, COLLAPSE, COMEBACK > A few decades after that, the nineties cigar boom hit. At its height, and as American smokers clamored for cigars to the tune of double-digit growth per year, dozens of people with a bit of cash and dreams of starting their own brand rushed into the country. Over 120 cigar factories opened in Santiago alone. In their desperation, many of the newcomers even drew upon questionable family history in the effort to make their lines seem prestigious and time-tested (Hey, great-great-uncle Pablo once swept the floor of a cigar factory, so we can say it's been the family business for 150 years!)

After the boom collapsed, those carpetbaggers lasted mere microseconds before sprinting for the proverbial hills, leaving their factories abandoned and any equipment to be snatched up by more prudent colleagues.

When they left, what remained were the dozen or so long-established players (along with the smattering of particularly smart neophytes who understood that the industry at its core was about quality, not image) kept doing what they did best: rolling premium cigars. And even though the boom itself had ended, it had birthed a new generation of cigar smokers who could better appreciate what the Dominican masters were doing.

The masters, in turn, could rely on their country's climate (similar to that of Cuba in the West), to help produce excellent tobacco. The most notable of the local crop is grown to the northwest of Santiago, in the Cibao Valley. Fed by the Yaque River, the plant is mild where it grows in the shade of the Cordillera Central and Cordillera Septentrional mountain ranges to the north, and stronger in the flatter, sun-baked areas to the south.

The fields themselves grow under a burning tropical sun, fenced by rows of tall corn which act as a windbreak. Given the value of the final crop and the care with which its tiny seeds are cultivated in the cigar makers' mesh-draped nurseries, it would simply not do to have them blow away. When the time comes, lines of workers will filter among the rows, plucking the leaves nearest the ground and carrying them into the curing barns to be strung from the rafters.

Inside the barns, the only light comes from chinks between the boards, but the heat is there—slowly transforming the leaves' original green shade to a brownish hue that represents gold to both the cigar makers and the thousands employed by them.

Despite their major share of the U.S. market, however, those *jefes* are still fighting for more of a foothold on the international market still dominated by Habanos S.A. In 1992, seeking to present a more unified front, they united together to form ProCigar, an association dedicated, in its own words, "to defend, protect and divulge the good name of the land of Cigar Country, number one exporter of premium cigars in the world."

But back to that first night of the first ProCigar festival. Onstage, before the smoke and lights and dancers turn the evening into a proper fiesta, the local giants stand as one to receive the audience's applause: José Seijas, Manuel Quesada, Hendrik Kelner, Daniel Nuñez (now retired), Guillermo León, and Juan Clemente. Despite their power within the industry, they all affect an air of humility; there's no flashiness in the way they dress or carry themselves, nothing glittering on hands tuned by years of cigar work. They stand there as a symbol of their nation's pride . . . icons of both its past and present.

FILLER UP

Cigar makers here import much of their wrapper and much of their binder leaf from Nicaragua, Connecticut, and other countries. Inside the Dominican Republic itself, they primarily grow three types of tobacco:

Piloto Cubano:
Produces a stronger, full-bodied taste

San Vincente:
A lighter leaf

Olor:
A downright mild strain of tobacco

The majority of these tobaccos end up as filler, where, in the hands of a master blender, they can be combined into a wide variety of strengths and flavors. Those who have been rolling cigars here for decades say the boom changed the taste profile of many Dominican sticks, from a pre-1990's mildness to a post-boom focus on complexity and strength—reflecting the changing tastes of many American cigar smokers.

CIGAR CELEBS

Perhaps in keeping with the tenets of the socialist revolution, Cuba has fostered no true cigar celebrities, with the singular exception of Don Alejandro Robaina. However, the same cannot be said for the Dominican Republic, where the best of the cigar makers—including many Cuban émigrés—quickly emerged as "cigar celebrities."

Today, these men are front and center in their companies' advertising, not to mention promotional events—even as many would offer a wry grin at the very idea, and joke that they don't exactly have matinee-idol looks.

The cigar royalty of the Dominican Republic includes José Sejas (general manager of Tabacalera de Garcia, creator of Mi Dominicana and Seijas Signature Series); Manuel Quesada (founder of MATASA, which produces Fonseca, among other cigars); Benjamin Menendez, who left Cuba in 1960 with his wife and three children, and would use his decades of cigar knowledge (learned in Havana's H. Upmann factory) in the service of a variety of companies, including General Cigar and Altadis U.S.A.; Avo Uvezian (creator of the Avo Cigar); Litto Gomez, cofounder, La Flor Dominicana, who with his wife, Ines Lorenzo-Gomez, created La Flor Dominicana's boutique cigar line; and the late Ramon Cifuentes, who left Cuba in 1960 with the cigar knowledge necessary to create a Dominican version of his Partagas cigars.

There are many others, of course, but that's another book entirely.

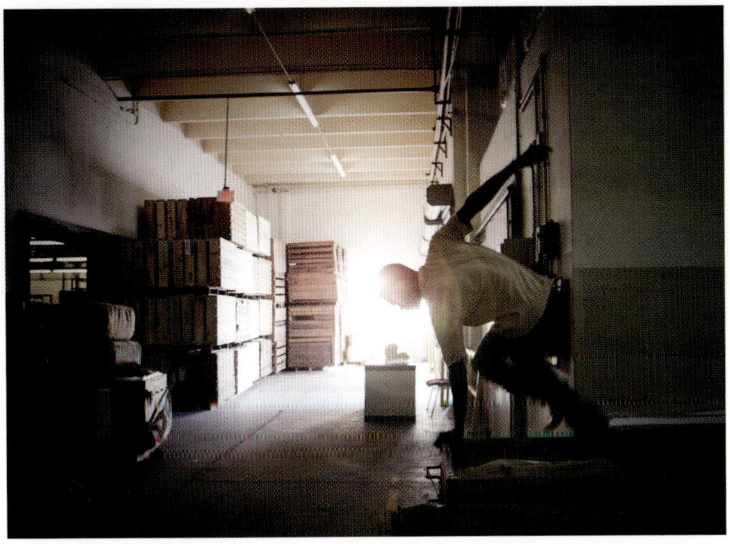
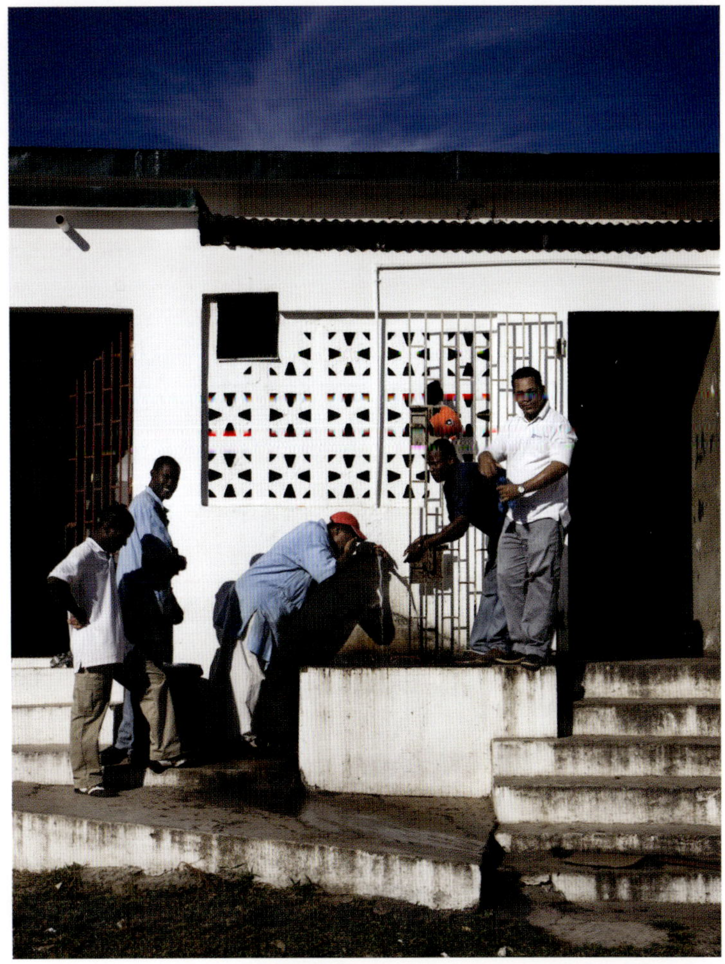
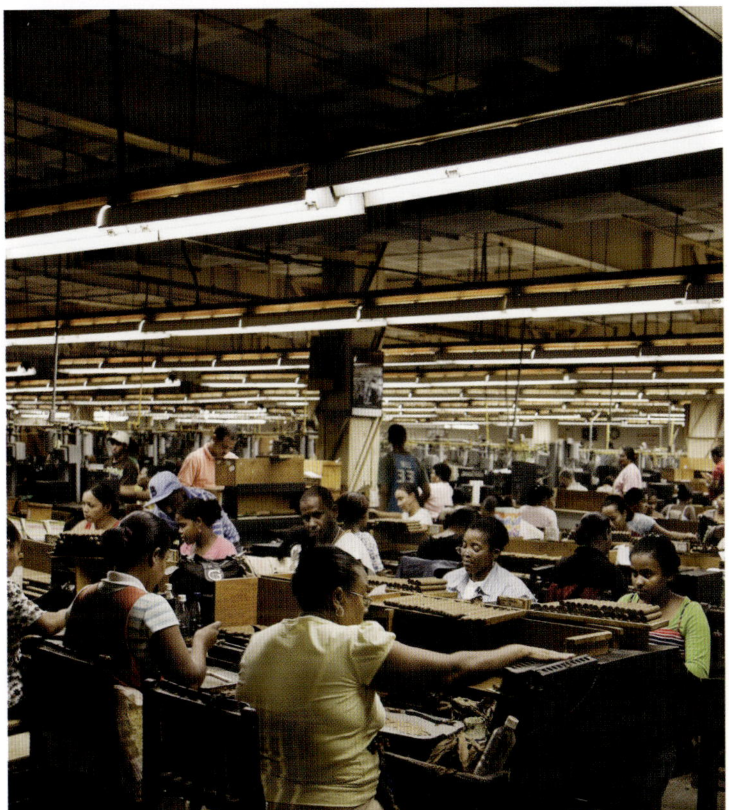
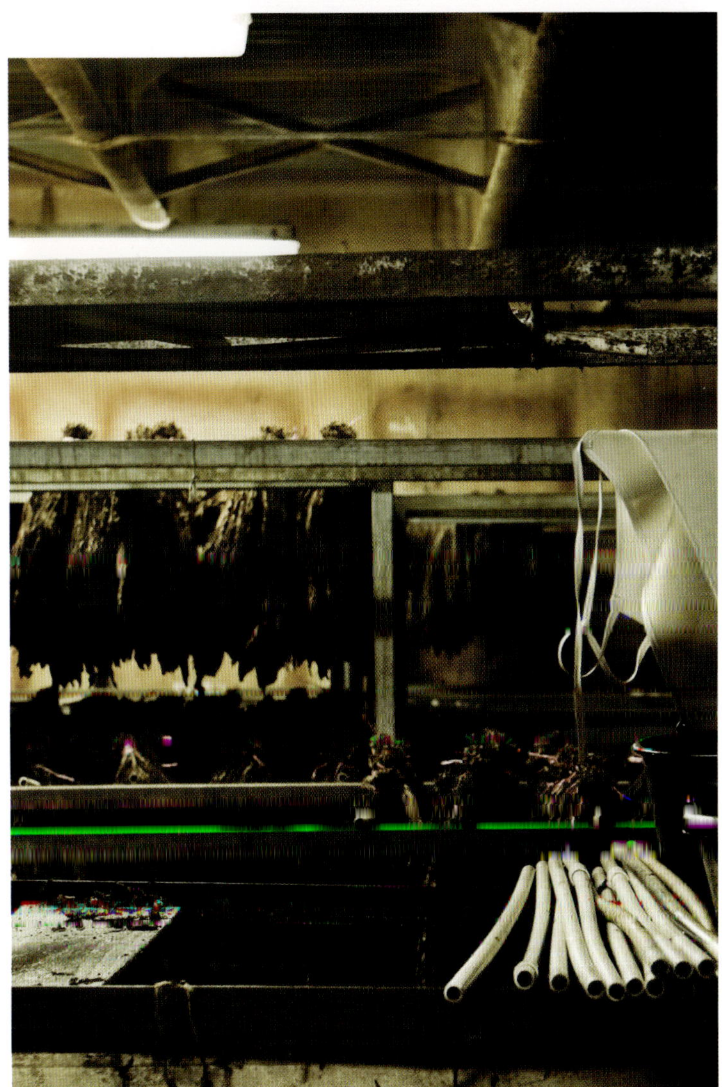
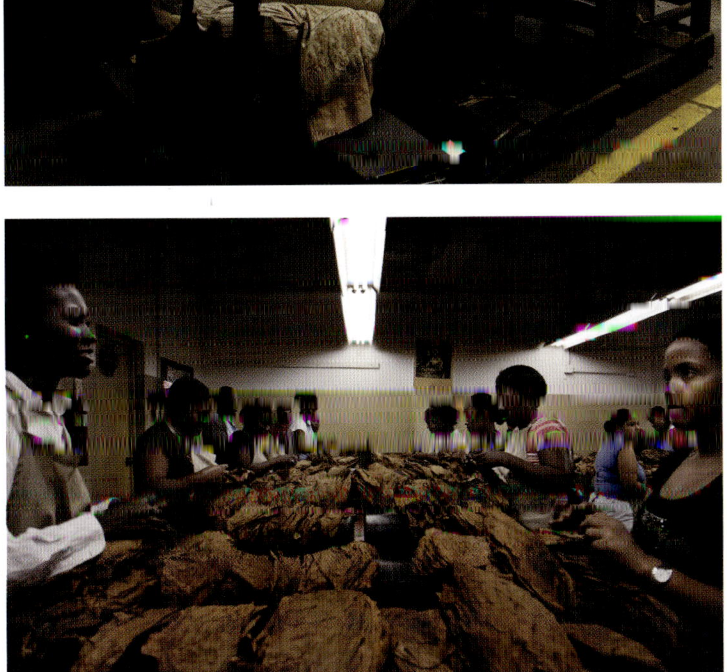

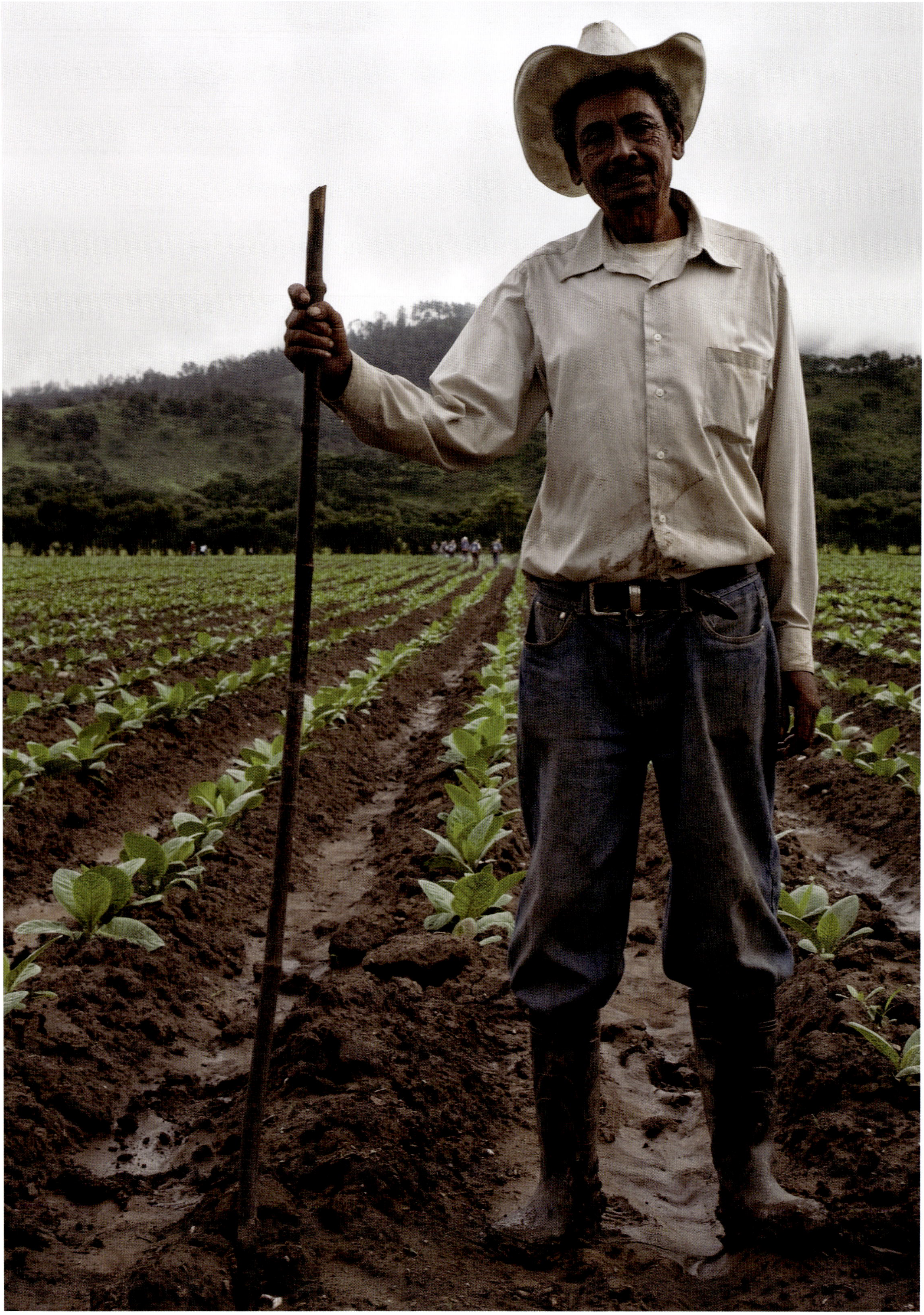

Honduras

This Central American country shares much in common with Nicaragua, its equally mountainous cousin to the south. Both grow tobacco in limited areas within their borders, both feature local cigar-growers (many of whom came here in flight from Castro's Cuba) who persevered and developed empires despite local upheaval, and both have produced leaf with a reputation that has only grown with years. It took some time, however, for Honduran cigar manufacturing to become an industry. In 1765, the Spanish began a tobacco trading post at Santa Rosa de Copán, both for the revenue and to draw settlers to the area. The town and the fertile soil around it were still drawing players over three hundred years later. A substantial share of the credit for the birth of Honduras's modern cigar industry, though, goes to the Cuban expatriates of the late 1950s and early 1960s, who came here after the Revolution to forge a new life.

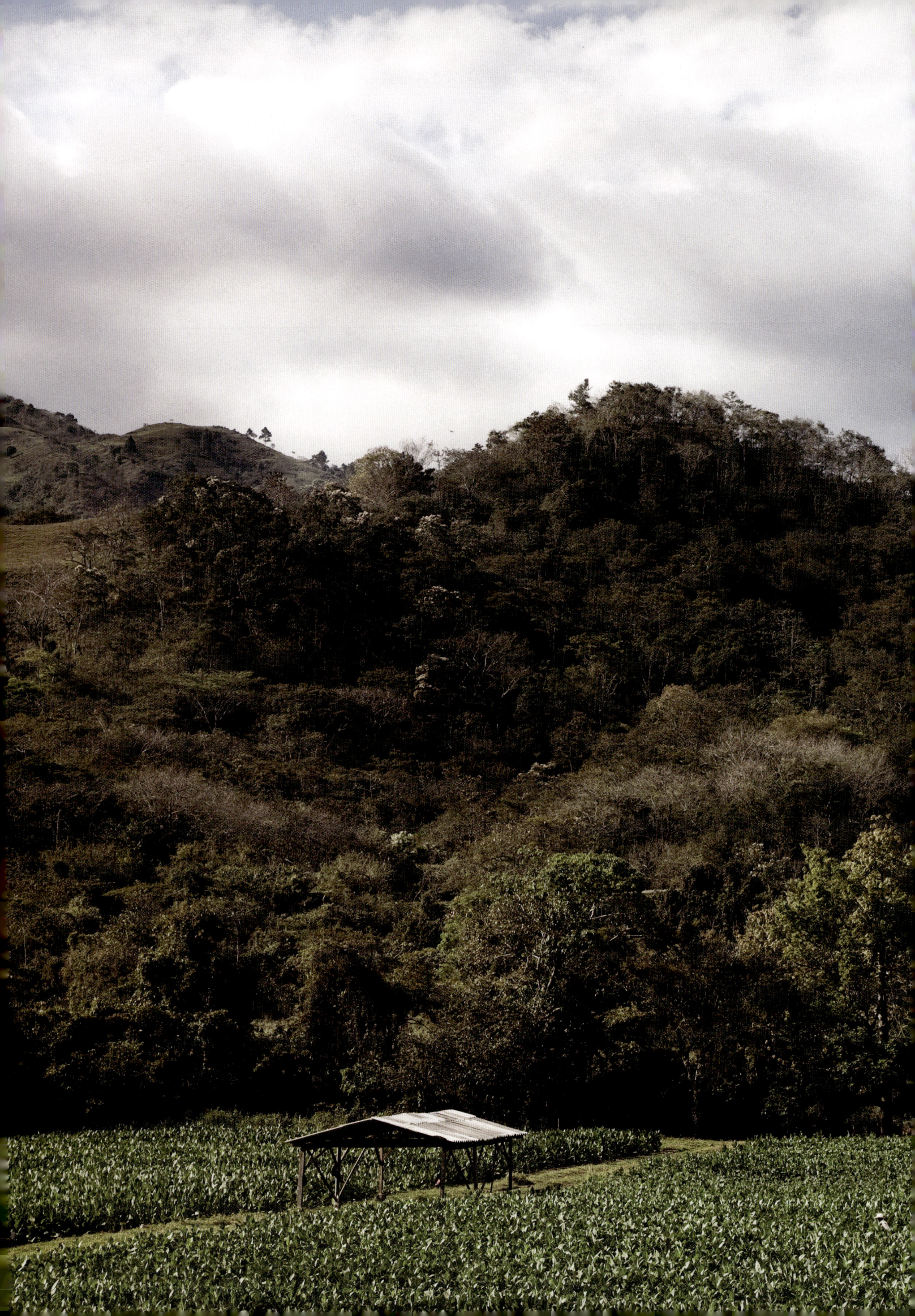

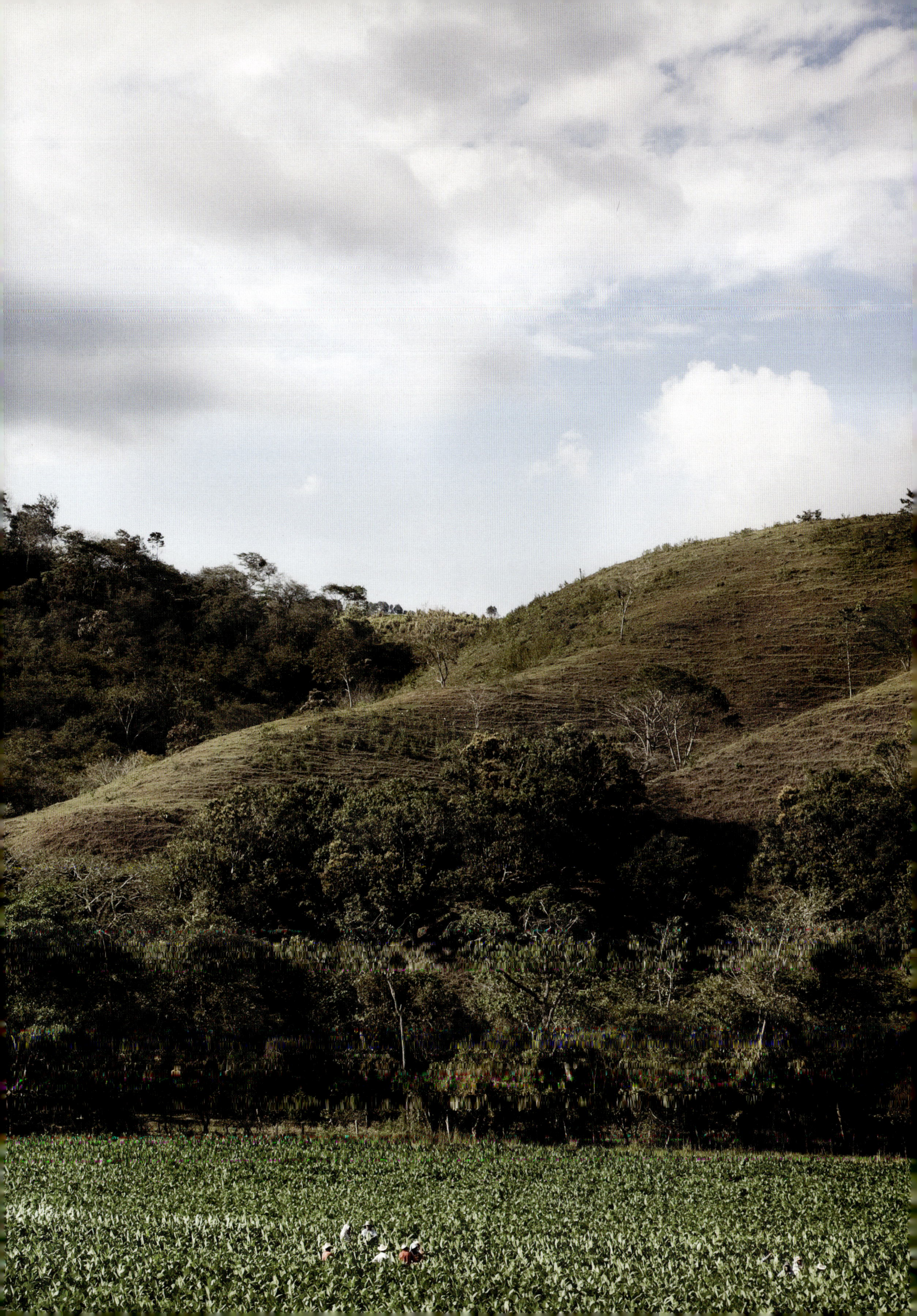

Many of them headed for the areas around Danlí, in the eastern part of the country, and what they found there was undeveloped land, to say the least. It lacked paved roads, never mind business-ready infrastructure; nonetheless, studies by the Honduran government's Ministry of Agriculture had shown that the land was more than capable of growing tobacco in large quantities. And so those Cubans settled down and extended roots both literal and metaphorical into the land.

Their initial struggles put the "hard" in "hardscrabble." Danlí may have been fertile, but this was not a land of plenty yet, and those first tobacco settlers became adept at using, and re-using, whatever materials were at hand in order to keep their farms and factories alive.

Many companies in Danlí have remained strictly independent concerns. Both Nicaragua and Honduras have wrestled with political demons over the last several decades (in the 80s, anti-Sandinista forces took positions in Danlí, using it as a base for incursions into Nicaragua; at the same time, the Honduran army battled left-wing elements and political opponents).

Some cigar makers' setups in Danlí serve as insurance against political unrest, with facilities that mirror their establishments an hour and a half away across the Nicaraguan border. Having factories and warehouses on both sides of the border makes the cautious cigar maker feel better positioned to ride out any storms of history. Today, Nicaragua remains cripplingly poor (it is, in fact, one of the most impoverished in the Western Hemisphere, with unemployment hovering around thirty percent) but stable.

COMING UP > Conditions in Honduras are optimal for strong, rich tobacco leaf. The country's three main growing regions (the Jamastran Valley, southeast of Danlí; the central Talanga Valley; and the areas west of Santa Rosa de Copán on the Guatemalan border) are thick with a loamy soil reminiscent of the Dominican Republic and Nicaragua, and famous for their Cuban-seed and Connecticut Shade tobacco. That, when combined with the damp mornings and bright afternoons of the growing season, translates into product of particular character: If Nicaraguan tobacco is notable for its strength, then its Honduran cousin is known among growers for its lighter, sweeter nature.

In modern-day Danlí the first thing one notices is the sheer number of cigar factories lining the two-lane road through town, sequestered behind imposing stone walls and steel gates. It seems that nearly every player in the industry has an outpost here; over the past few decades, a multitude of companies have moved in to take advantage of the country's tobacco-cultivating culture—one that extends back several centuries to the Maya (when Columbus arrived here on his third voyage, in 1502, he yet again found tribes torching up the local leaf).

Long before the tobacco arrives in Danlí for processing, though, much of it begins life in the Jamastran Valley, a few miles away and reachable via a two-lane winding road, interrupted by a police checkpoint. A few hundred yards past the bored officer (who fixes drivers with a signature dose of official glare), the low buildings of Danlí fall away to a patchwork of shanties lined with roadside food stalls and throngs waiting for the bus. Past that, there are only the fields, stretched out between the low green hills.

At the height of the growing season, the soil is thick with nutrients. Workers' battered bicycles line the dirt track leading to the main road, and the workers themselves kneel to their tasks between the rows. Occasionally, one *jefe* or another will be present, leaning against the side of a mud-spattered SUV and surveying the first step of a worldwide undertaking.

And, in that spirit, cigar-making here continues apace. Some 45.85 million Honduran cigars were imported into the U.S. in the first six months of 2008, a trend that has been moving upward for five years in a row. In Honduras's factories, workers roll dark tobacco leaves from those rich, misty fields into fresh cigars. Across the country, men in white sit in the warrens of La Flor de Copana and contemplatively roll tobacco-smoke on their educated tongues. They know what you know, and what the Spaniards and the Mayans before them knew: the soil here is rich . . . the tobacco good.

Those survival skills came in handy in 1998, when Hurricane Mitch swept over the country and devastated nearly three-quarters of the tobacco crop, in addition to causing some $3 billion in infrastructure damages. Slowly, with the same deliberation they used in building their small empires the first time around, the farmers pieced their shattered lives and facilities back together.

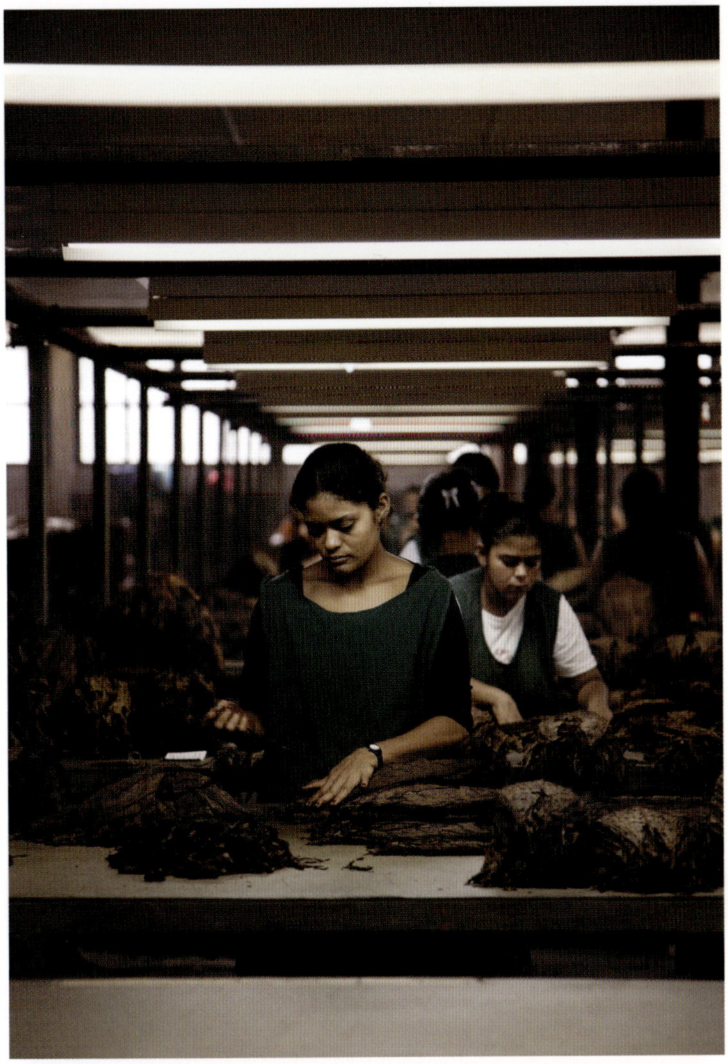

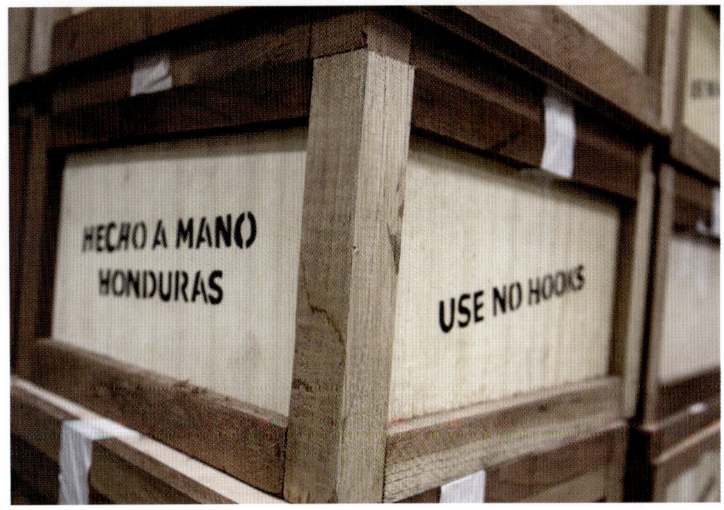
HECHO A MANO
HONDURAS
USE NO HOOKS

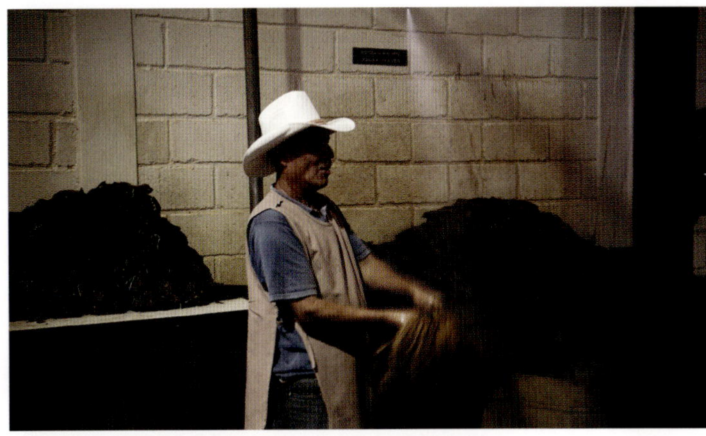

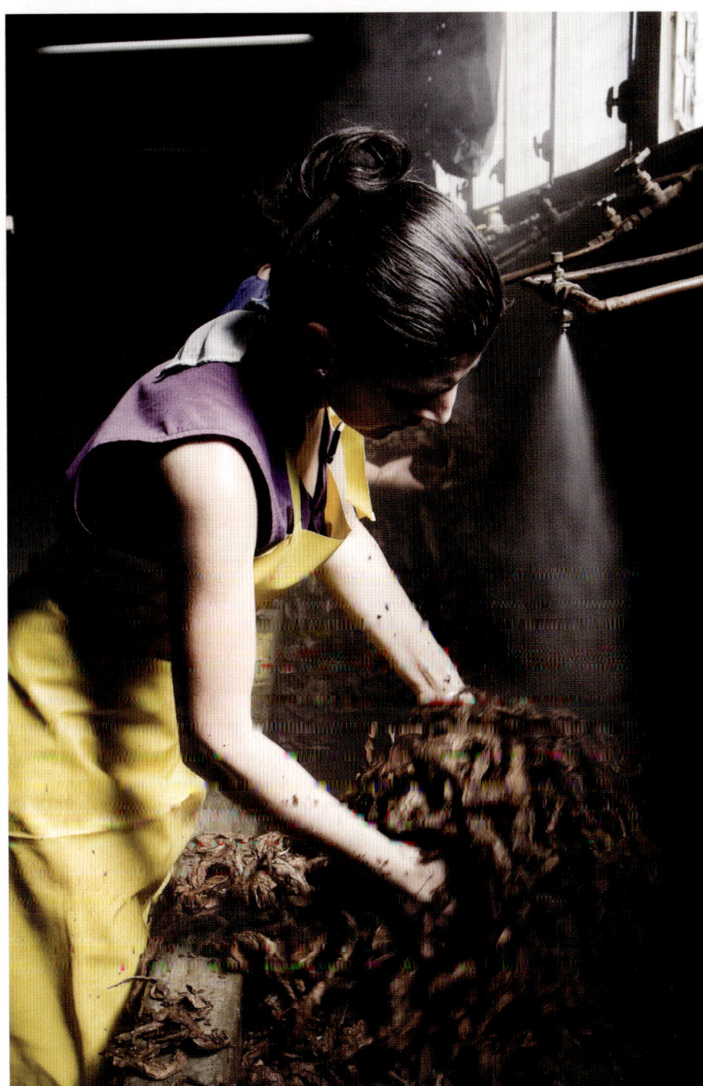

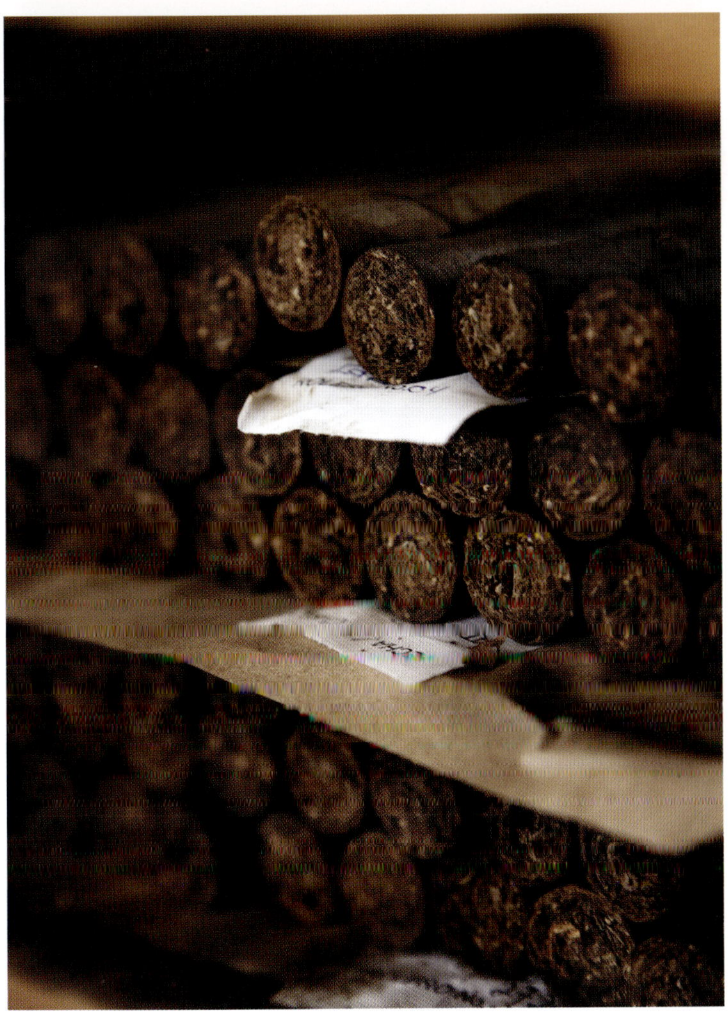

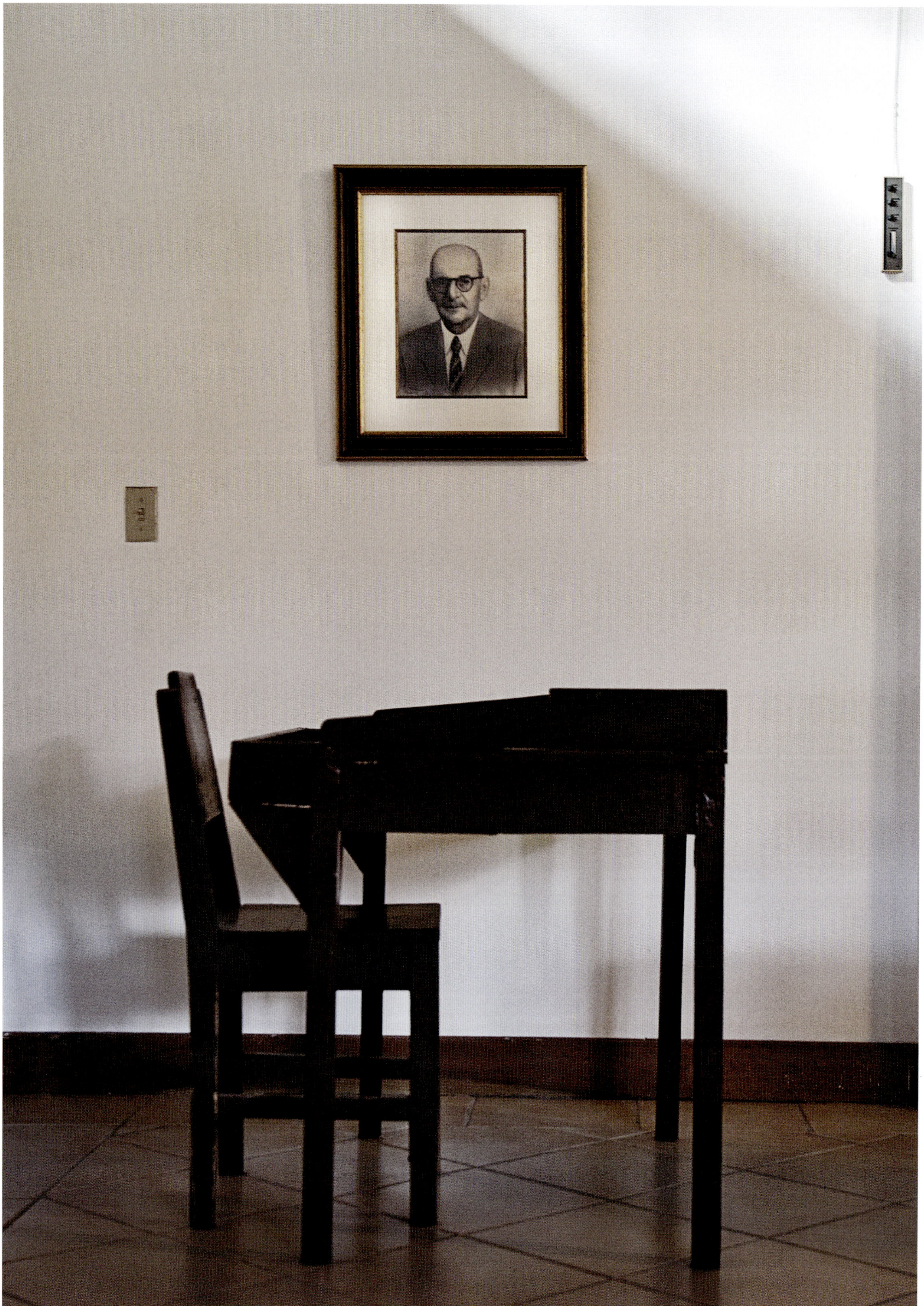

Nicaragua

To say that this Central American country has come a long way from its civil conflicts of the 1970s and 1980s is something of an understatement. The highway between the capital, Managua, and the highlands cigar town of Estelí bustles with monster trucks loaded with fresh cut logs, brightly painted school buses filled with villagers, men in white hats on horseback, and locals selling everything from nuts to parrots from small roadside stands. In Estelí itself, a tall white church looms over the colorful chaos of the central square, and the only signs of the violence of past decades, when this city was pounded by artillery fire from the surrounding ridges, are the shrapnel holes in buildings' bright stucco.

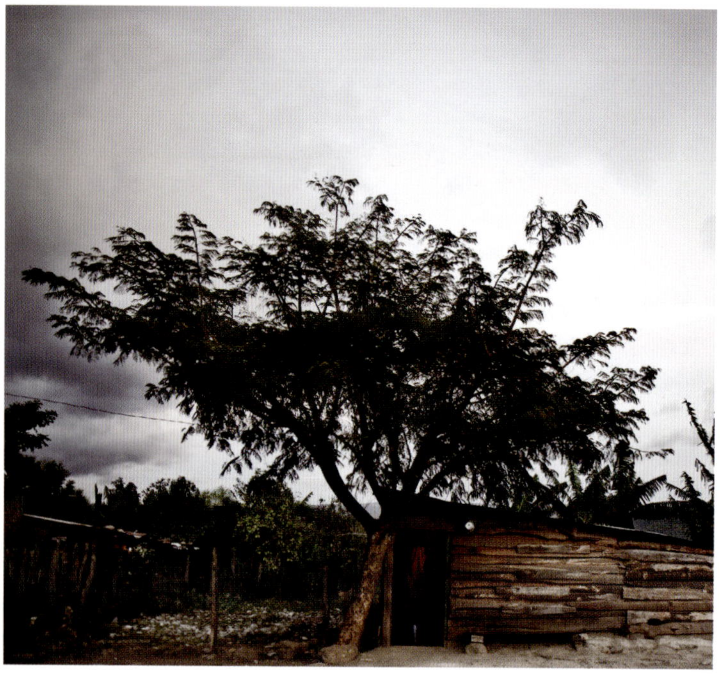

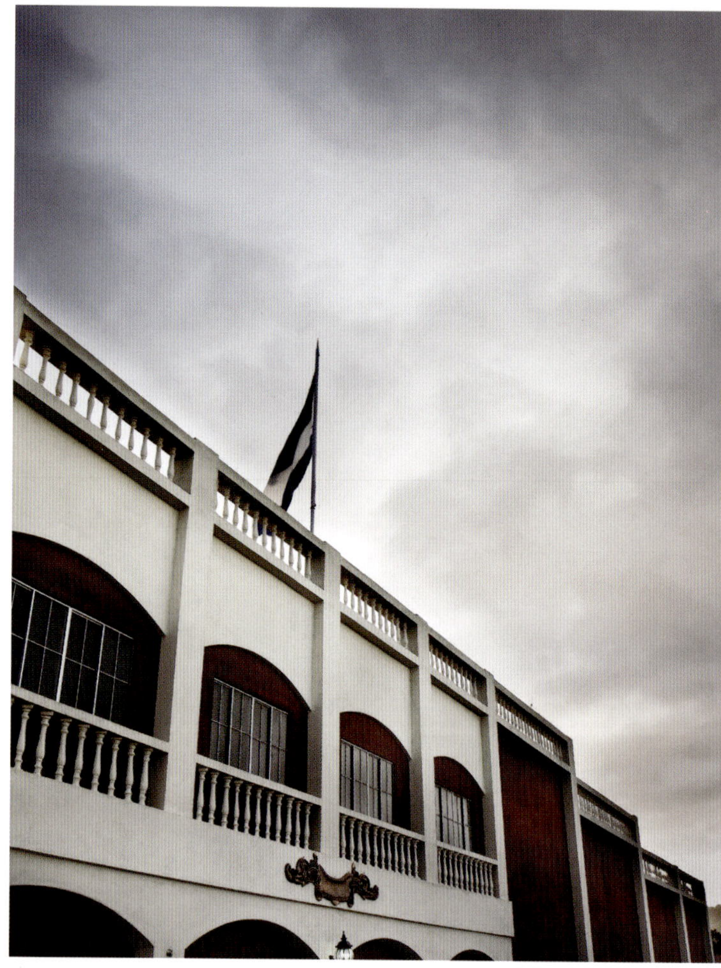

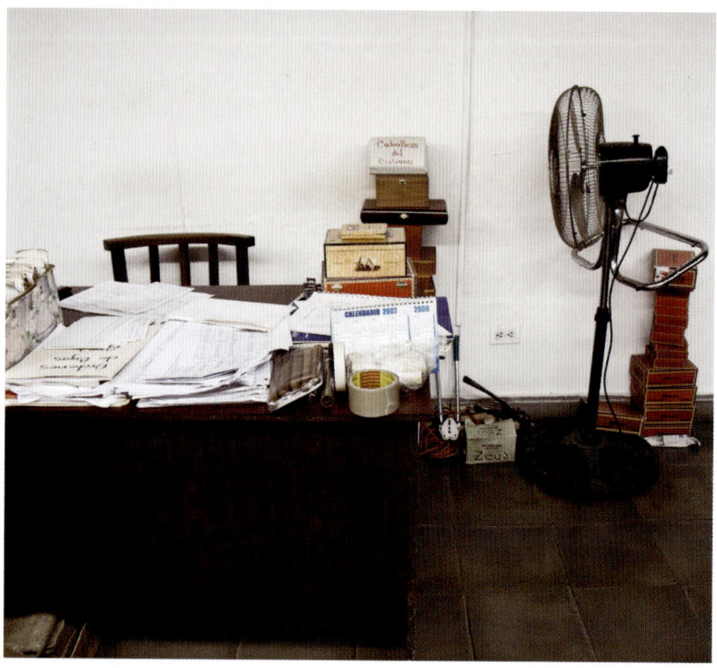

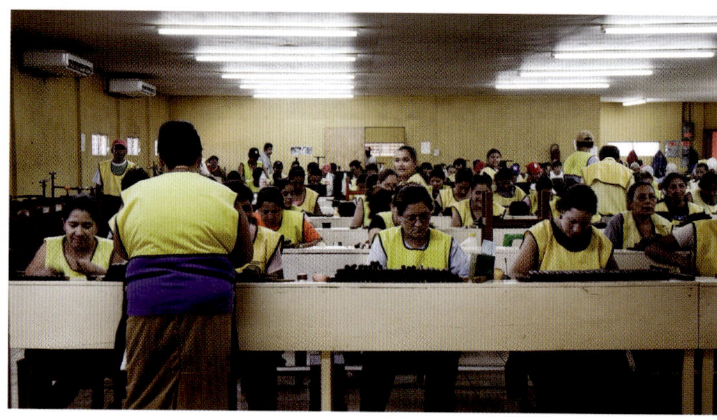

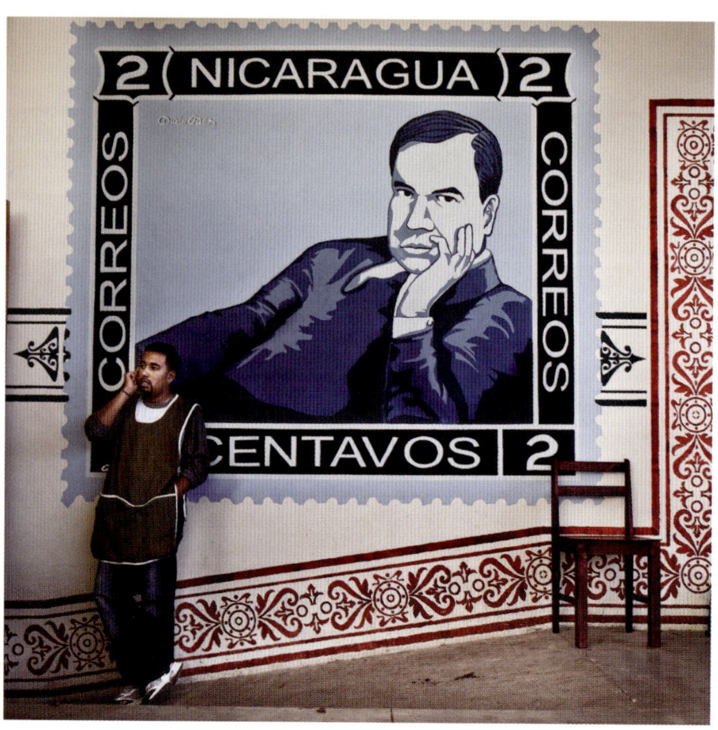
2 NICARAGUA 2
CORREOS
CORREOS
CENTAVOS 2

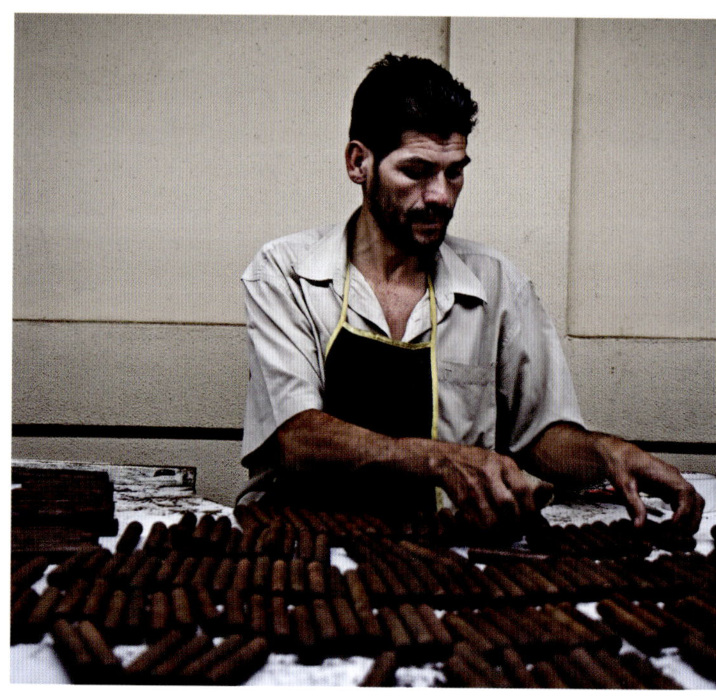

The visitor looking for a cigar break can sit on the old rough-hewn stone stoop of his hotel in the late evening, maduro smoking in hand, and watch the day wind down: factory workers ambling home or stuffed five to a stuttering Honda; kids skittering after a soccer ball in the street; dogs nosing the rubble in search of food.

With peace and stability has come the rise, in this hilly hamlet, of a small cigar empire: At least five major cigar makers occupy compounds within a fifteen-minute drive of the central church, producing the majority of the country's annual 300 million–plus sticks.

At six in the morning, an air-raid siren will wail (its flat bellow silencing the roosters who have spent the pre-dawn hours crowing unopposed) and streams of workers will make the return journey to the cigar factories that employ the majority of the townspeople.

In a darker era, owners took pains to establish factories and warehouses on the Honduran side of the nearby border—facilities that many maintain today. But even as the tides of civil war destroyed the country's infrastructure and eventually swept over the owners' properties (the Padrón family factory burned in the late 1970s, and the government confiscated the Plasencia family holdings), and even after the American embargo a few years later cut back their access to supplies and raw material, few abandoned Nicaragua entirely.

FAMILY BUSINESS > They had ample reason to stay. Nicaragua is a hotbed of volcanic activity (as your plane swoops into Managua, mountains belching pale steam are visible in the distance), resulting in nutrient-rich soil that produces tobaccos of notable complexity and strength. The three primary growing regions are Estelí, Condega, and the Jalapa Valley (in addition, a large island known as Ometepe, in a lake near Managua, has also been noted for its tobacco cultivation).

One local cigar maker, whose family hails from Cuba, claims that the tobacco here rivals that found even in Vuelta Abajo. Others aren't quite willing to make such a bold statement, but nobody can deny that these tobaccos have boosted Nicaragua's reputation as a supplier of fuller-flavored cigars that suit the American audience's appetites.

Unlike the Dominican Republic, however, which in the mid-1990s saw a massive influx of neophyte cigar makers looking to establish a reputation and generate a quick buck, Nicaragua and its fifty-year tradition of cigar making never saw a spike in aspiring *jefes*. A few passionate types, however, did venture down here with a dream of creating their own cigar company, bouncing up the hilly road from Managua despite the threat of Kalashnikov-wielding bandits.

Among those young cigar makers were the Drew Estate boys, Jonathan Drew and Marvin Samel. The college buddies founded the company in 1995 as a New York City cigar store before deciding to try their hand at the manufacturing side of the business. Drew rolled his first cigars in a tiny Estelí storefront (formerly a motel) inherited from Nick Perdomo Jr., president of Tabacalera Perdomo S.A. and another local legend. Today, Drew Nica, the company's massive factory on the outskirts of town, produces some 70,000 cigars a day, including Acid (a flavored cigar line popular among twentysomethings), Liga Privada (a personal favorite), and Chateau Real.

Other longtime cigar makers were able to get a fresh start in Nicaragua, which (along with Honduras) served as a refuge for Cuban families fleeing their native island in the wake of Fidel Castro's takeover.

One such family, the Padróns, had been growing tobacco for more than a century in Cuba's Vuelta Abajo when Castro's revolution forced their current patriarch, "Don" Jose Orlando Padrón, to emigrate to Miami. Initially armed with only a few dollars, he managed to build a new cigar company, which includes Padrón's current factory in Estelí. Over the course of thirty-eight years in Nicaragua, the Padróns endured everything from the depredations of the Sandinistas to the U.S. embargo (during which production shifted entirely to Honduras, where the family had opened a small factory in 1977) to a devastating outbreak of blue mold. Their cigars eventually gained acceptance in the American market in the early years of the cigar boom.

"Don" Jose Orlando's son, Jorge Padrón, started working in the family business in his early teens. Today, he oversees the company's operations as its president, supervising the production of lines including the Padrón Anniversary and the Padrón Serie 1926.

Padrón isn't the only multi-generation cigar business in town, however. On Estelí's southern edge, where the hilly streets start to give way to the gently rolling hill country, sits the *fábrica* commonly referred to as "the cathedral of tobacco." With its narrow stained-glass windows and central courtyard featuring a quietly burbling fountain, the Plasencia family's cigar factory is, in many ways, the culmination of five generations' work (it was built in partnership with Swiss tobacco brand Dannemann and modeled after the latter's first factory in São Felix, Brazil). As a clan, the Plasencias lost everything to Castro, then nearly everything to the Sandinistas. Yet Nestor Plasencia Jr. and his father continue their work, experimenting with new lines such as the Plasencia Reserva organic cigar, as well as operating another facility across the Honduran border in Danlí.

Across town from the Plasencia factory, on the outskirts of Estelí, sits the massive compound that houses Central America Tobacco, producer of Toraño cigars. Its owner, Carlos Toraño, is yet another who lost his family's Cuban tobacco business to the revolution. In his case, though, the loss was even more personal. His father had given money to Castro while the latter was fighting in the hills, only to see the family's assets seized soon after the island became an ostensible socialist paradise.

Having lost everything, the family scattered to the far corners of the tobacco world. Toraño himself ended up in Miami, where he sold computer systems briefly before reentering the tobacco business in 1974. After starting out as a grower, he decided to launch his own brand in 1994, starting with Carlos Toraño Dominican cigars. Owning a factory gave him control over the process; today, his massive facility produces, in addition to his own lines, cigars for clients including CAO and Gurkha.

Another massive factory (at more than 80,000 square feet, it's so large that workers call it *il monstro*) sits just to the south; its owner, Tabacalera Perdomo S.A. president Nick Perdomo Jr., supervises its operations with the same eagle-eyed style he brought to his former job as an air-traffic controller in Miami. His family, too, has a history with the Cuban cigar industry; his grandfather rolled cigars at the H. Upmann factory, while his father did the same at the Partagas fábrica.

In 1992, Perdomo Jr. decided that making cigars would be preferable to making sure tourist-filled 747s landed on time, and started his company in Miami. Three years later, he moved to Estelí, at first producing cigars out of the small storefront later used by Jonathan Drew. In 1999, buoyed by years of profits, he opened *il monstro,* rolling notable cigars for his own and clients' labels such as the CAO L'Anniversaire, the Perdomo Habano, and the Perdomo Reserve.

Other factories in Estelí are equally *monstro*.

Originally started in 1995, Nicaraguan American Tobaccos S.A., or NATSA, is a *fábrica* whose growth mirrors that of the country's cigar scene. Within a sprawling compound in Estelí, under the watchful eye of renowned cigar maker Frank Llaneza, hundreds of cigar rollers perform their magic on brands including the Siglo Limited Reserve and Juan Lopez.

Founded by Juan Francisco Bermejo Sr., who fled Cuba after Castro's takeover and spent decades plying his craft throughout the cigar world, NATSA soon became Nicaragua's largest producer of premium handmade smokes, primarily cigars for Lew Rothman's J.R. Cigar retail operation and Cigars by Santa Clara brand. Rothman also had an ownership stake in the factory, one that transferred to Altadis U.S.A. when that company purchased J.R. Cigar in 2003.

That was three years after Bermejo Sr. passed away, his life having been the very definition of perseverance through hardship. After his death, responsibility for the factory's brands transferred to his son, Juan "Triki" Bermejo Jr., who monitored production until injuries he sustained in a car accident necessitated that other people step in.

Frank Llaneza had helped with Bermejo Sr.'s business operations at crucial moments over the years, so it must have seemed very kismet for him to lend his blending skills to some of the increasingly modern factory's most notable creations and bring his decades of knowledge into the rollers' room.

Those decades of knowledge—shared in large part by the country's other cigar masters in residence—along with the richness of the soil, transform Nicaragua into that rarest of places: a pure and simple cigar haven, the ideal place to sit on your hotel steps and breathe smoke while watching the sun set over quiet hills.

A FLAVORFUL SMOKE

Nicaragua's three primary tobacco-growing regions, Estelí, Condega, and the Jalapa Valley (as well as the island of Ometepe) produce full-bodied, flavorful, and rich tobacco used in cigar makers' blends throughout the Caribbean Basin—even those companies without a factory located in the country. The Siglo Limited Reserve, created under the watchful eye of master blender Frank Llaneza, Padrón, and Joya de Nicaragua, are some of the country's best.

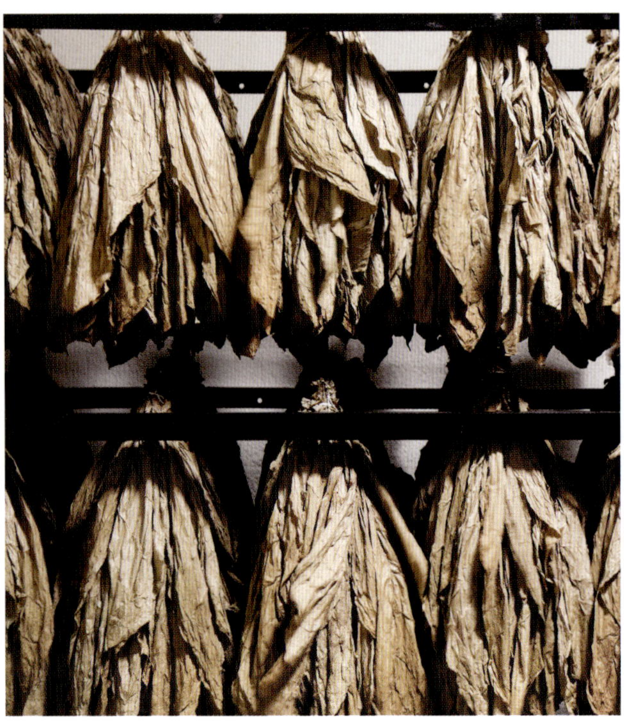

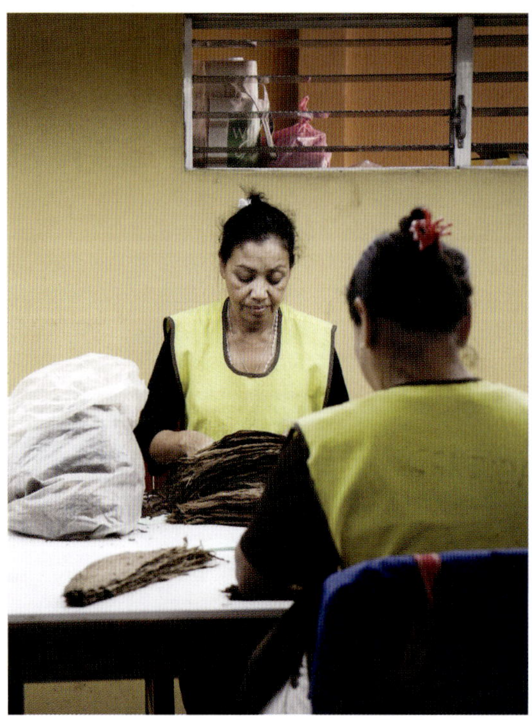

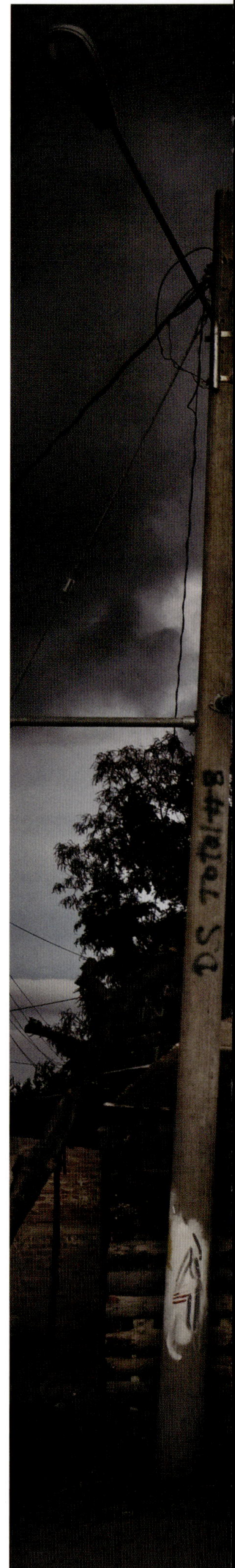

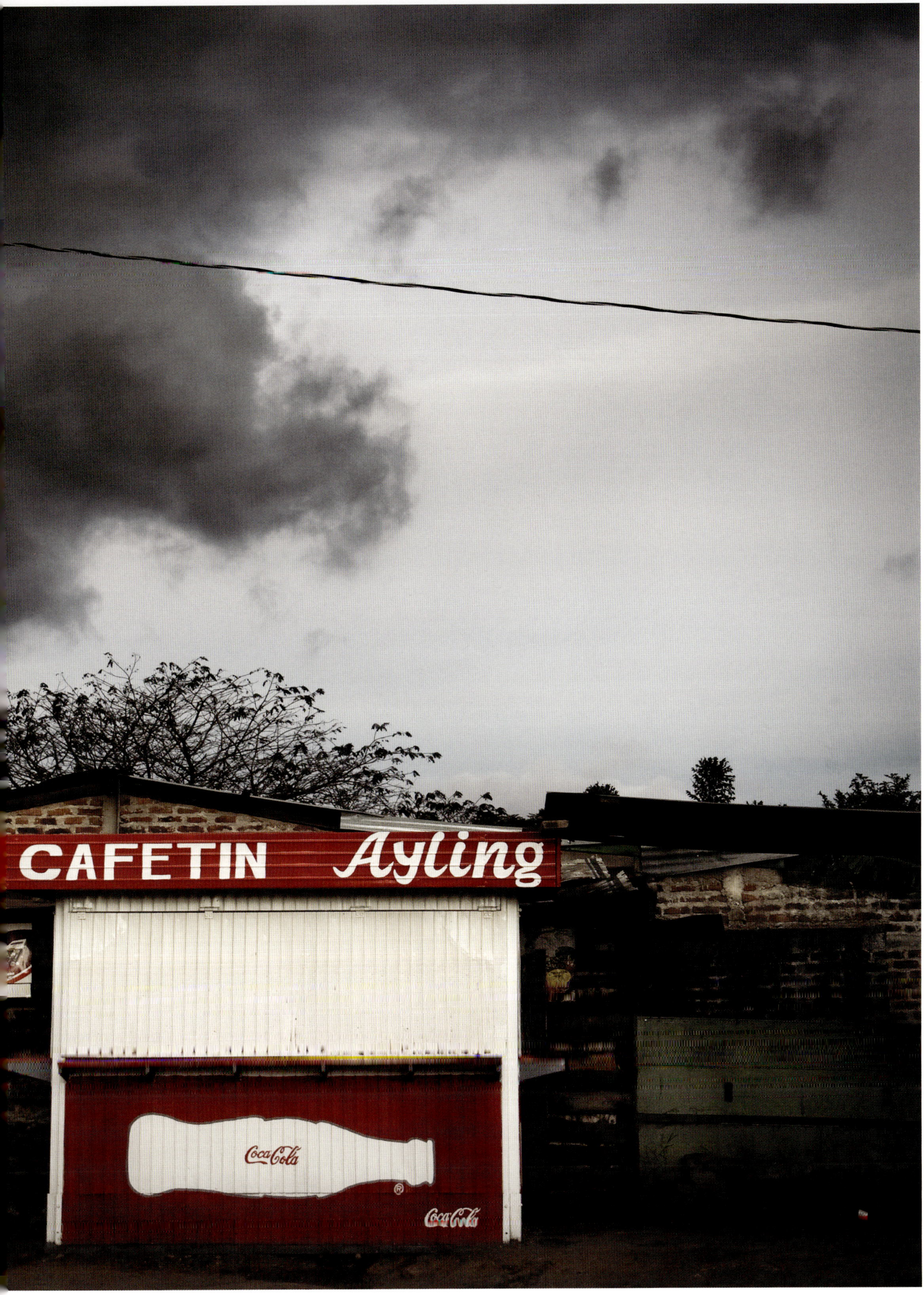
CAFETIN Ayling
Coca-Cola
Coca-Cola

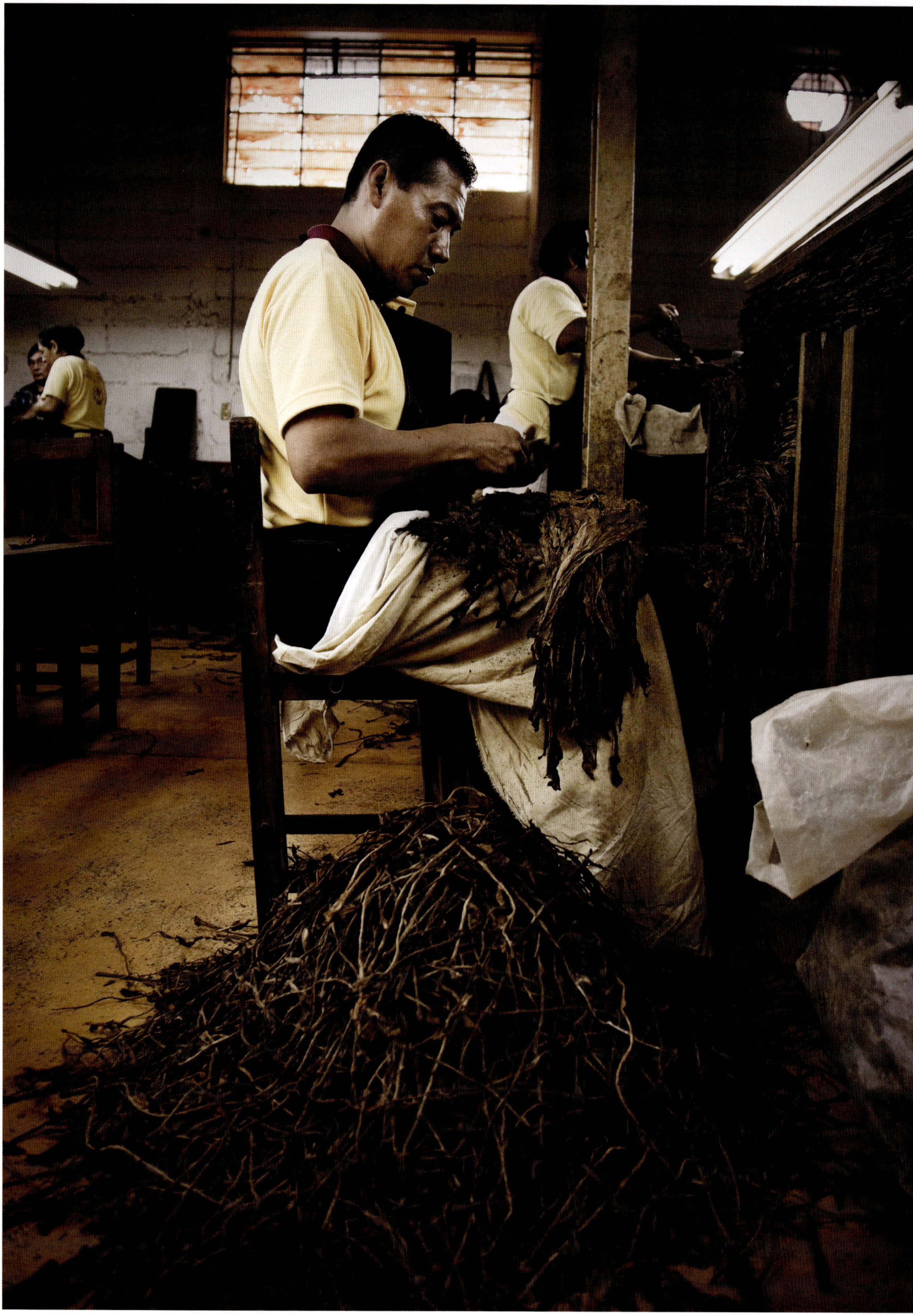

Mexico

Deep in the Mexican valley of San Andrés Tuxtla, and at the back end of a wide tobacco field, rises a barren hill of dirt and broken rock: a burial mound for the bygone cultures that once worked this fertile land. A few hundred yards away sit the seventeen high tech curing barns of the current family used to process leaf for their Te-Amo brand of cigars, their metal sides glinting in the sun. That one juxtaposition frames the past and future of Mexico as tobacco country. Centuries ago, the Maya cultivated their smoking crop just a few hours south of here, and likely traded it with their neighbors. Today, in the southern part of what has become the state of Veracruz, boutique cigar makers within this volcanic, lake-filled valley (an area famous for San Andrés Negra tobacco, rich and dark) craft iconic puro cigars. If every cigar-world nation has its "Cuba"—the area where weather and soil combine to create a worthy tobacco-cultivating area—then this is Mexico's.

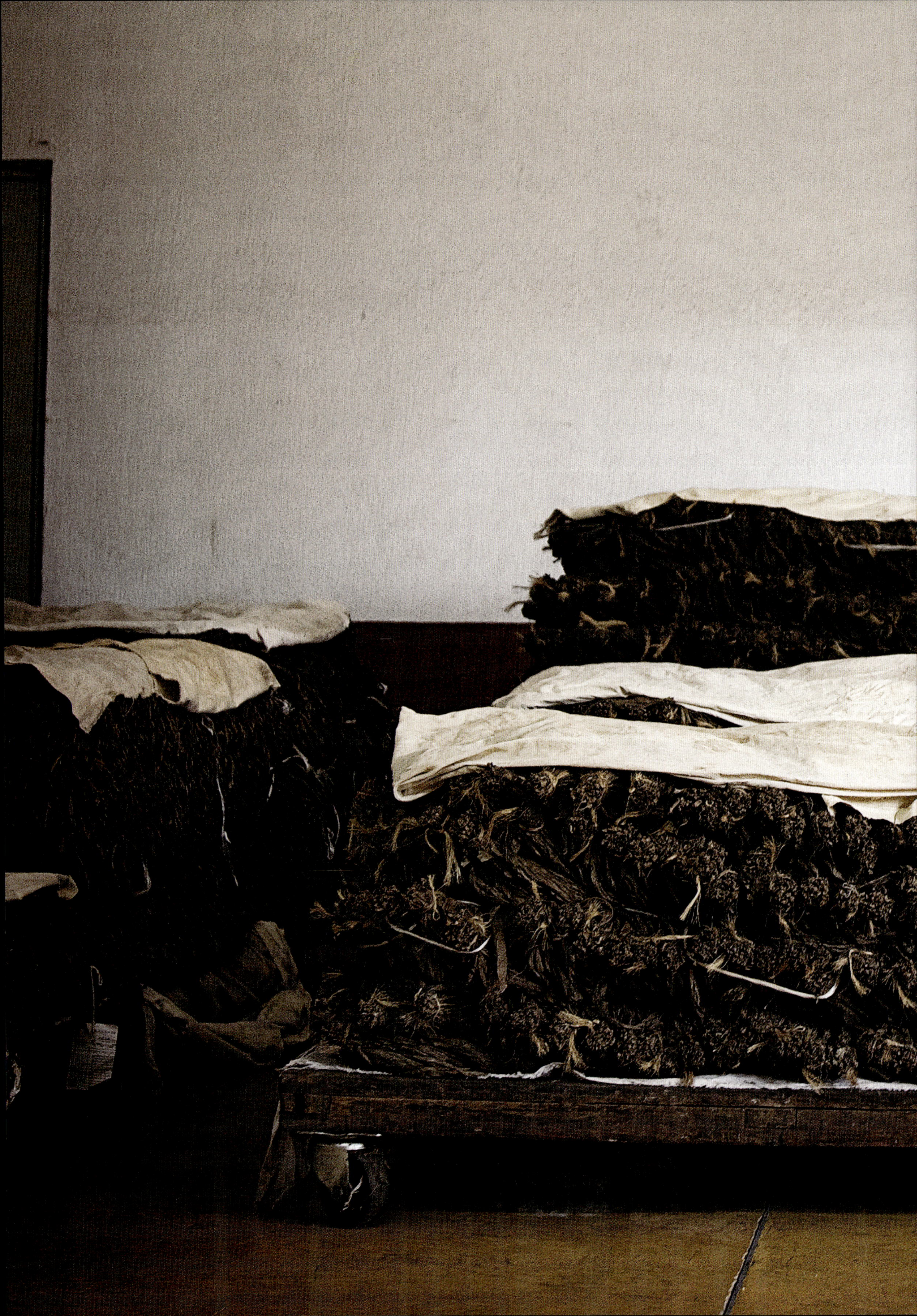

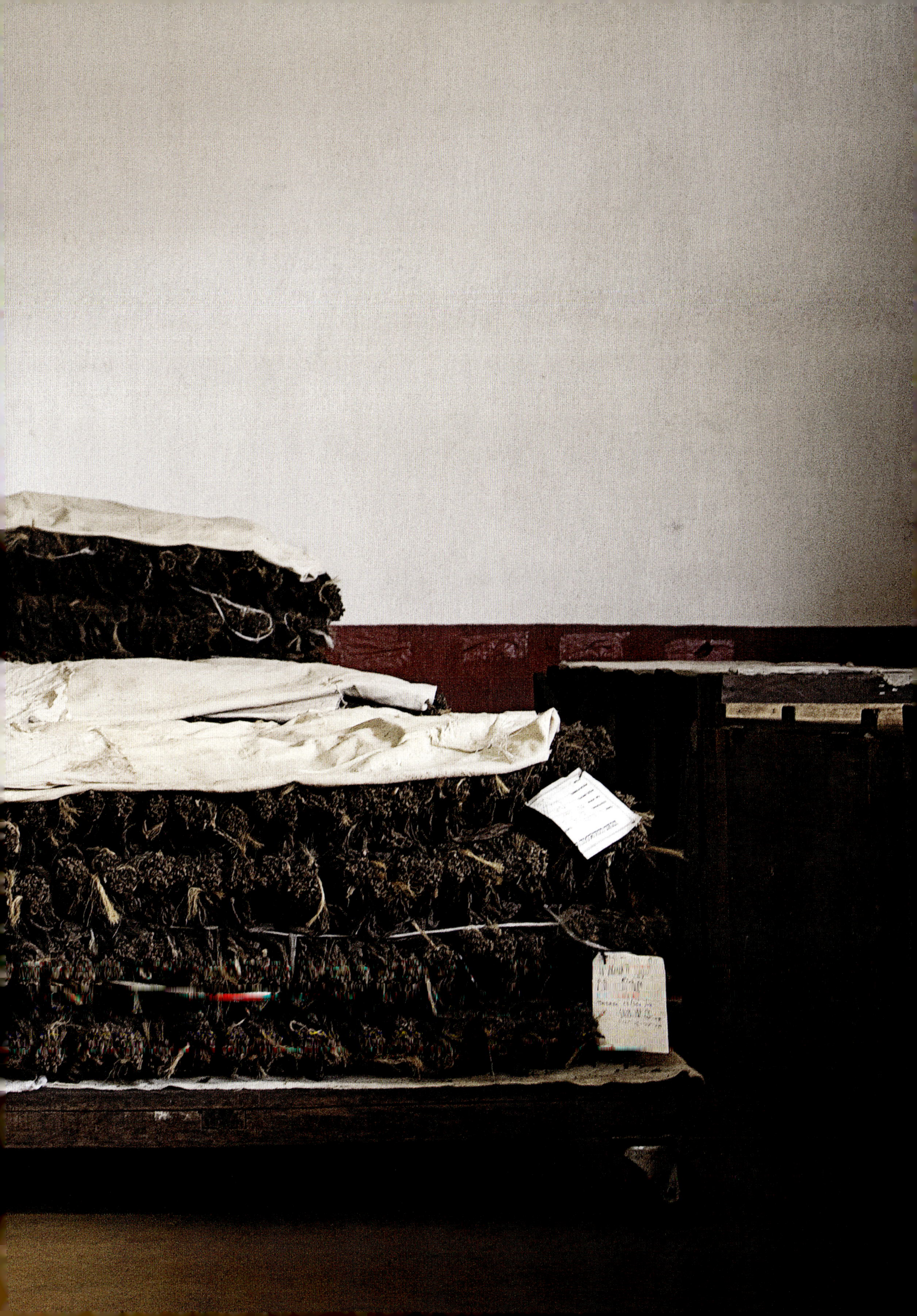

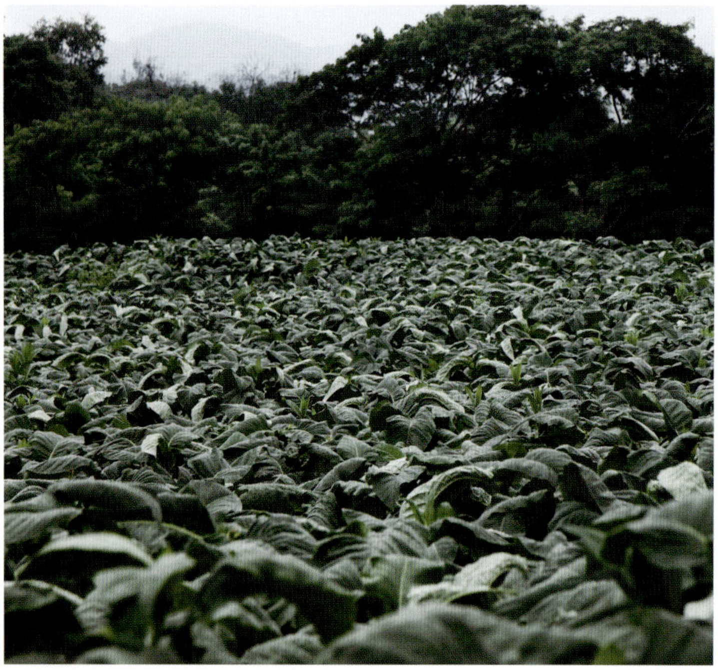

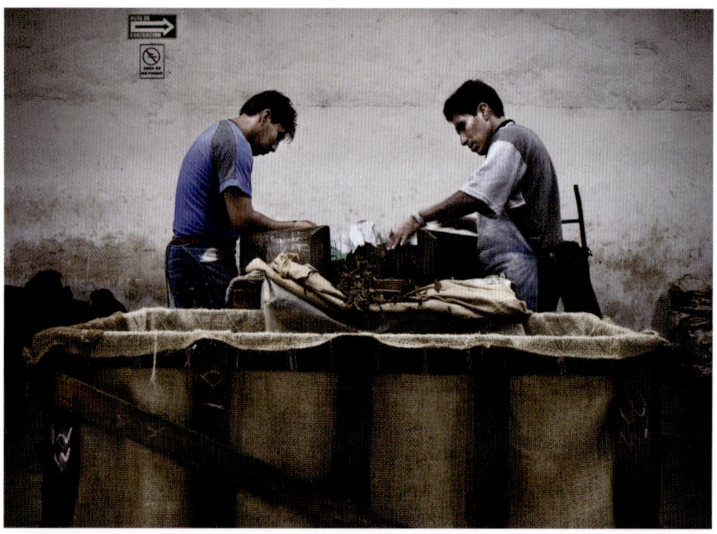

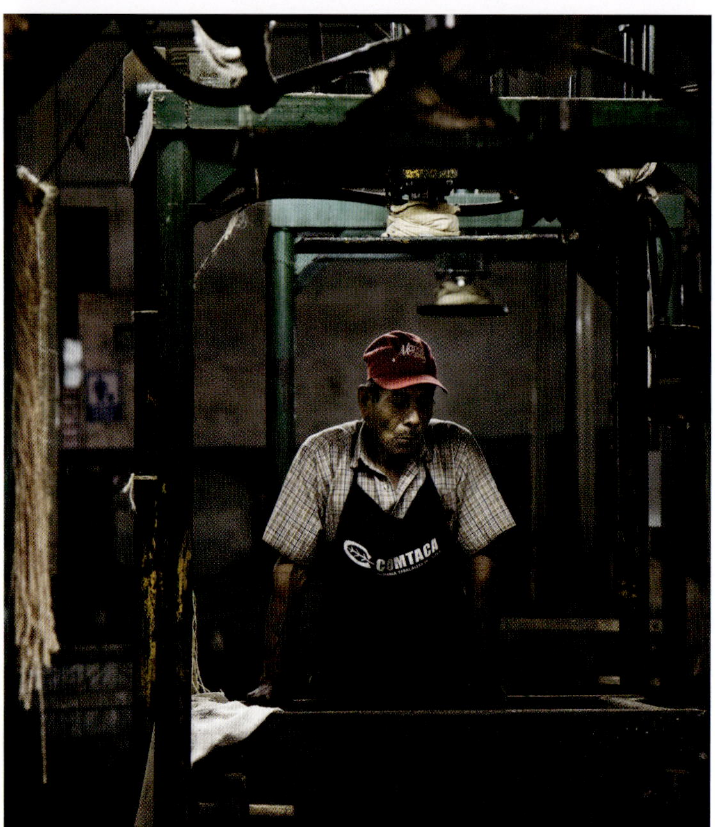
COMTACA

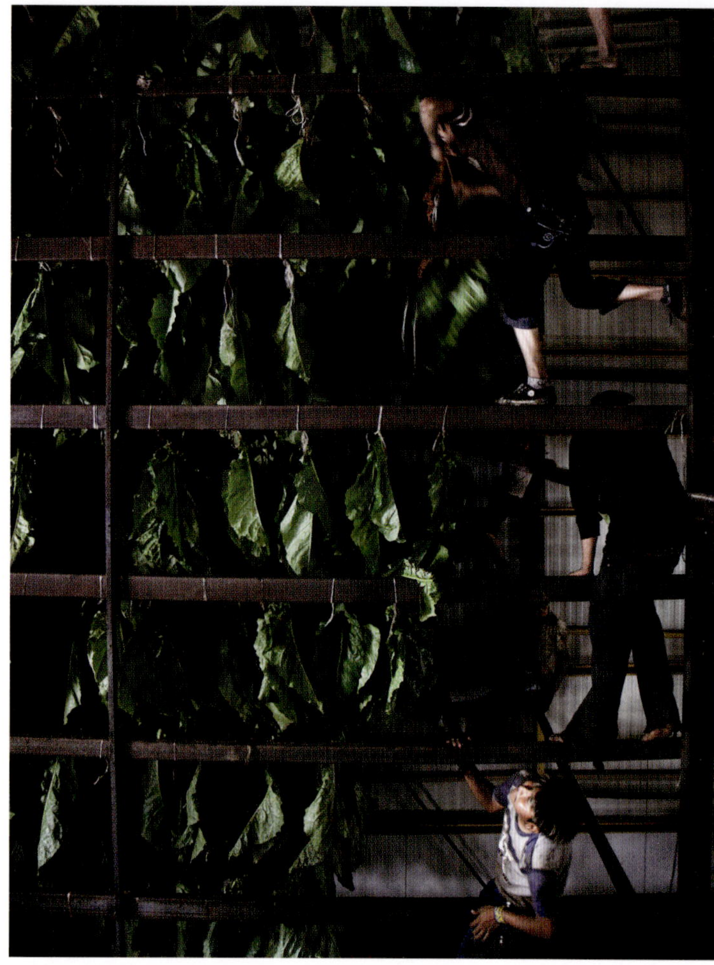

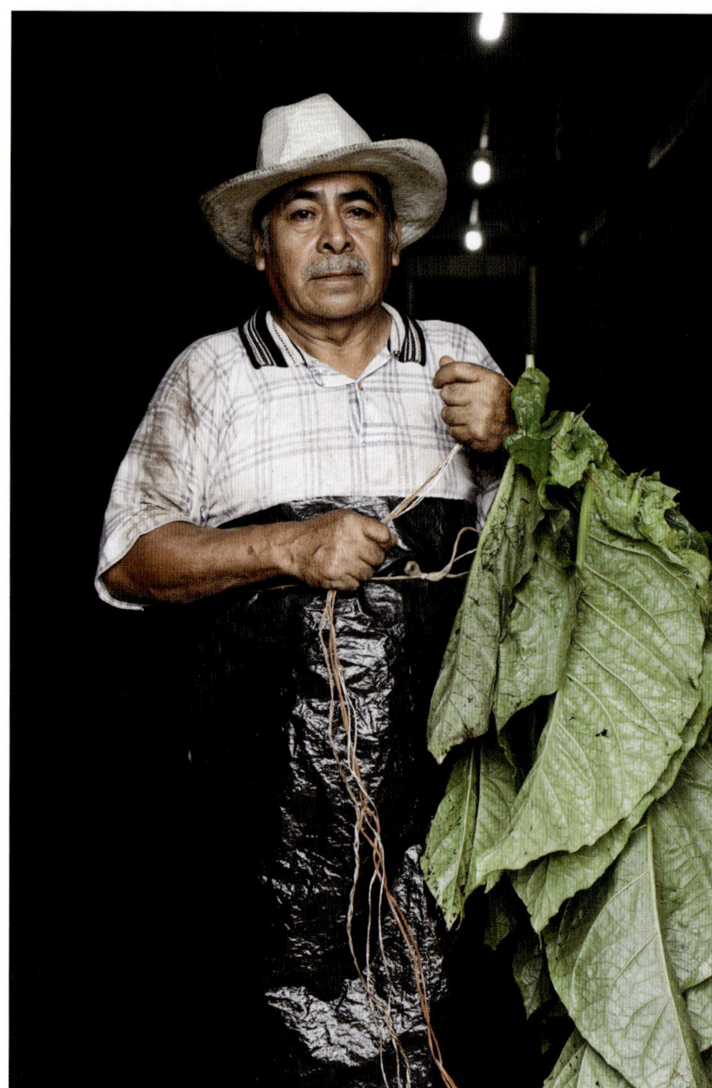

At the height of the wet season, San Andrés Tuxtla blooms in a thousand shades of green. The Turrent family grows San Andrés Negra, Sumatra, Corojo, and Connecticut wrapper here, and the hills and valleys seem carpeted with broad tobacco leaves speckled with mist. For years, cigar makers in other countries used Mexican tobacco as a vital component in their blends; but it was largely Mexican cigar makers themselves who used the local leaf in a puro cigar.

THE CABDRIVERS' CIGAR > The modern high-water mark for the Mexican cigar was the 1960s and '70s. In the decades after the Cuban embargo, cigar lovers in the U.S. scrambled to find a suitable brand that would satisfy their smoke cravings without necessarily breaking their wallets. A segment of them discovered Te-Amo, a Mexican brand crafted by the Turrent family (which had been growing tobacco in San Andrés Tuxtla since the 1880s) and today stands as the country's largest cigar maker through their company, Nueva Matacapan de Tabacos S.A. de C.V.

In the grittier New York City of thirty years ago, distinctive red-lettered Te-Amo signs sprung up on the front of seemingly every tobacco store between the Bronx and Staten Island. The stick itself quickly became known as the "cabdriver's cigar," an inexpensive working-class smoke that could be enjoyed by anyone between shifts.

Then came the cigar boom, and with it a market flooded with competitors that could match or even beat Te-Amo's prices. At the height of the boom, the Turrent family's boat was lifted along with everyone else's; cigar sales rose to some twelve million sticks annually. Then sales fell off; by 2006 the number of Te-Amo cigars sold had declined nearly twelvefold to around a million.

But the Turrents' business, under patriarch Alberto Turrent IV, displayed the same sort of fortitude in the face of falling sales that had sustained the family through a century in southern Mexico. They hung on; and having reached bottom in 2006, the company's sales resumed a slow climb upward. Partnered with Altadis U.S.A., they came into the twenty-first century ready to become a higher-profile operation, complete with 700 workers and 400 hectares under cultivation.

MODERN TIMES > Now, to the high-tech curing barns. Giant machines bolted to their sides provide the sort of ultra-precise climate control that can only be approximated through the use of windows and shutters in older barns. Inside, a small army of workers, wrapped in plastic against the damp, string fresh tobacco leaves onto long poles, which they then lift three stories above the ground and slot into metal rafters. In another barn, meanwhile, fire pits in the floor will provide the smoke and heat to blacken the dangling wrappers to an appropriate tint.

Further along in the process, the tobacco ends up at a nondescript warehouse off the village square, a warren of concrete rooms loud with the hum of wheels as more workers maneuver pallets of leaves through the low spaces. From there, tobacco will travel to their yellow-walled main *fábrica*, Nueva Matacapan Tabacos. The Turrents take justifiable pride in their space, and crowds of tourists will occasionally bus into the enclosed parking lot for factory tours, leaving their vehicle under the watchful eyes of both a shotgun-toting gatekeeper and the Virgin de Guadalupe, in statue form and festooned with plastic flowers.

Inside, the rollers at their long tables work diligently to make Te-Amo cigars, offered in three different blends (identified as the Dominicana, Nicaragua and Honduras); the family also produces, with five different aged tobaccos, the A. Turrent Six Generations cigars.

Unlike many boutique *fábricas,* Turrent's seems dedicated to keeping its prices at an absolute minimum for hand-rolled premium cigars—a philosophical nod to the era when Te-Amo made its name by appealing to the everyman.

Stand there long enough, and you'll notice the filler leaves being rolled into themselves before being integrated into the cigar. This technique, originally from Cuba, is called *entubado,* and the Turrent rollers practice it skillfully—although it also means the overall cigar takes a quarter as long to make. Tubing is believed by many cigar makers to accomplish two ends: it packs more tobacco into each cigar and it channels the heat and smoke from the lit tip down the shaft more efficiently, leading to a more flavorful smoking experience.

UP AND COMERS > Veracruz is dotted with small cigar makers trying to make a name in the U.S. Numbers vary, but anywhere from a handful to a few dozen storefront cigar factories have risen in Mexico, producing puros for either local consumption or limited export to the U.S., Europe, or Asia.

Now that the cigar boom has passed, and with it some of the snobbery that helped drive down sales of competitively priced Mexican cigars, the cigar makers here see a chance to seize some additional market share—not to mention some respect. Cigar manufacturers in other countries, whether they're willing to shout it from the rooftops or not, have become fans of using Mexican tobacco in their brands; but what would make the Turrents and other local players even happier is to have American shelves loaded with their own cigars, just like in the old days.

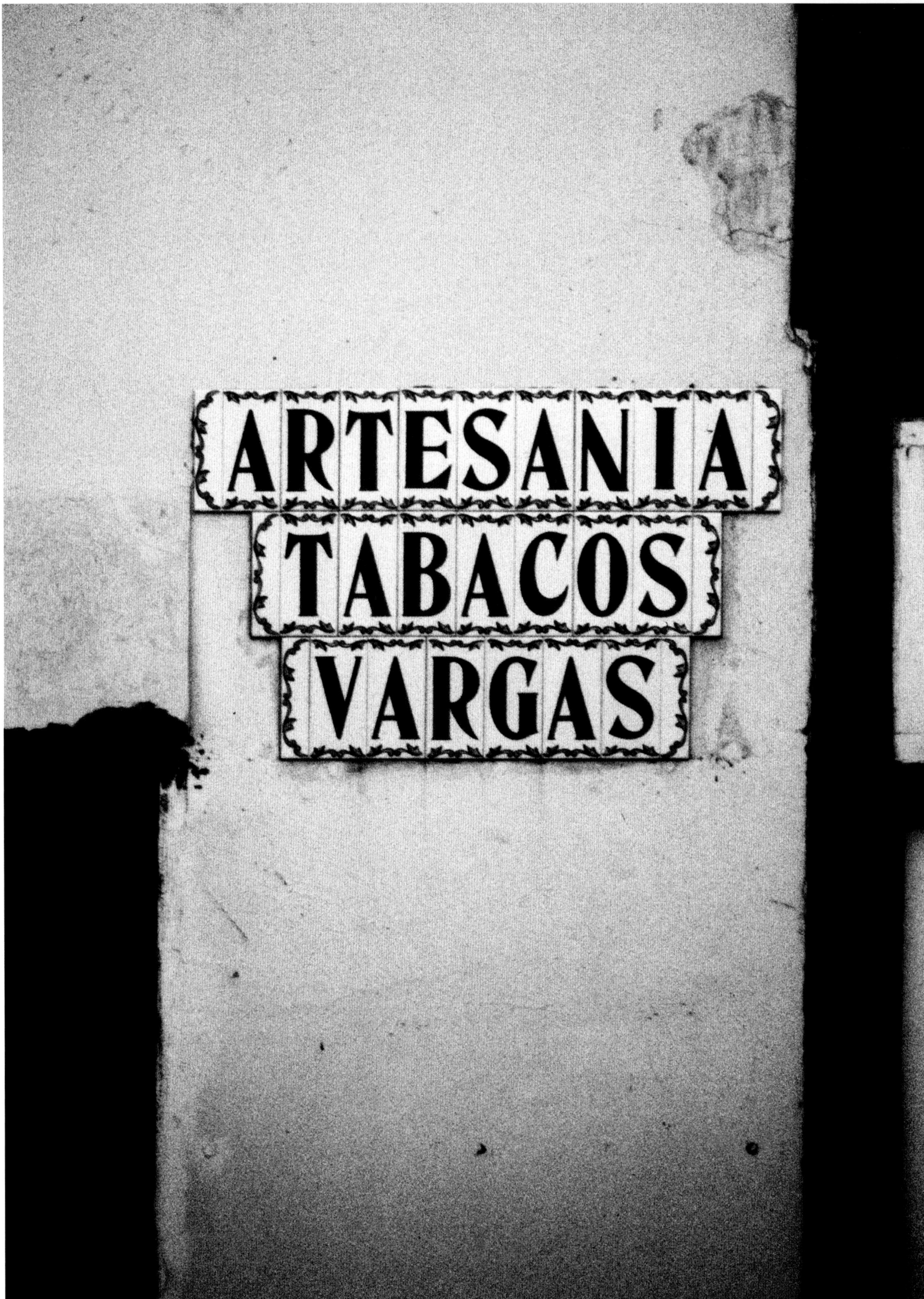
ARTESANIA
TABACOS
VARGAS

The Bahamas
Canary Islands
Connecticut
Cameroon
Ecuador
Jamaica
Italy
Brazil
Miami
Indonesia
& the Philippines

Cuba, the Dominican Republic, and other countries in Central America and the Caribbean Basin hold a vaunted place among cigar smokers, but other nations have also contributed mightily toward the taste and experience of hand-rolled cigars.

1. CONNECTICUT (USA)

Although not exactly a tropical climate, a small section of the Connecticut River Valley (just beneath the state's northern border) has developed a well-deserved reputation for growing some of the finest wrapper leaves in the world. It also happens to be the only place in the United States devoted to premium cigar leaf, despite the thousands of acres given over to "blonde," or cigarette tobacco, in the southern United States. Tobacco is also grown to the west in Connecticut's Housatonic River Valley.

The tobacco here is Cuban seed, and either shade-grown beneath cheesecloth tents or left to sprout under the full sun. Over 2,000 acres of the valley are devoted to it, less than a tenth of what was under cultivation 80 years ago, and the number of curing barns that dot the landscape has been declining over the decades. While the crop sells for upward of $60 per pound, the high costs of everything from fertilizer to labor make it a low-margin crop for farmers, who may be more tempted to sell to the developers swallowing up thousands of acres of surrounding farmland.

Still, with tobacco having been grown here for centuries (the Native American tribes in the valley were smoking it long before settlers arrived), and with demand for premium wrapper leaf continually strong, it's unlikely that Connecticut's "Tobacco Valley" will disappear anytime soon.

2. THE BAHAMAS

To nearly everyone, the Bahamas equals sun, ludicrously tanned bodies, and casinos right out of the James Bond flick *Casino Royale*. To a select few, though, it also means cigars—particularly at Graycliff, a former sea captain's mansion–turned-Inn, where a cadre of rollers in a basement room produces small batches of the eponymous house cigar. The brainchild of owner Enrico Garzaroli, who started the Inn in 1971, the hand-rolled sticks have gained a reputation among cigar makers who prefer boutique brands. From the original Red Label blend, created by Cuban master Avelino Lara (famous for once serving as Fidel Castro's personal roller and possibly creating a little-known cigar brand called Cohiba), the line has grown to encompass several other cigars. Oenophiles take note: Graycliff features an epic wine cellar; at 270,000 bottles (including a 1727 Riesling) it is the third-largest in the world.

3. CANARY ISLANDS

This seven-island archipelago off the coast of Morocco once served as a waypoint for explorers headed for the New World to plunder (and bring back tobacco). Some four hundred years later, another migration occurred in the opposite direction, as cigar families fleeing the Cuban Revolution crossed the Atlantic to set up shop there.

Three of the islands (Tenerife, Gran Canaria, and La Palma would eventually house factories) produced premium brands, including Don Diego and Montecruz, that became leaders in the U.S. market for a period in the 1970s. A decade later, however, a spike in union trouble and labor costs, paired with difficulties in obtaining tobacco (particularly Cuban) from across the Atlantic withered these brands' American presence. Today, however, some small brands such as Vargas and Baretto have survived.

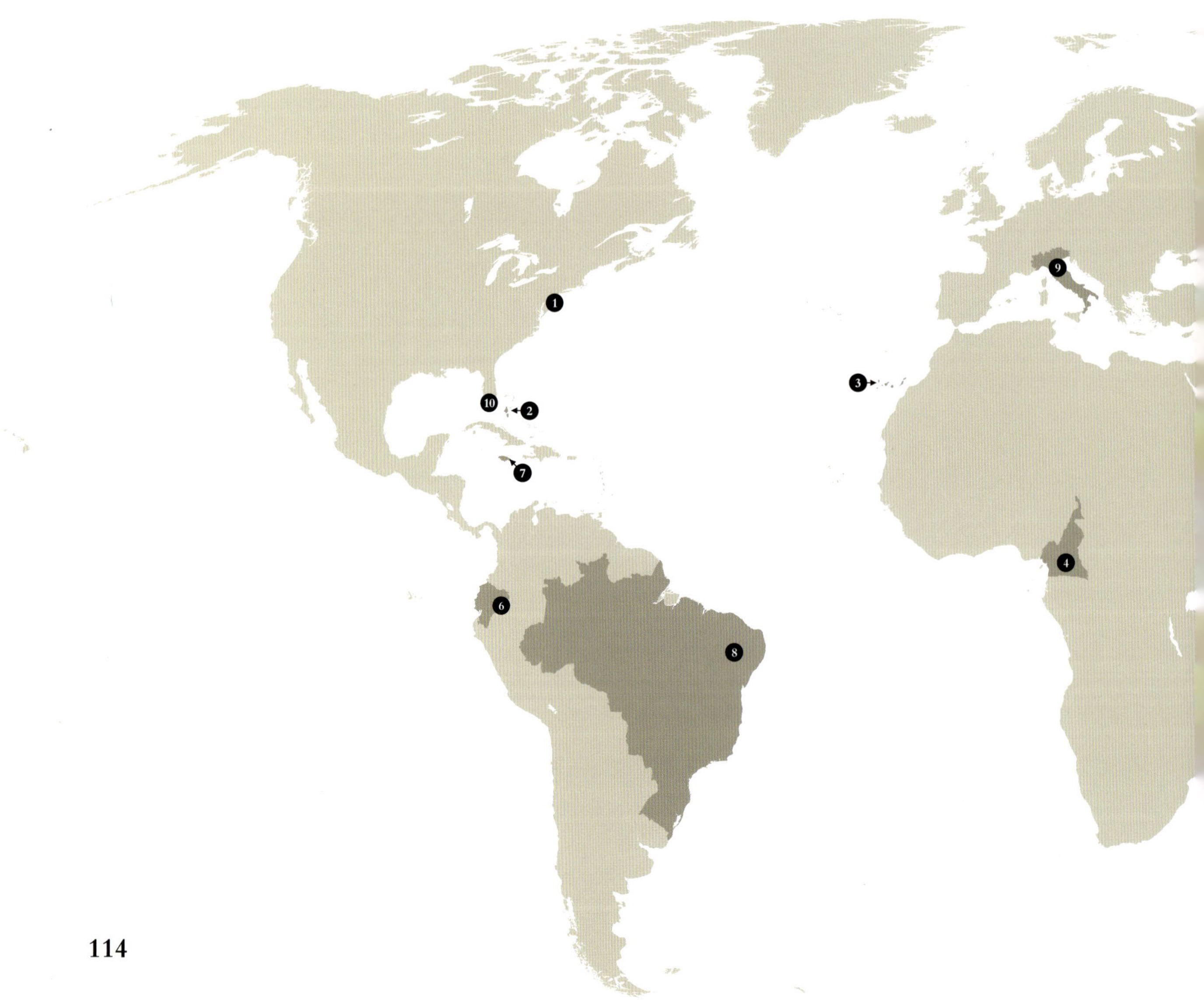

4. CAMEROON

From the 1950s through 1993, the production of these sweet and complex Sumatran-seed wrapper leaves in Cameroon was firmly in the hands of French conglomerate SEITA, S.A. It was easy to see why the company invested such time and money in the Bertoua region (in the eastern part of the country, somewhat close to the border with the Central African Republic), as it produces a tobacco lusted after by many cigar makers.

That was before a toxic combination of company in-fighting, regional instability, and high costs led to the end of that particular setup. In the aftermath, many companies had to resort to Indonesian tobacco in order to find something that fit their desired taste profiles.

Then, into the African vacuum stepped Richard Meerapfel, whose family's interests in the tobacco-selling business extend back over a century. In 1995, he began tobacco-growing operations in Cameroon and Central African Republic through CETAC, S.A. (Compagnie d'Exploitation des Tabacs Centrafricain), a joint venture between him and a few African partners. Although Meerapfel passed away in 2003, many credit him with preserving the legacy of Cameroon wrapper.

5. INDONESIA & THE PHILIPPINES

Spanish explorers from the New World brought tobacco to the Philippines, where in short order, it became immensely popular among the local peoples, who cultivated it for export to Asia and Europe and collected enormous profits for their trouble. Spanish rulers, of course, wanted those boatloads of cash for themselves, and instituted a tobacco monopoly in the late eighteenth century. The locals promptly started farming the crop illegally, and smuggled it with peerless effectiveness until the Spanish canceled the monopoly in 1881.

That year, the cigar companies in Manila established the Compania General de la Tabacos de Filipinas, and started the Philippines' largest cigar factory, La Flor de la Isabela; the brand named after the factory remains the most famous of the locally produced cigars. Today, the tobacco (a very mild variety) is grown primarily in northern Luzon, the nation's largest island.

Neighboring Indonesia is perhaps most famous for its local version of Sumatra-seed tobacco, which is also grown for wrapper in many places outside of Asia; tobacco from Java finds its use as filler and wrappers. While much of the tobacco grown here ends up in cigarettes, the overall industry helps support millions of farmers.

6. ECUADOR

A mountainous country with a warm tropical climate ideal for tobacco production, Ecuador features a small cigar industry that primarily focuses on producing Sumatran- and Connecticut-seed wrappers as well as some binder. The volcanic soil provides all the nutrients the plants need, and the country's wealth of cloud cover provides a shade-grown effect without the farmers needing to resort to draping their fields with acres of cheesecloth.

7. JAMAICA

Yeah, mon. This Caribbean nation is known for more than one kind of plant; for more than three centuries, tobacco has been grown all over Jamaica, particularly around Kingston. The native leaf grown here produces a very mild smoke, however, and few blenders have used it in their cigars, preferring the stronger and more complex tobaccos of the Dominican Republic and elsewhere.

Despite the fact that the country never developed the same sort of cigar culture as Cuba, Jamaica's central location in the Caribbean (just south of Cuba) has made it ideal—at least geographically—for cigar production, and some major players have taken stakes in the island's growing smoke industry. Much of the credit for this goes to Great Britain, which during World War II decreed that investments had to be made only within the Commonwealth. This meant that many Cuban cigar makers, rather than losing the Britons as a source of revenue, moved their operations 100 miles south across the water.

By the late 1980s, the local cigar industry had become the fourth-largest exporter of premium cigars to the U.S. market. Larger players stepped onto the scene, including Consolidated Cigar (the predecessor of Altadis U.S.A.), which owned a quarter of Jamaica Tobacco Manufacturing Co. along with Robert L. Gore (scion of the family that created the locally made Royal Jamaica, a popular brand in the United States after the Cuban embargo). A number of other popular brands were also created on the island. However, the dip that followed the glut of the 1990s cigar boom curtailed the island's production and, coupled with high production costs, forced many companies to curtail their enterprise on the island.

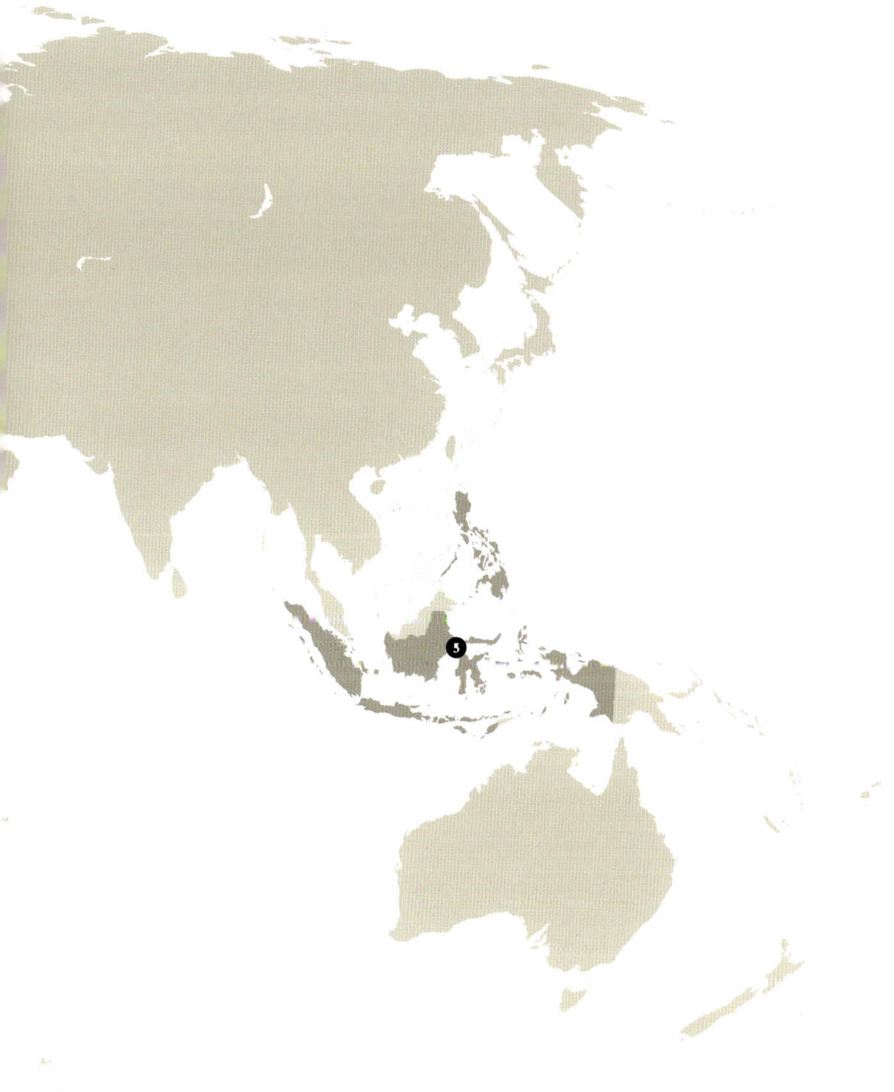

8. BRAZIL

Soon after Pedro Alvares Cabral "discovered" Brazil for Portugal in 1500, European colonists began using land here to raise a particularly dark and strong type of tobacco, along with sugar, as a cash crop; and much of it, after being fermented in the colonial capital of Bahia, was shipped back to the Old World for use in snuff and chewing tobacco. Brazil's northeastern regions, with their frequent dry spells and heavy rain season, were ideal for growing quality leaf.

By the late 18th century—a few decades before Brazil's independence from the Portuguese—cigars were being rolled here in earnest. Fast-forward to the beginning of the twentieth century, and Brazil had workers producing some 120 million cigars annually. Then that number began to dip: Instead of rolling cigars, the country started exporting the tobacco. By the time of Castro's revolution, when the cigar-makers fleeing Cuba suddenly needed to find new sources of strong and heavy tobacco, Brazil was primed to send its crops all over Latin America to become part of the blend in premium cigars.

Two notable tobaccos grown in Brazil are Mata Norte and Mata Fina. Incredibly expensive for cigar-makers to purchase in bulk, Mata Fina (which shares a name with the region in which it's grown) is an aromatic but milder tobacco, especially compared to the full-bodied Mata Norte, which is grown in an area north of Cruz das Almas and whose leaves are left to dry in the sun after harvesting. In addition to native Brazilian varietals, growers here take advantage of the weather to plant Sumatra and Cuban-seed tobaccos for wrapper.

Within Mata Fina, several sub-varieties of tobacco are produced, including Mata Sul, which is more mild-bodied, and Mata São Gonçalo, wrapper grown around the hamlet of São Gonçalo dos Campos.

While other regions of Brazil grow cheaper tobacco for machine-made cigars, these leaves often find their way into premium blends. Today, a variety of the finest cigars, ranging from the Brazilian puro Dona Flor to the full-bodied CAO Brazilia, the Carlos Toraño Signature and the Alec Bradley Trilogy Maduro, all boast the flavorful kick that is Brazil's tobacco signature.

9. ITALY

"You see, my mule don't like people laughing." Clint Eastwood clenches his jaw around the Toscano, its tip and his eyes blazing. "He gets the crazy idea you're laughing at him."

Fifteen feet away, the gunmen sitting on the fence—seconds away from being on the receiving end of Eastwood's bullets—tense in naked fear. Then the shooting starts—and once it ends, the cowboys find themselves added to the rising body-count of director Sergio Leone's *Fistful of Dollars* (1964).

Perched in a corner of Eastwood's mouth throughout Leone's Man With No Name trilogy, the thin Toscano Originale became an iconic prop. However, irrespective of Eastwood's influence, the cigar has maintained a substantial following of present-day smokers who enjoy its Kentucky-grown tobacco. A Toscano being savored by a speeding Vespa rider is a common *"la dolce vita"* sight in *Firenze*, *Milano* and *Roma*.

After harvesting, the tobacco leaves are dark-fired and twice fermented using a proprietary process before an aging period in cardboard boxes. Even after the cigars have been hand-rolled, these medium filler smokes frequently undergo another required aging period of up to twelve months before shipment. This process is only one part of what makes Toscano Originale unique; the other comes from the tradition of cutting the cigar in half (denoted where the band is placed mid-cigar), effectively creating two cigars out of each one.

First manufactured in Florence in the early nineteenth century, the Toscano was traditionally held by state monopoly, except for a short period in 2004-06 when it came under control of ETI (Ente Tabacchi Italiani) and then British American Tobacco. After that, the cigar again fell under Italian ownership, specifically the Maccaferri Group, headed by the Maccaferri family of Bologna.

Today, the company produces twenty-two types of cigars other than the Originale, including the longer aged Riserva, via factories in Lucca and at Cava de' Tirreni near Salerno, and a pre-manufacturing facility near the small town of Foiano della Chiana. Production at the original Lucca factory, itself once a convent for Dominican nuns, has been moved to a modernized facility on the town's outskirts.

10. MIAMI (USA)

Arguably the one of most cigar-friendly town in the States, for decades Miami has provided a haven not only for cigar manufacturers, but also generations of smokers who practically live in its wide variety of cigar stores, lounges, and clubs. After the Cuban Revolution, many cigar-makers fleeing Castro's regime found their way here—sometimes after a brief stint in the Canary Islands or other places—and then used the greater metro area as a base of operations while they replanted their empires in the Dominican Republic and other Caribbean Basin countries, as well as South American countries, notably Brazil.

Cigars had been manufactured in Florida for decades before that point, of course; Key West and Tampa had once been major cigar-making cities, with around 250 factories dotting the streets of Tampa's Ybor City at the beginning of the twentieth century. But Ybor City faded as the world's cigar capital, as manufacturers found less-expensive alternatives for mass manufacturing in other countries.

Despite that migration, however, Florida remained close to the hearts and minds of the cigar-makers, who opened modest fronts primarily in Miami's Little Havana district to carry their more exclusive lines and give any cigar tourists the thrill of a behind-the-scenes view.

To that end, families such as the Padróns opened cigar stores/lounges just off of the famed Calle Ocho; others opened small factories, including General Cigar Company's El Credito Cigar Factory, Jose "Pepin" Garcia's El Rey de los Habanos, Casa Felipe, Reyes Family Cigars, and the Fabrica de Tabaco Padilla, overseen by Cuban-American artist and master cigar-blender Ernesto Padilla. Often staffed with a mere handful of rollers, these factories nonetheless produce some of the industry's most iconic boutique brands, from the Don Pepin Garcia and Tatuajes to La Gloria Cubana Artesanos de Miami.

In other words, even while Miami will never produce remotely close to the number of cigars of a Nicaragua or Dominican Republic, it nonetheless remains a spiritual home of sorts for the stars of the cigar industry and cigar lovers from around the world.

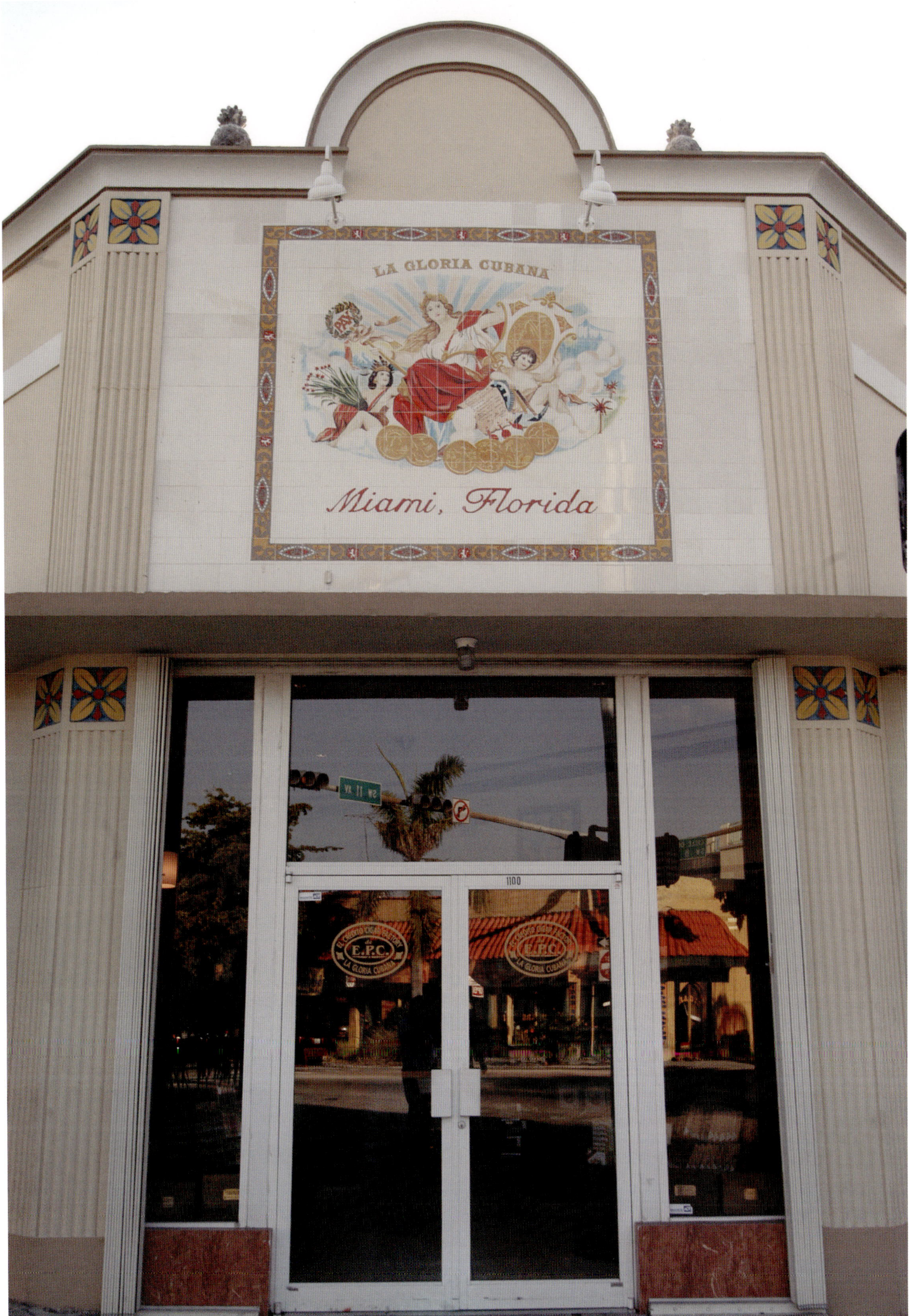
LA GLORIA CUBANA
Miami, Florida
E.P.C.
LA GLORIA CUBANA
1100

Cigars & Stars

> As I mentioned in the preface of this august volume, celebrities have always been an integral part of the cigar landscape. Along the byways of my career, I've had the pleasure of smoking with old-school stars such as Milton Berle and James Coburn, sports figures like Michael Jordan and a roster of actors including Pierce Brosnan, Johnny Depp, Andy Garcia, Whoopi Goldberg, Samuel L. Jackson, Kurt Russell, Gregory Hines, and Sly Stallone—to name a few. Seriously, that's the short list.

During my time at the store in Beverly Hills, many of the Golden Era TV and Hollywood legends were still alive—James Stewart, George Burns, Dean Martin, Bob Hope, etc. And if they smoked cigars, they undoubtedly passed through the shop at least once.

One such Old Hollywood fixture was Milton "Uncle Miltie" Berle, the first major TV star who guest hosted the short-lived (1969–1970) but wildly influential syndicated TV series *Playboy After Dark*. Although well in his advanced years when I knew him, Berle possessed an acerbic tongue, a keen wit, and perfectly timed schtick—but mostly I liked him because he was dirty. He loved telling crass jokes and stories, many of which centered on his *schmeckle* (word had it that Berle was quite . . . endowed. For that mental image, you're welcome).

You could also see right away that Berle had a tough side, an artifact of his childhood spent as a Jewish kid in a five-story Harlem walk-up. If Berle hadn't become an entertainer, you could easily imagine him following in the footsteps of his contemporary, Meyer Lansky.

Berle had a fondness for double corona–size cigars, which he said reminded him of his dick—then again, why anyone would want to smoke his own dick was beyond me. Hey, I went with it.

So late one morning, Berle called up the store himself and ordered two boxes of DCs, following that up with a request that I personally bring them over to the Friar's Club (then on Little Santa Monica) around lunchtime, which I knew meant that he would feed me. I wasn't above such considerations at the time, or now for that matter.

A buddy of mine was in the store with me when I got the call. Overhearing the conversation, he asked if he could tag along. I said, "Sure."

After all, what was the harm?

As noontime approached—and seeing that it was a nice day outside—we decided to hoof it over to the Friar's Club. Milton was in the upstairs dining room when we arrived. When we got to the top of the stairs, he greeted me with a firm handshake, and looking over at my blond friend, said, "Zigmundt, what's with bringing a goy to a Jew club?" (Berle refused to call me "Aaron," "Sigmond," or even my preferred "Sig," instead insisting on calling me "Zigmundt"—a derivation of my last name with a decidedly Yiddish lilt.) At first, I thought he was joking about my friend, but it was a half-joke at best. Upon hearing Berle's jibe, my WASPy compadre meekly proffered something approximating, "If it helps, I had a Jewish great-grandmother on my father's side . . ."

To which Milton quipped, "Who gives a fuck?"

I could barely contain my laughter.

We sat down at a semicircular booth that surveyed the whole dining room. Once seated, I gave Milton his two boxes, the contents of which he promptly opened and dumped into giant Ziploc bags already filled with cigars.

At the conclusion of the meal, Milton offered me a cigar, which I accepted. Then he turned to my friend and said, "Goy, you smoke?" To which my buddy—clearly regretting his decision to come here more and more by the second—replied with a monotone and monosyllabic "Yes." With that, Berle produced a Cuban Montecristo tubo and lobbed it across the table.

Everyone began to cut and light their cigars. Upon spying how I was enjoying my post-lunch constitutional, Berle looked at me and said, "You are smoking that thing all wrong. Watch me. This is this is how Sid Caesar used to smoke a cigar, how George Burns smokes a cigar, how I smoke a cigar; you young *pischers* haven't a clue how to smoke a cigar."

At this, my friend chuckled. Uh-oh.

Upon hearing him laugh, Berle burst out, "What's so funny? You're not even smoking." My friend tried to explain that the tube he had given him was in fact lacking a cigar—empty.

Upon hearing this, Berle lunged across the table (keep in mind he was eightysomething at the time), grabbed the tube out of my friend's hand, and hurled it across the dining room, where only stupid luck prevented another guest from being hit.

Berle snapped, "When you sit at Milton Berle's table, in the Milton Berle Dining Room, at the club that Milton Berle founded, you smoke a fucking cigar and learn to speak up!" His face was bright red. One of his posse, another octogenarian who nonetheless looked capable of kicking my twentysomething ass, quietly whispered: "Milton, why so *fershlugginer*?"

The rest of us finished our cigars in silence, my friend never receiving a replacement for his. Upon finishing my smoke, I thanked Mr. Berle for lunch and went back to the store. I was not invited back . . . ever.

If anyone's had better luck with wrangling and engaging celebrities, though, it's *Playboy,* whose renowned Interviews and 20 Questions have allowed generations of men to (at least half-truthfully) claim, "I'm just reading it for the articles." The magazine is also noted for its long-standing dedication to punctuating its feature stories with not only photography, but also illustrations and fine paintings. In deference to this *Playboy* tradition, Robert Risko (whose work in *Vanity Fair* and *The New Yorker* has raised him to the pantheon of iconic illustrators/caricaturists such as Edward Sorel, Arnold Roth, and Al Hirschfeld) will bring to life, over the following pages, some of the cigar world's most iconic celebrities doing what they do best: making cigar smoking look damn cool.

"A cigar is a great thing when you don't want to speak."

MILTON "UNCLE MILTIE" BERLE

“Given the choice between a woman and a cigar, I will always choose the cigar.”

GROUCHO MARX

“I got cigars and smoked them that day in order to look older and kept a cigar in order to seem like an older actor.”

ORSON WELLES

“I haven’t been sick a day since I was a child. A steady diet of cigars and whiskey cured me.”

W.C. FIELDS

“If I’d taken my doctor’s advice and quit smoking when he advised me to, I wouldn’t have lived to go to his funeral.”

GEORGE BURNS

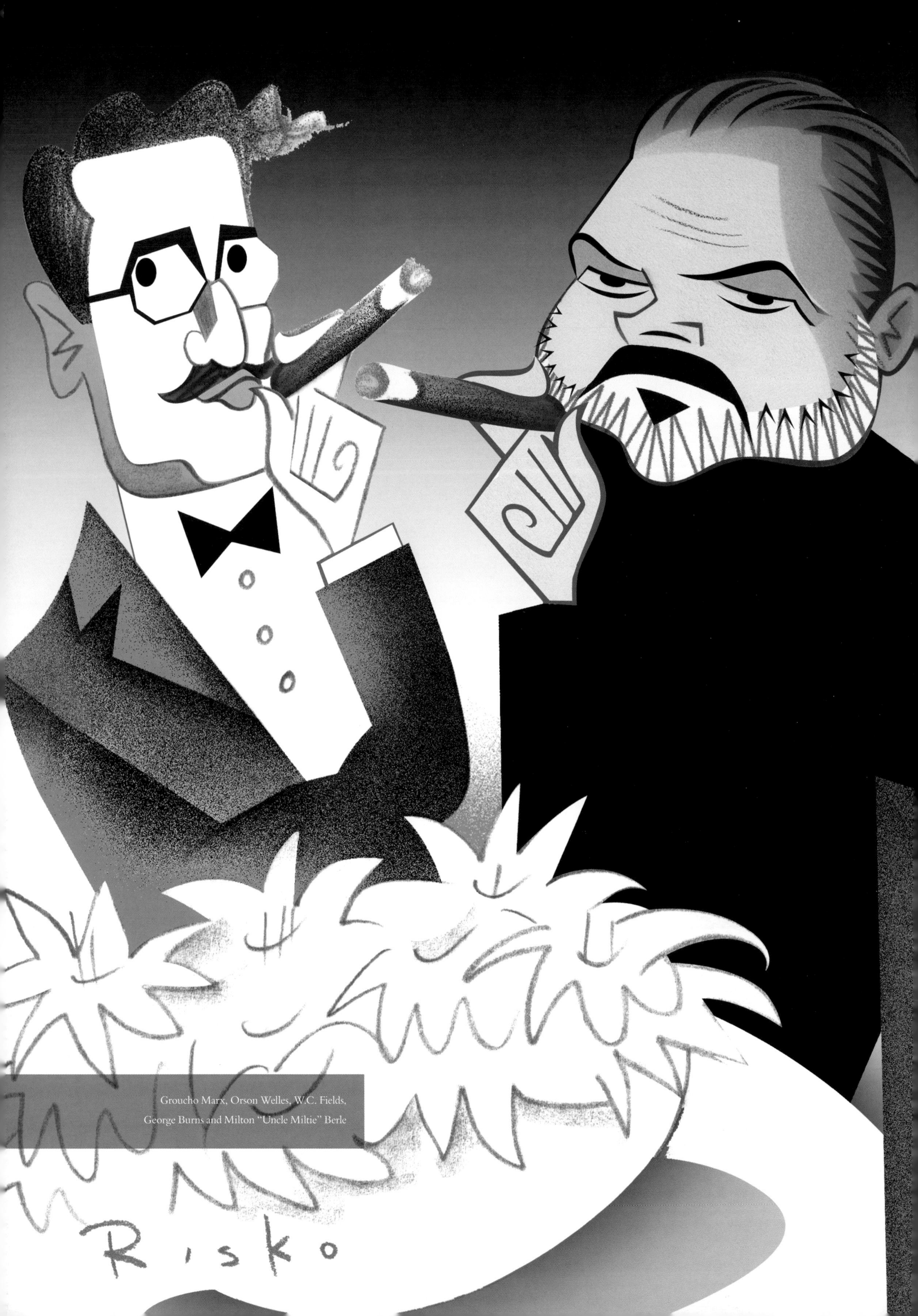

Groucho Marx, Orson Welles, W.C. Fields,
George Burns and Milton "Uncle Miltie" Berle

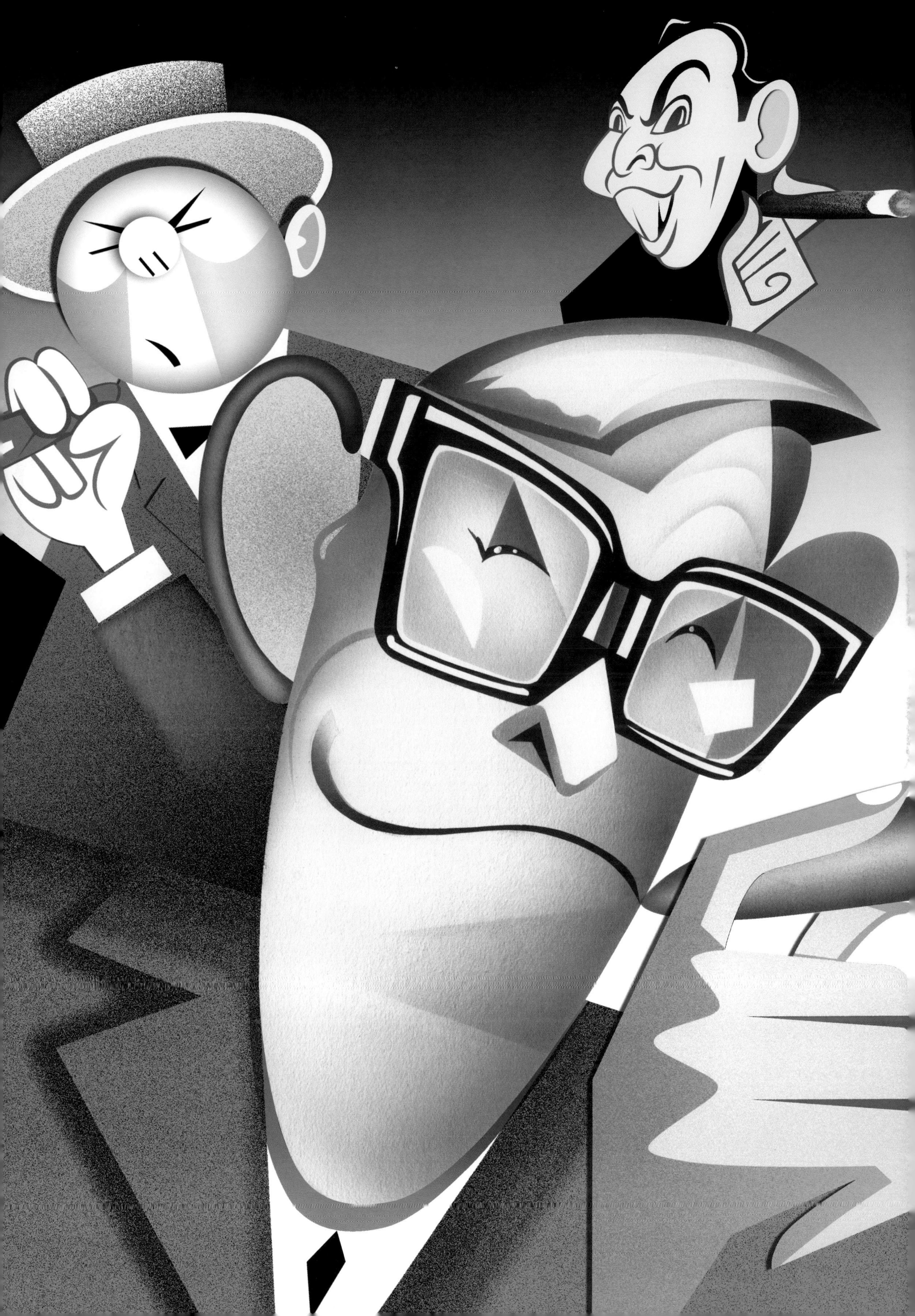

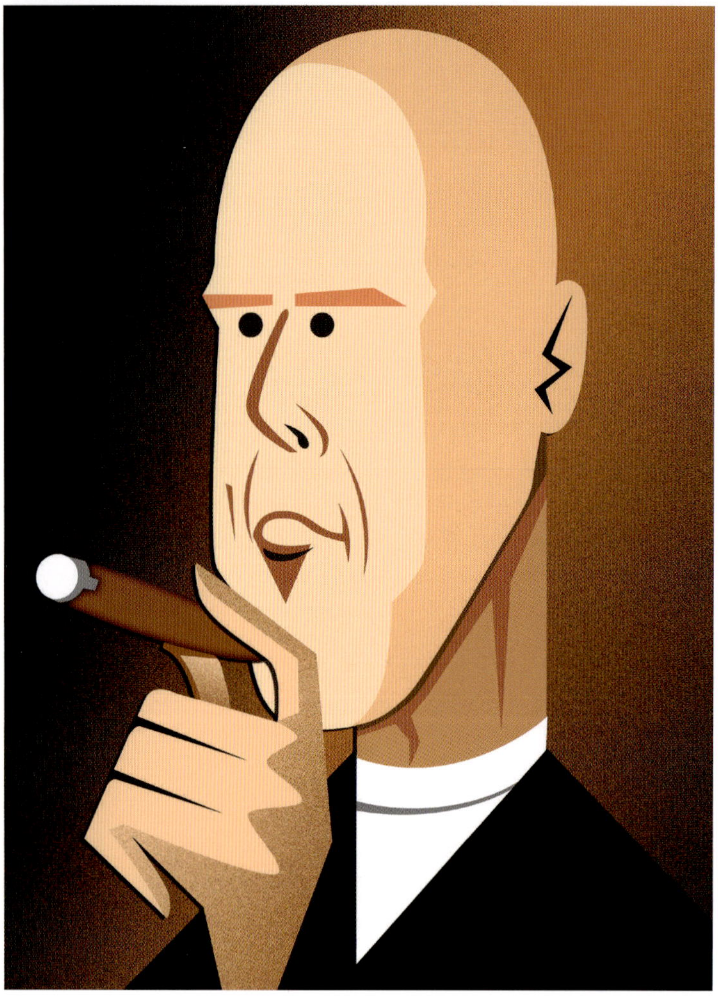

BRUCE WILLIS

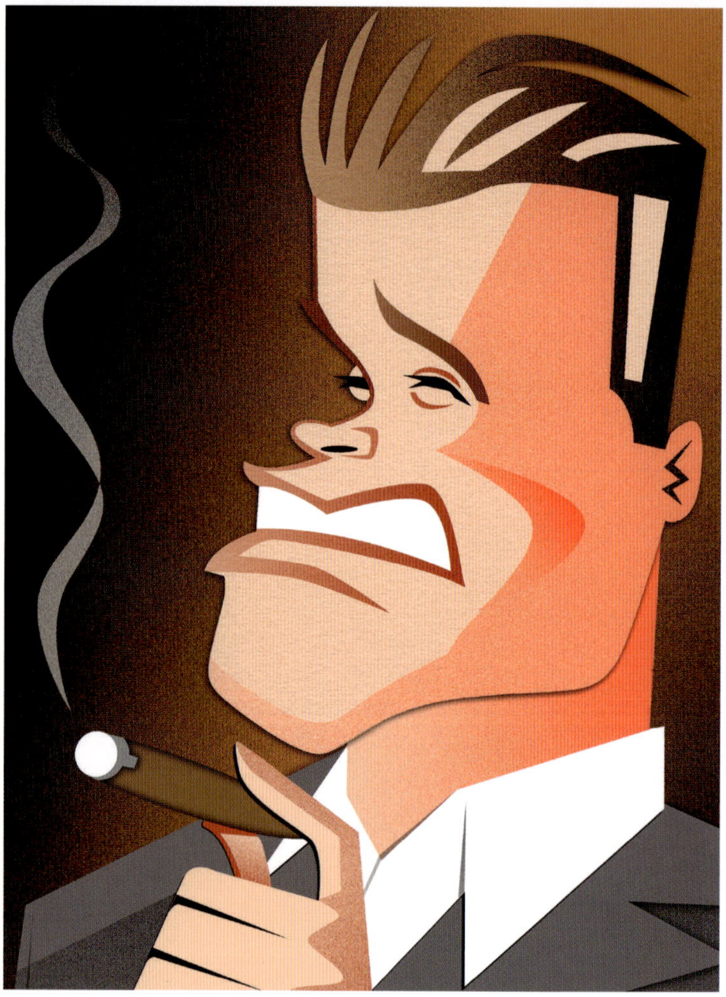

ARNOLD SCHWARZENEGGER

"Taking in and blowing out smoke? And now you see girls smoking cigars. It got to be such a fad. Girls on the covers of magazines, smoking cigars. Give me a break."

JAMES COBURN

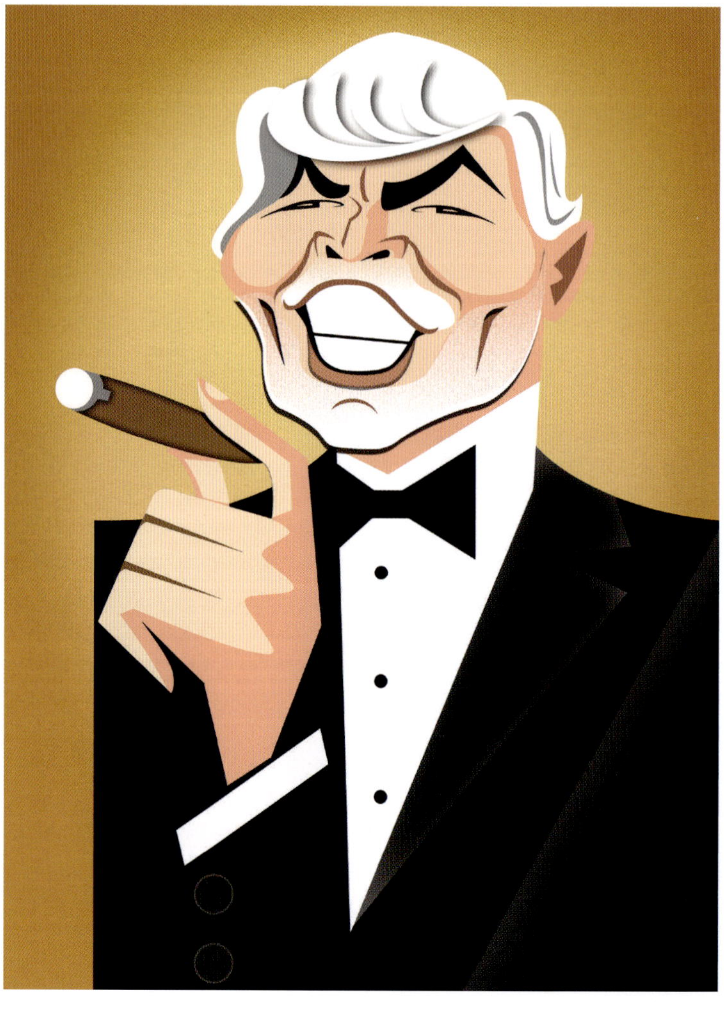

“I never got sick of smoking anything. I inhaled everything, and I smoked them by myself.”

SAMUEL L. JACKSON

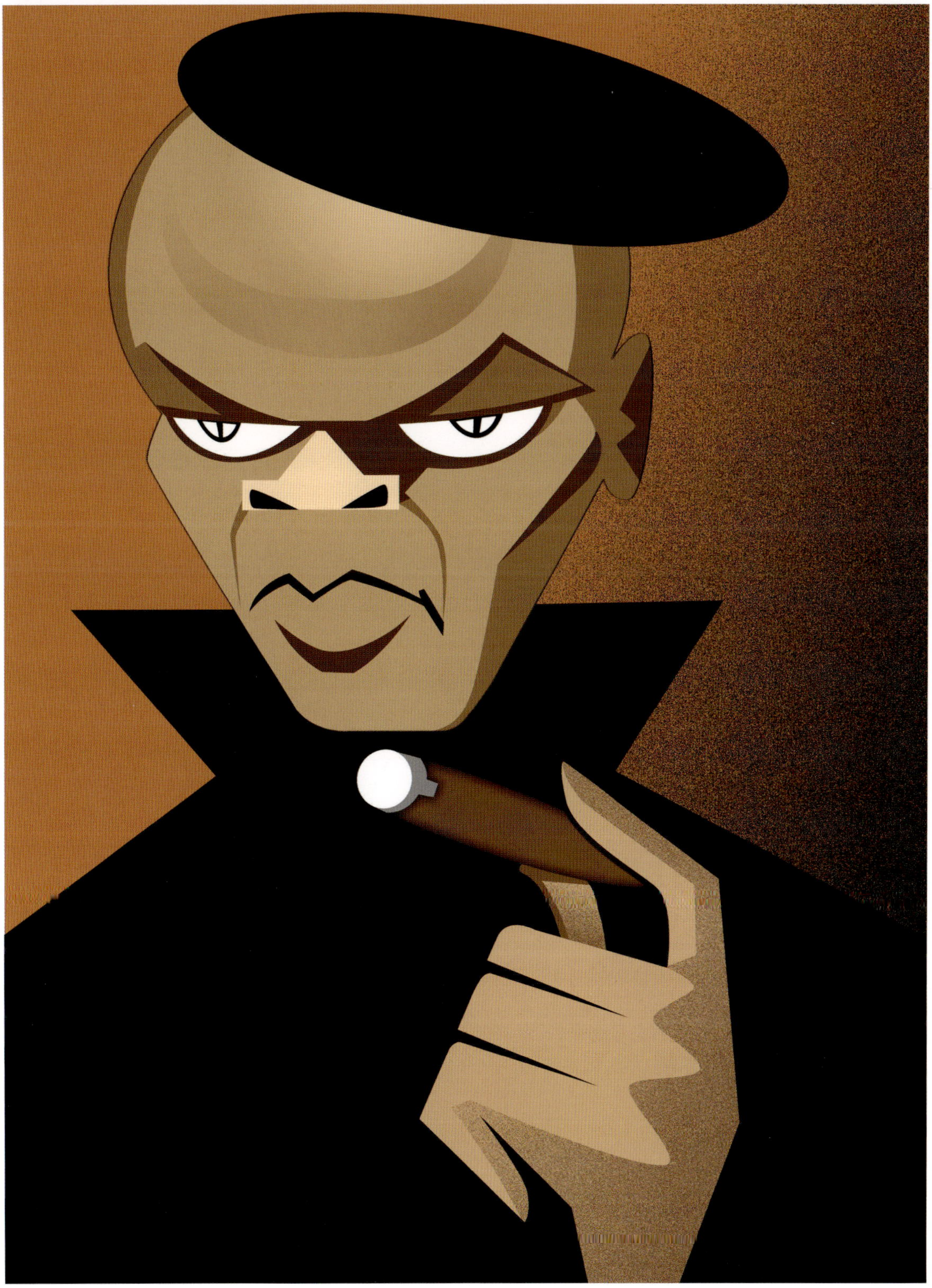

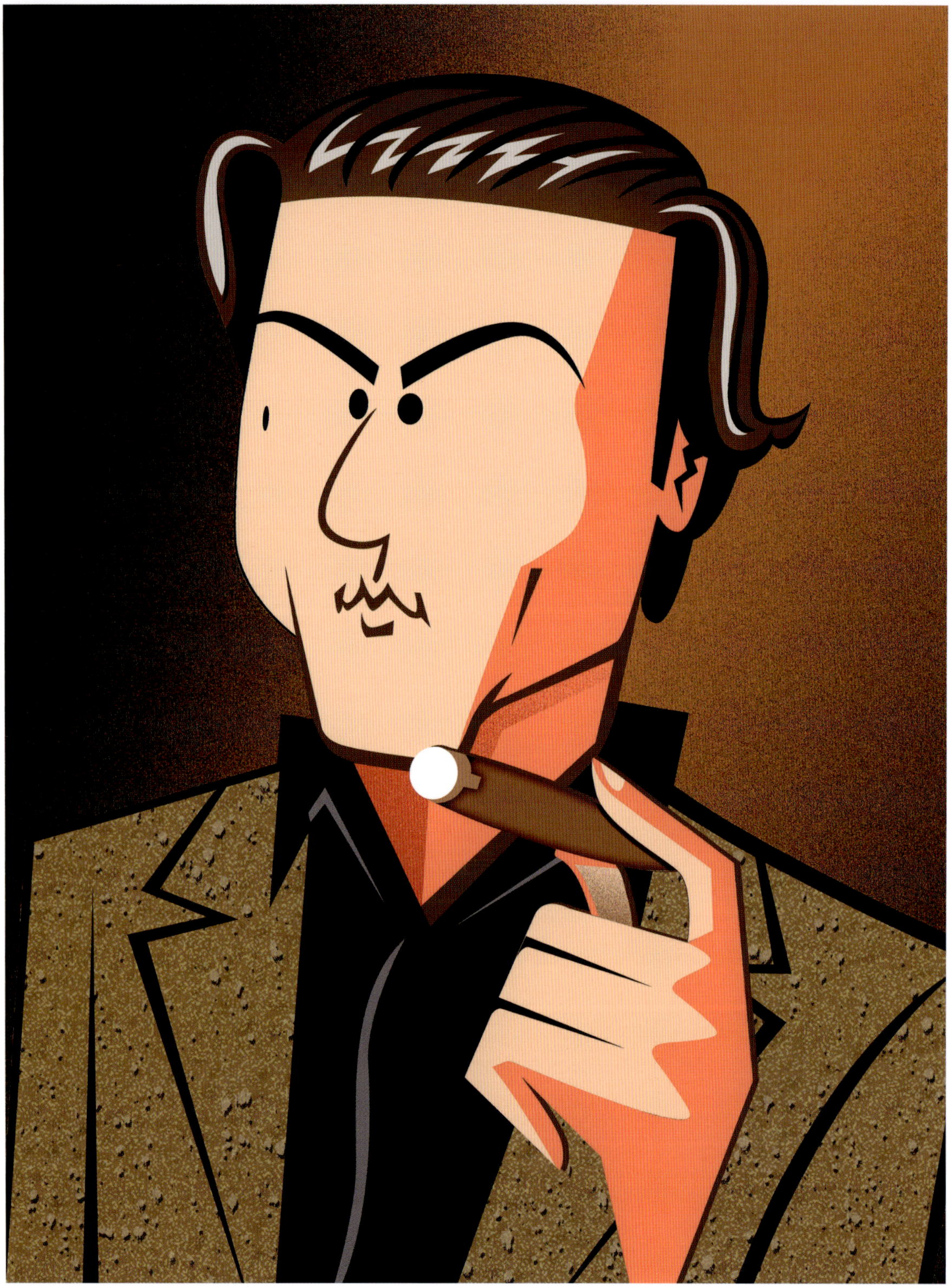

ROBERT DE NIRO

JACK NICHOLSON

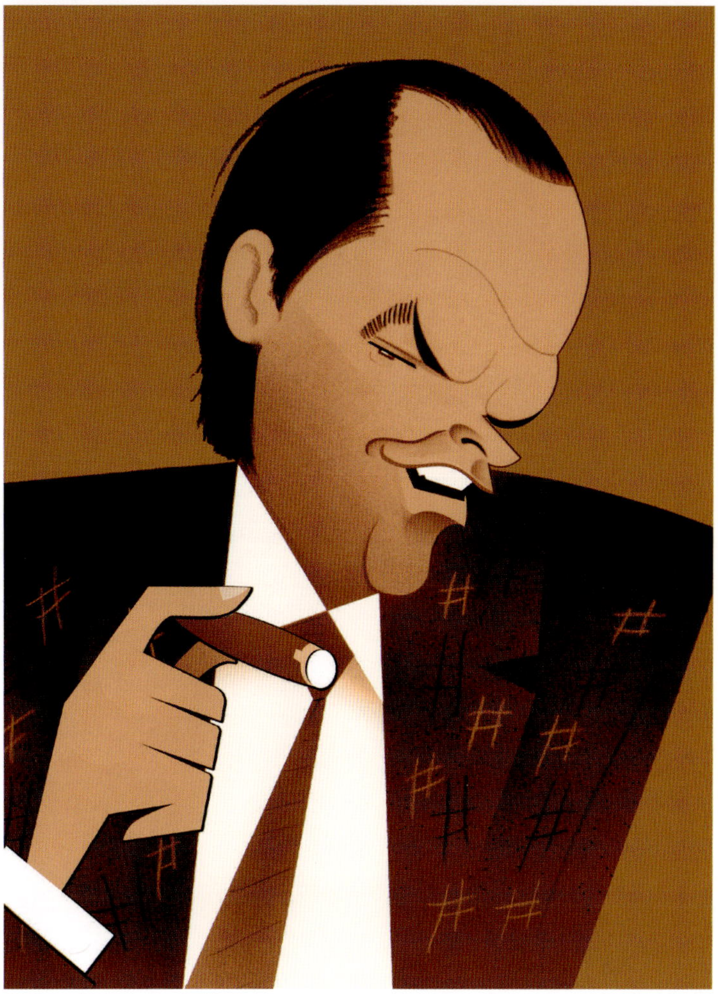

JAMES GANDOLFINI

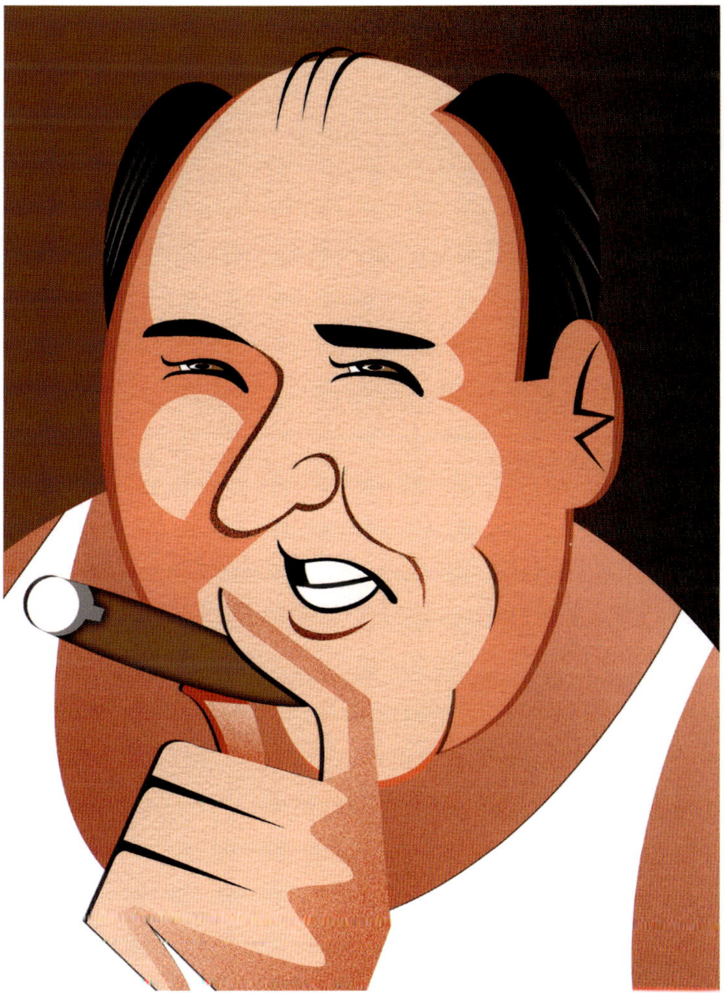

DENNIS HOPPER

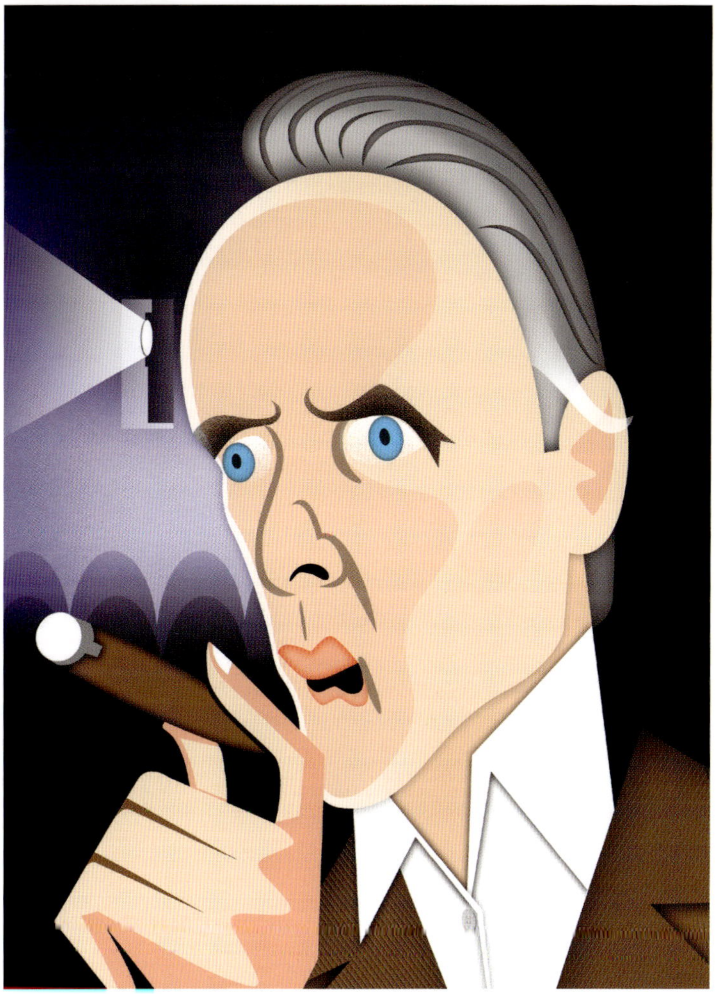

"There is nothing better than a cigar after winning a championship. Nothing."

MICHAEL JORDAN

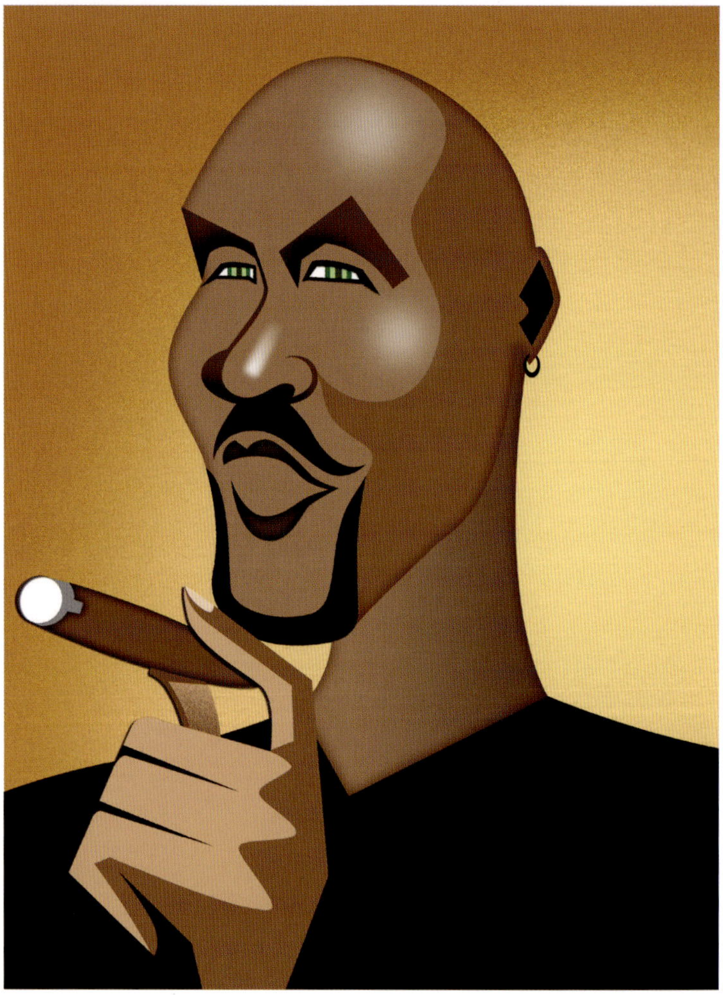

ROBERTO CAVALLI

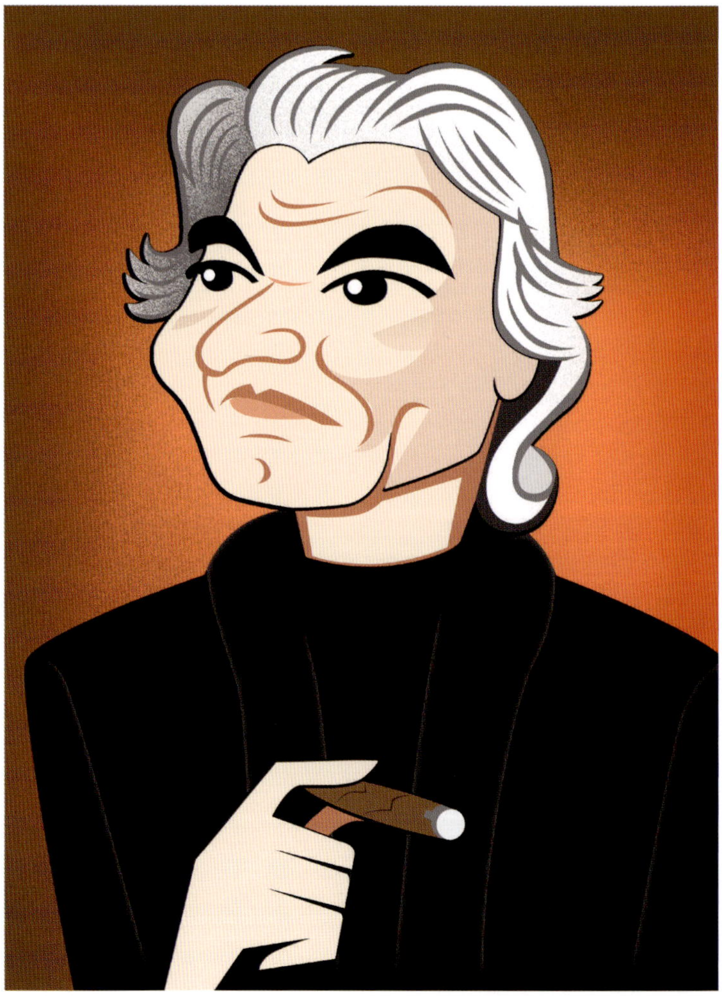

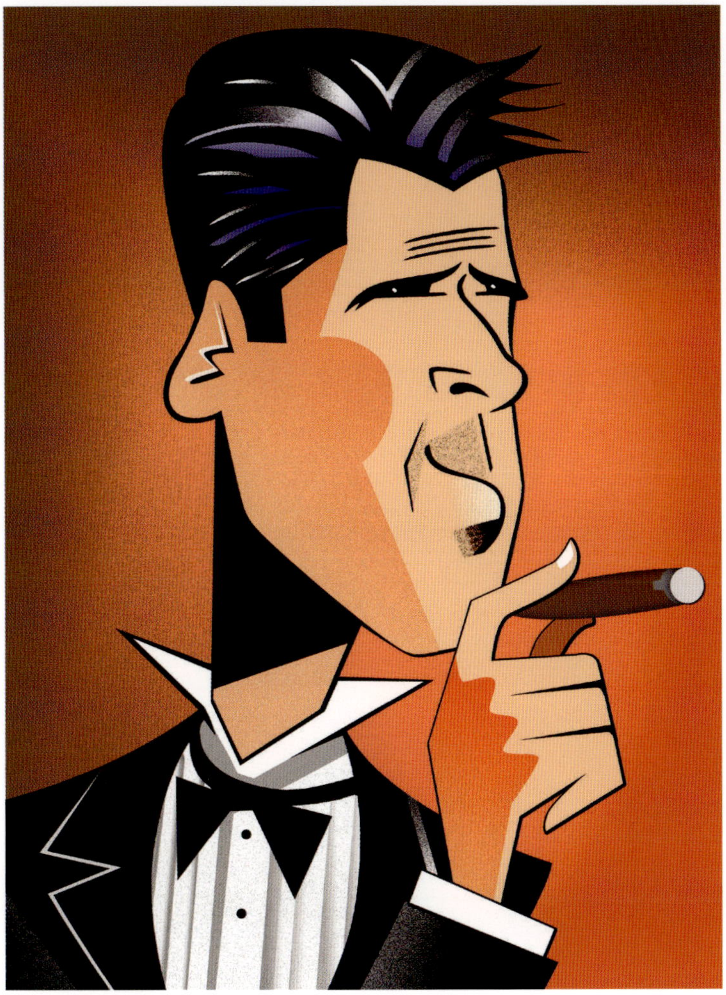

PIERCE BROSNAN

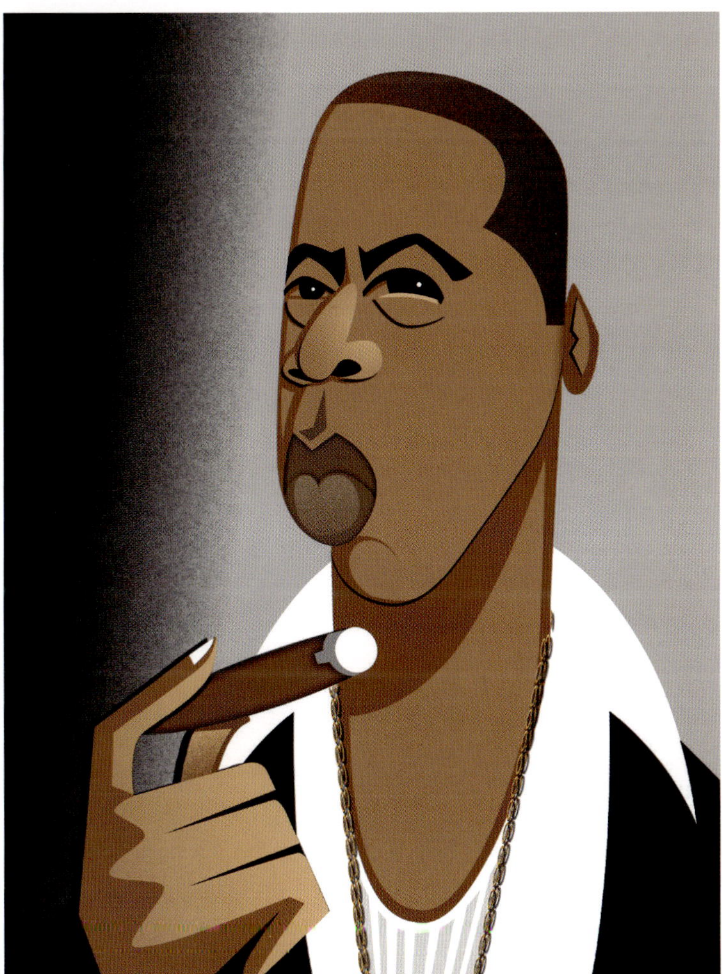

"You got your big cigar going, a nice glass of cognac, you feel like you've made it."

JAY-Z

"I love to smoke. I wish I had more than two hands so I could hold more cigars."

JOHNNY DEPP

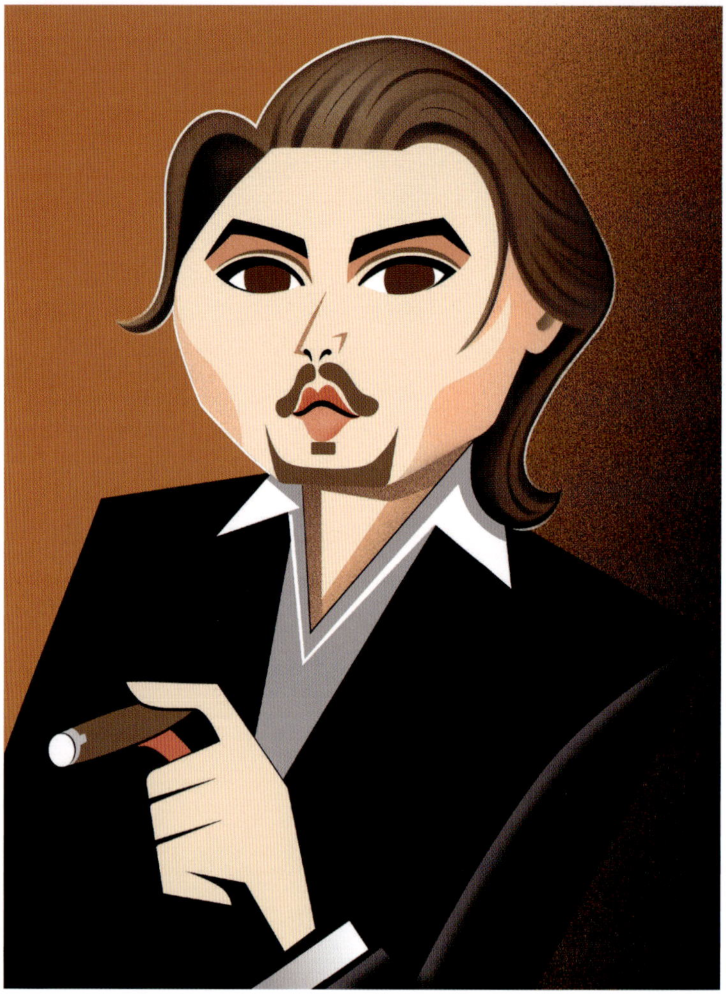

SEAN "DIDDY" COMBS

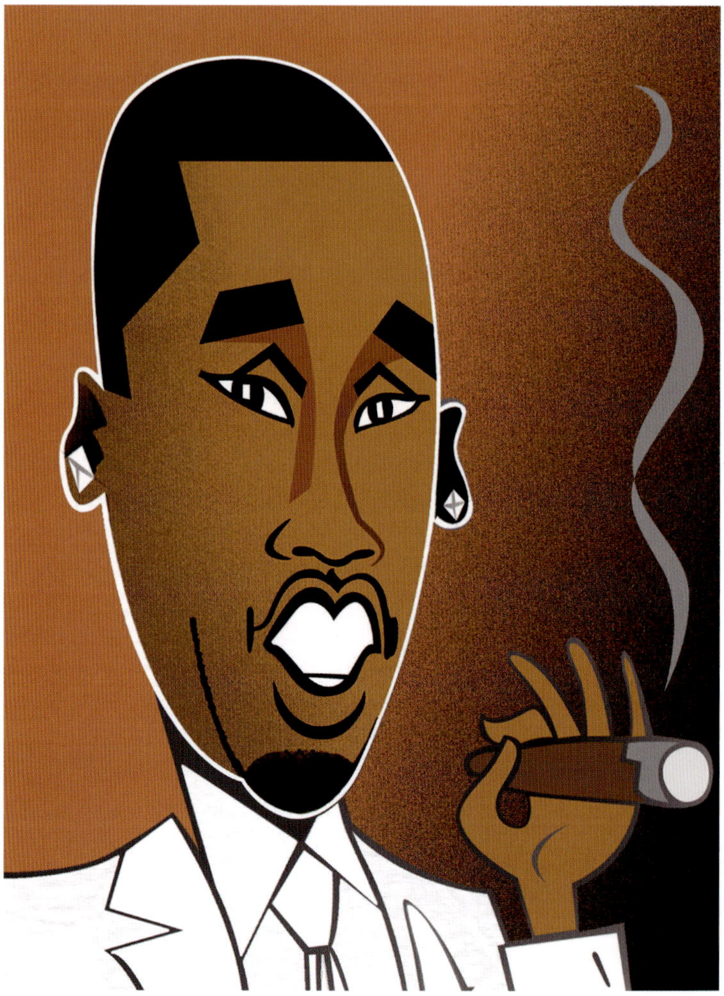

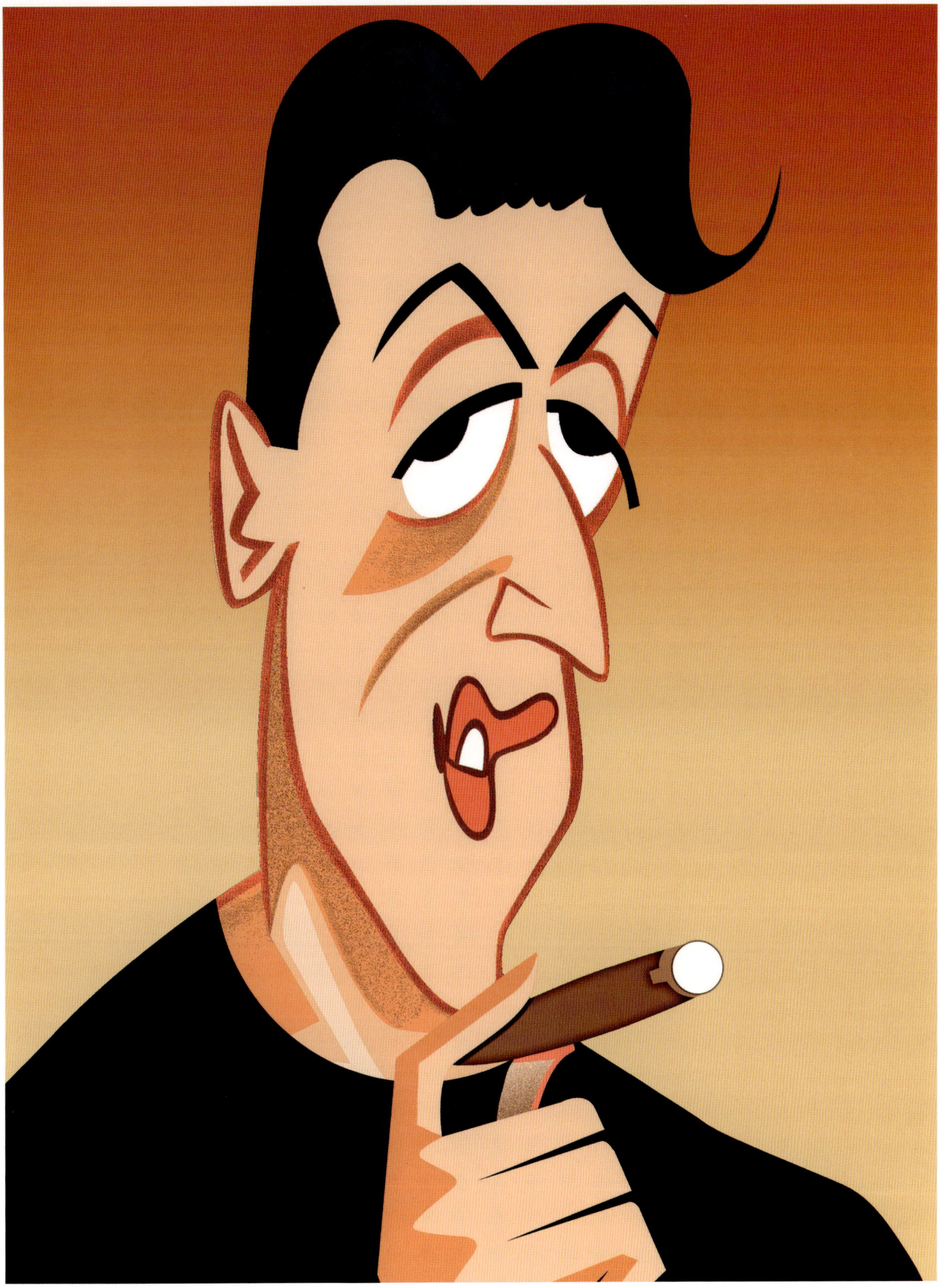

"I believe that a good cigar, a glass of wine and a good conversation is as close to euphoria as you can get in a legal sense."

SYLVESTER "SLY" STALLONE

Other Cigar Quotes

"On a cold winter morning, a cigar fortifies the soul."
STENDHAL

"Gentlemen, you may smoke."
KING EDWARD VII

"I am sure there are many things better than a good cigar, but right now, I can't think of what they might be."
RICHARD CARLETON HACKER

"The most futile and disastrous day seems well spent when it is reviewed through the blue, fragrant smoke of a Havana cigar."
EVELYN WAUGH

"What this country needs is a good five-cent cigar."
THOMAS MARSHALL (U.S. VICE PRESIDENT)

"Here, have a cigar. Light it up and be somebody."
PETE KELLY'S BLUES

"The cigar numbs sorrow and fills the solitary hours with a million gracious images."
GEORGE SAND

"If you kiss a cigar, it will kiss you back. If you treat it like a dog, it will turn around and bite you."
GEORGE BRIGHTMAN

"A good Cuban cigar closes the door to the vulgarities of the world."
FRANZ LISZT

"I vow and believe that the cigar has been one of the greatest creature comforts of my life—a kind companion, a gentle stimulant, an amiable anodyne, a cementer of friendship."
WILLIAM MAKEPEACE THACKERAY

"Sometimes a cigar is just a cigar."
SIGMUND FREUD

"If I paid ten dollars for a cigar, first I'd make love to it, then I'd smoke it."
GEORGE BURNS

"If you smoke too much, you will become drunk as with a strong wine . . . I found this out for myself."
BARTOLOMÉ DE LAS CASAS

"Cheap cigars come in handy; they stifle the odor of cheap politicians."
ULYSSES S. GRANT

"By the cigars they smoke, and the composers they love, ye shall know the texture of men's souls."
JOHN GALSWORTHY

"Cigar smoking knows no politics. It's about the pursuit of pleasure, taste, and aroma."
ANONYMOUS

"To smoke is human; to smoke cigars is divine."
ANONYMOUS

"I've never met someone with a lit cigar in hand and two in pocket that I would not call friend."
ANONYMOUS

WOMEN & CIGARS

"A good cigar is as great a comfort to a man as a good cry to a woman."
EDWARD BULWER-LYTTON

"If your wife doesn't like the aroma of your cigar, change your wife."
ZINO DAVIDOFF

"A WOMAN IS ONLY A WOMAN, BUT A GOOD CIGAR IS A SMOKE."
RUDYARD KIPLING

"There are two things a man never forgets–his first love and his first cigar."
JOHN BAIN

"A WOMAN IS JUST A SCRIPT, BUT A CIGAR IS A MOTION PICTURE."
SAMUEL FULLER

"Cognac and cigars . . . it's like finding the perfect woman. When you've got her, why go chasing after another?"
MICHAEL NOURI

"Women are jealous of cigars... they regard them as a strong rival."
WILLIAM MAKEPEACE THACKERAY

EPICUREAN QUOTES

"After a truly good meal, an outstanding cigar is still the most satisfying after-dinner activity that doesn't involve two human beings."
BRAD SHAW

"A good cigar is like tasting a good wine: you smell it, you taste it, you look at it, you feel it—you can even hear it. It satisfies all the senses."
ANONYMOUS

"Eating and sleeping are the only activities that should be allowed to interrupt a man's enjoyment of his cigar."
MARK TWAIN

"I smoke in moderation. Only one cigar at a time."
MARK TWAIN

"My rule of life prescribed as an absolutely sacred rite smoking cigars and also the drinking of alcohol before, after, and if need be during all meals and in the intervals between them."
WINSTON CHURCHILL

"I drink a great deal.
I sleep a little, and I smoke cigar after cigar.
That is why I am in two-hundred-percent form."
WINSTON CHURCHILL

LITERARY QUOTES

Lady Bracknell: Do you smoke?
Jack: Well, yes, I must admit I smoke.
Lady Bracknell: I am glad to hear it. A man should always have an occupation of some kind.
OSCAR WILDE, *The Importance of Being Earnest*

"HE SAT DOWN, TUCKED THE TIGER-SKIN ROBE AROUND HIS LEGS AND LIT A CIGAR. 'HOW IS IT YOU DON'T SMOKE? A CIGAR IS NOT JUST A PLEASURE—IT'S THE CROWN AND HALLMARK OF PLEASURE. AH, THIS IS LIFE!' "
LEO TOLSTOY, *Anna Karenina*

"I promised myself that if ever I had some money that I would savor a cigar each day after lunch and dinner. This is the only resolution of my youth that I have kept, and the only realized ambition which has not brought disillusion."
SOMERSET MAUGHAM, *Summing Up*

"Lastly (and this is, perhaps, the golden rule), no woman should marry a man who does not smoke."
ROBERT LOUIS STEVENSON, *Virginibus Puerisque*

"There's peace in a Larrañaga, there's calm in Henry Clay."
RUDYARD KIPLING, *The Betrothed,* fifth couplet

POEMS

TO MY CIGAR

Yes, social friend, I love thee well,
In learned doctors' spite;
Thy clouds all other clouds dispel,
And lap me in delight.

CHARLES SPRAGUE

SUBLIME TOBACCO!

Divine in hookahs, glorious in a pipe,
When tipped with amber, mellow, rich, and ripe;
Like other charmers, wooing the caress
More dazzlingly when daring in full dress.
Yet thy true lovers more admire, by far,
Thy naked beauties—give me a cigar!

LORD BYRON, *The Island,* Canto II

PART III

WHAT A PAIR: *SMOKES & DRINKS*

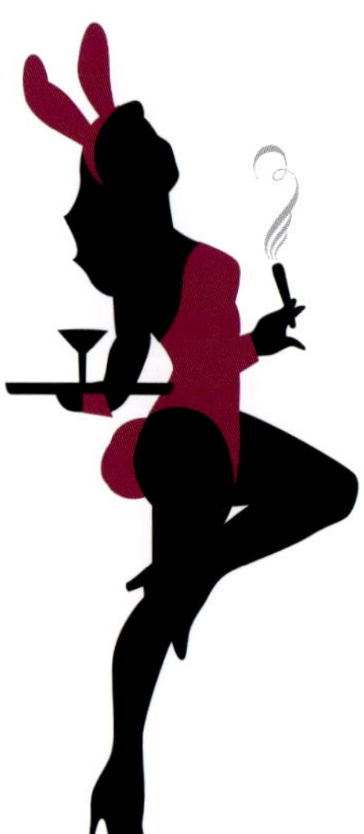

I've been known to enjoy a libation (or five), and like to think I have a better-than-basic knowledge of wine and spirits; however, I don't have a Ph.D. in the subject. I just like to knock back what I enjoy.

As to my personal tastes, I've always said, "I could give up drinking if it weren't for tequila, wine, and cognac." That remains very true.

However, since spirits (as well as wine, beer, and coffee) and cigars are rather inseparable pairs, I thought I would defer to my friend Adrian Bartoli, who has spent the better part of his post-collegiate life making observations on such things.

After settling into your chair at the local cigar-friendly establishment, a cigar perched comfortably between the index finger and thumb of your left hand, you notice something discomforting: an empty right hand. What to do?

You could always light up a second cigar: one for each hand. But while this solution seems to present a pleasant symmetry, two-fisted smoking is seen as a bit of a faux pas. Try it, and you'd likely need a third hand to give the one-finger salute to people complaining about your excessive clouds of smoke.

Fortunately, there is one tried-and-true alternative for those unoccupied fingers: a drink.

But what potion is most appropriate? The traditional choice would be to pair that cigar with a fine brandy, preferably one from the Cognac region of France. There is a time-honored practice of gently blowing the smoke from your cigar into a snifter of fine cognac, letting the flavors mingle for a brief instant therein before inhaling the smoke again.

Yet for every supporter of cognac, someone will opine that rum offers a better choice, or that nothing compares to a tumbler of single-malt Scotch whiskey.

The truth is that there is no single answer to this question–it is largely a matter of personal preference. That being said, applying certain guidelines to your selection will both assure a good smoke and make you look like a sommelier of cigars at the same time.

When it comes to smokes and spirits, flavor pairing works on a few fundamental concepts. You want to match up flavors that complement each other, avoid flavors that antagonize each other and minimize flavor duplication or overlap.

Flavor compatibility seems fairly intuitive: sweet and salty, for example, go together quite well. The flip side is flavor antagonism: when was the last time you saw a huge demand for turkey cannoli?

But what is flavor duplication? You are probably quite familiar with it, actually. Whenever you mix two of the same flavor, your taste buds become oversaturated and a bit desensitized; add several spoonfuls of sugar to a morning cup of coffee, and the accompanying donut will taste less sweet.

The flavor-duplication principle lies behind a misconception on the part of some cigar-smokers, in which they assume that a cigar with a particular flavor profile should be matched with foods or drinks that contain the same profile; that bittersweet chocolate should go with a cigar that offers chocolate-like taste notes. Alas, this isn't the case (try a handful of almonds to bring out the chocolate flavors in your smoke).

You won't often be eating a meal while simultaneously smoking a cigar, but rare is the connoisseur who torches up without at least occasionally having a drink nearby—and in this scenario, the rules of flavor still apply. With so many combinations of drinks and cigars, it's worthwhile to spend a little time on each of the different types of beverages you could encounter on a smoke break.

THE BIG C'S: COFFEE AND COGNAC > There are many reasons to extol the virtues of combining coffee and cigars. Indeed, in certain circumstances the pairing of flavors can be ideal. However, a number of cigars also feature taste notes of coffee; thanks to flavor duplication, this means that puffing while sipping your morning cup of Caffé Americano can rob an excellent-smoking cigar of much of its flavor. You can avoid this by pairing that cup of java with a cigar that has mineral qualities.

Cuban coffee, strong and sweet, couples particularly well with a cigar. Whenever I'm sitting in their offices, cigar makers always ask, first, "Would you like a cigar?" followed by, "Would you like a coffee with it?" The answer to both questions is inevitably "yes," and they always join me. These connoisseurs can't all be wrong.

So coffee does have a place in the world of cigars—one that goes beyond the major pick-me-up of combining nicotine and caffeine.

Cognac, by contrast, is the archetypal drink pairing for cigars, and its reputation is extremely well-deserved. That fabled spirit falls into four quality grades:

V.S.: *Stands for Very Superior, and spends at least two and a half years in wood before seeing the light of day.*

V.S.O.P.: *Stands for Very Superior Old Pale, and is aged for a minimum of four years (you'll occasionally also see V.V.S.O.P.—which throws in an extra Very). The milder flavors of this cognac can pair nicely with milder cigars.*
X.O.: *Aged in oak for a minimum of six (and upward of 20) years, this "extra old" cognac (the producer's most-aged) has traditionally been paired with stronger cigars.*
Vieille Réserve/Hors d'âge: *While technically this cognac doesn't have to be older than an X.O., that's almost always the case; hence "hors d'âge," or "beyond age." Nearly every cognac (and some Bordeaux) house has their own specific contribution to this very special category, such as the Rémy Martin Louis XIII, Hennessy Richard, Pierre Ferrand Ancestrale, and Très Vieille Reserve Lafite-Rothschild.*

Many cigar and spirit lovers seek out older cognacs, such as X.O. blends, for all their smoking needs, and match the characteristics of the individual blends to the cigars. Milder cigars will do well with cognacs from houses like Rémy Martin or Hine, while more robust cigars will benefit from more concentrated blends, such as Hennessey or Pierre Ferrand.

Cognac has been so popular for pairing with cigars that several "cigar blends" have been manufactured for exactly this purpose. These blends are somewhere between a V.S.O.P. and an X.O. in age and character, and try to serve as an all-purpose drink for all types of cigars. If you have room for only one bottle of cognac in your liquor cabinet, a "cigar blend" is a reasonable choice–and if you can find it, that one bottle should be the Pierre Ferrand Cigare Blend Reserve Havana. This extremely rare bottle of twenty-five-year-aged cognac suits a range of cigars. Another is the Hine Cigar Reserve.

BEER & STOUT > Who'd have thought? Beer and stout can be excellent accompaniments to a fine cigar, but that fact seems hardly recognized among smoke and drink connoisseurs. True, the Belgian lambics simply cannot harmonize with cigars and should be avoided; likewise, dark and malty porters and stouts, while initially appearing synergistic, tend to blunt cigars' natural flavors and should be disregarded for specific pairings.

That said, a lighter beer with a more pronounced bitterness, such as a fine India Pale Ale (IPA), will bring out the hidden flavor in milder cigars.

RUM > Given that rum and cigars are made in the same part of the world, they would seem to be a natural match.

Indeed, some rums will pair readily with cigars. But many of the flavor notes that rums display, such as vanilla, spices, citrus, and honey, are the very ones that we enjoy in cigars, which can play right into the hands of our old friend, flavor duplication.

When pairing with rum, consider avoiding milder or stronger cigars; the ideal choice is a medium-bodied cigar with strong notes of nuts and leather. For best results, puff while sipping a Havana Club Añejo 7 Años or Montecristo twelve-year aged rum.

PORT AND SHERRY > A fortified wine from Portugal, Vinho do Porto (or, as we know it, "port") is made by adding brandy to a sweet wine. As you might expect, the combination is an excellent one. The sweet fruit of the port pairs well with the savory, smokier flavors of heavier cigars, even as the alcohol helps cleanse the palate. Straightforward ruby ports ideally pair with bold-flavored cigars (think a Dominican puro or full-bodied Nicaraguan), while tawny ports (which have been aged in wood for several years) are better paired with light- to medium-bodied cigars, such as those from Honduras.

Sherry, a fortified wine similar to port, can likewise be a great choice when carefully paired with a cigar. Avoid sweeter sherries (oloroso or cream sherry) as they will deaden the flavor of your cigar; better are drier sherries such as Terrantez (a sherry from Madeira in Portugal), which pairs exceptionally well with spicier cigars. For medium-bodied cigars, try a dry Amontillado sherry.

TEA > Tea can be an excellent choice to accompany a fine cigar. To boil it down: avoid the fruit infusions (raspberry tea, etc.) as they will dull the flavor of the cigar. Unsweetened black teas are an excellent choice for milder Dominican and Costa Rican cigars, as they will mask any bitterness and help coax the tobaccos' subtle flavors out into the open.

A highly complex cigar, such as Cuban or Nicaraguan, is best matched with fresh green and white teas and their subtle mixture of astringency and sweetness. The exceptions to this rule are Pu-erh tea (aged green tea) and Lapsang souchong (smoked leaf tea), the strong and distinctive flavors of which do not easily pair with cigars.

WHISKEY > Considered by many the red-haired stepchild of the spirits world, whiskey (or whisky) actually represents a remarkably diverse collection of spirits, each

determined by the type of grain used in its fermentation:
Blended: *Derived from mixing two or more whiskeys, commonly either a single-malt whiskey with a neutral spirit or an unmalted grain whiskey.*
Bourbon: *Distilled from a mixture of chiefly corn, as well as other grains.*
Canadian: *Made typically from rye—hence its U.S. moniker, "rye whiskey."*
Single Malt: *Wholly distilled from a single type of malted grain (traditionally barley) at a single distillery.*

In general, the best choice for a cigar pairing is a single-malt Scotch, but the best selection can often be difficult. Broadly speaking, the single malts from the Orkney Islands (e.g., Highland Park) or the Lowlands (such as Glenkinchie) will pair best with modern-style mild- to medium-bodied cigars.

Single malts from the Speyside (like Glenrothes) or the Islay area (like Lagavulin) will pair best with stronger, woody cigars, bringing out the smoke's more leathery highlights. Lastly, Scotch from the Highland region goes nicely with a fruitier Honduran cigar (such as The Macallan 18).

WINE > Pairing wine and cigars can actually be quite difficult. With so much variation between the different types of wine and cigars, finding a match is challenging. Fuller-bodied red wines seem to work best with cigars, such as Australian Shirazes, Spanish Riojas and California Zinfandels. This is not to say that white wines deserve total exclusion; some French Alsatian wines, and select Champagnes such as Bollinger R.D., will pair quite nicely—should you want to imitate Tony "Scarface" Montana in the hot tub with a cigar and a glass of bubbly.

One of my favorite cigar-friendly wines is the M. Cosentino Cigarzin, a California vintage zinfandel first released during the 1990s cigar boom, and created specifically to be paired with cigars; I am pleased to say that the most recent vintages hold up quite nicely.

There is also Randall Grahm's Le Cigare Volant wine, produced by Bonny Doon. Although not always easy to pair with a specific cigar, the fact that this vino has a "cigare" in the name makes it a nice cigar-dinner complement (plus, it goes particularly well with grilled beef or lamb).

SMOKING RANGE

The bottom line is simple: When it comes to pairings, drink whatever will help you get the most enjoyment out of your cigar. Of course, this will require a bit of experimentation on your part—but with the guide below as a starting point, you can head out prepared to maximize your pairing experience:

MILD CIGARS: black tea, India Pale Ale, Highland Park whiskey, Rémy Martin cognac

MEDIUM-BODIED CIGARS: tawny port, aged rum, Glenkinchie whiskey, Hine cognac, soda with bitters

FULL-BODIED CIGARS: Hennessy cognac, Glenrothes whiskey, ruby port, Armagnac

NOTABLE SMOKE SHOPS & CIGAR BARS

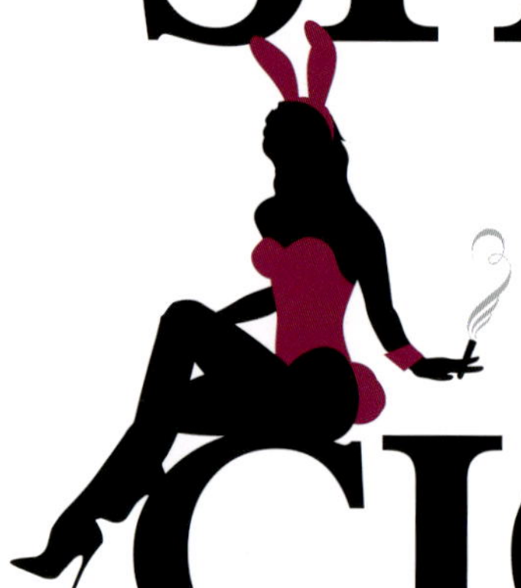

A select guide to fine tobacconists, cigar bars, and other smoke-friendly establishments for the international playboy: New York, Miami, Chicago, Las Vegas, Los Angeles and other U.S. cities, Nova Scotia, Quebec, Ontario, Manitoba, Alberta, British Columbia, Hong Kong (China), Shanghai, Beijing, Moscow, Amsterdam, Paris, London, and Havana.

UNITED STATES

NEW YORK

Stores

Barclay Rex
70 E. 42nd St.
212-692-9680

Barclay Rex
570 Lexington Ave.
212-888-1015

Barclay Rex
75 Broad St.
212-962-3355

The Cigar Inn
1314 First Ave.
212-717-7403

The Cigar Inn
1016 Second Ave.
212-750-0809

Davidoff of Geneva
The Shops at Columbus Circle
10 Columbus Circle
212-823-6383

Davidoff of Geneva
535 Madison Ave.
212-751-9060

De La Concha
1390 Avenue of the Americas
212-757-3167

J.R. Cigar
562 Fifth Ave.
212-997-2227

Nat Sherman
12 E. 42nd St.
800-MY-CIGAR

OK Cigars
383-A West Broadway
212-965-9065

Bars

Beekman Bar & Books
889 First Ave.
212-758-6600

The Carnegie Club
156 W. 56th St.
212-957-9676

Circa Tabac
32 Watts St.
212-941-1781

Club Macanudo
26 East 63rd St.
212-752-8200

Grand Havana Room (private)
666 Fifth Ave.
212-245-1600

Hudson Bar & Books
636 Hudson St.
212-229-2642

The Johnson Club Room (private) at Nat Sherman
12 E. 42nd St.
800-MY-CIGAR

Lexington Bar & Books
1020 Lexington Ave.
212-717-3902

The Pen-Top Bar & Terrace at The Peninsula Hotel
700 Fifth Ave.
212-956-2888

The Terrace at Sutton Place Bar
1015 Second Ave.
212-207-3777

The Velvet Cigar Lounge
80 E. 7th St.
212-533-5582

MIAMI

Stores

Absolute Cigar Shop
22 SW 8th St.
305-374-9999

Ciboney Cigars
9600 SW 8th St. #7
305-207-4445

Cuba Caiman Cigars
3810 SW 8th St.
305-529-2470

Cuba Tobacco Trading, Inc.
1528 SW 8th St.
305-649-2717

Genuine Tobacconist
14236 SW 8th St.
305-226-9994

King's Treasure Tobacco, Inc.
401 Biscayne Blvd.
305-374-5593

Magic City Cigars
89 NW 1st St.
305-372-1774

Mike's Cigars
1030 Kane Concourse
Bay Harbor Islands
305-866-2277

Puros Fine Cigars
10792 Coral Way
305-222-2217

Shisha International
1225 Washington Ave.
305-532-1511

Smoke Shop 2
130 SE 3rd Ave.
305-358-1886

Lounges

Aromas of Havana
14781 Biscayne Blvd.
305-940-0988

Deco Drive Cigars
1136 Collins Ave.
305-673-6071

Deco Drive Cigars West
1650 Meridian Ave.
305-674-1811

Deco Drive Cigars East
1436 Ocean Dr.
305-672-9032

The Havana Club (private)
200 South Biscayne Blvd., 55th floor
305-405-7663

Havana Smokers Cigar Lounge
4203 Ponce de Leon Blvd.
305-441-2915

La Bodeguita del Medio
3138 Coral Way
305-441-7016

Sabor Havana
2309 Ponce de Leon Blvd.
305-444-1764

Sabor Havana
2600 NW 87th Ave., Suite 3
305-436-8860

CHICAGO

Stores

Blue Havana
856 W. Belmont Ave.
773-242-8262

Cigar King
8016 N. Lincoln Ave.
Skokie, IL
847-675-2447

Cigars and More
314 S. Milwaukee Ave.
Libertyville, IL
847-918-9999

8 to 8
300 East St. Charles Rd.
Villa Park, IL
630-993-1234

Iwan Ries & Co.
19 So. Wabash
312-372-1306

Jack Schwartz Importer
141 W. Jackson Blvd.
312-782-7898

La Casa del Tobacco
1937 W. North Ave.
773-384-5225

Up Down Tobacco
1550 N. Wells St.
312-337-8025

Lounges

Humidor of Downers Grove
949 Burlington Ave.
Downers Grove, IL
630-241-3399

LAS VEGAS

Stores

Casa Fuente
The Forum Shops
3500 Las Vegas Blvd. South
702-731-5051

Colosseum Cigars
Caesars Palace
3500 Las Vegas Blvd. South
702-866-1234

Cigars by Freyboy
Luxor Hotel
3900 Las Vegas Blvd. South
702-262-4444

Davidoff of Geneva
Venetian Hotel and Casino
3377 Las Vegas Blvd. South
702-733-5999

Davidoff of Geneva
MGM Grand Hotel and Casino
3799 Las Vegas Blvd. South
702-933-2105

Davidoff of Geneva
Mandalay Bay Hotel and Casino
3950 Las Vegas Blvd. South
702-737-0326

LOS ANGELES

Stores

2nd Street Cigars & Gallery (La Plata Cigars)
124 West Second St.
Downtown L.A.
213-452-4427

The Big Easy
12604 Ventura Blvd.
Studio City
818-762-3279

Buena Vista Cigar Club & Lounge
9715 South Santa Monica Blvd.
Beverly Hills
310-273-8100

Ceniza Cigar Lounge
260 E. Colorado Blvd.
Pasadena
626-795-4664

Cigar Warehouse
15141 Ventura Blvd.
Sherman Oaks
818-784-1391

Hi Time Wine Cellars Smoke Shack
250 Ogle St.
Costa Mesa
949-650-8463

J Restaurant & Lounge
1119 South Olive St.
Downtown L.A.
213-746-7746

The Lone Wolf Cigar Co.
223B Broadway
Santa Monica
310-458-5441

Newport Tobacco
533 Newport Center Drive
Fashion Island
Newport Beach
949-644-5153

Wally's
2107 Westwood Blvd.
Los Angeles
310-475-0606

Clubs

Grand Havana Room (private)
301 North Canon Drive
Beverly Hills
310-446-4925 corporate office
310-385-7700 club

Nazareth's Fine Cigars
350 N Canon
Beverly Hills
310-271-5863

OTHER U.S. CITIES

Stores

The Briar Shoppe
2412 Times Blvd.
Houston, TX
713-529-6347

Churchill's Fine Cigars
5041 N. 44th St.
Phoenix, AZ
602-840-9080

Club Humidor
11745 I-10 W., Ste. 140
San Antonio, TX
210-558-7700

Diebel's
Club Plaza
426 Ward Parkway
Kansas City, MO
816-931-2988

Havana Connections
11616 W. Broad St.
Richmond, VA
804-364-5711

L J Peretti
2 1/2 Park Square
Boston, MA
617-482-0218

Leaf & Bean
3525 Washington Rd.
McMurray, PA
724-942-6670

Lighten Up Cigars
480 Lancaster Ave.
Frazier, PA
610-251-9117

Rain City Cigar
5963 Corson Ave. South
Seattle, WA
206-767-3619

Rich's Cigar Store
820 SW Alder St.
Portland, OR
503-228-1700

Smoke Inn
801 Village Blvd.
West Palm Beach, FL
888-766-5371

The Tobacco Shop of Ridgewood
10 Chestnut St.
Ridgewood, NJ
201-447-2204

Up in Smoke
7707 N. MacArthur Blvd.
Suite 140
Irving, TX
972-556-0115

Ye Olde Pipe & Tobacco Shoppe
2017 E. Camelback Rd.
Phoenix, AZ
602-955-9542

CANADA

NOVA SCOTIA

Smoke on the Water
Bishop Landing
1475 Lower Water St.
Halifax
902-425-5857

QUEBEC

Cigar & Compagnie
6981 Boul. St-Laurent
Montreal
514-277-0014

J.E. Giguere Ltee
59, Rue Buade
Quebec City
418-692-2296

La Casa Del Habano
1434 Sherbrooke West Rez De Chaussee
Montreal
514-849-0037

Societe Cigare
575 Grande-Allee Est., #202
Quebec City
418-640-2591

Stogies Lounge
2015 Crescent
Montreal
514-848-0069

Vasco Cigars
1327 Rue Ste Catherine Ouest
Montreal
514-284-0475

ONTARIO

B. Sleuth & Statesman Inc.
130 King Street West
Box 28 The Exchange Tower
Toronto
416-363-7575

Celebrity Tobacco & Gifts
Trafalgar Village Mall
117 Cross Ave Unit B/2
Oakville
905-849-3845

Cigar Bodega
205 Main St.
Unionville
905-513-1810

Cigar Studio
4 Willingdon Blvd.
Toronto
416-237-1810

Gordon's Cigar
5858 Ferry St.
Niagara Falls
905-358-7425

La Casa Del Habano
141 Yorkville Ave.
Toronto
416-926-9066

La Casa Del Habano
358 Ouellette Ave.
Windsor
519-254-0017

The Smoking Cigar
1699 Bayview Ave.
Toronto
416-545-0063

Thomas Hinds Tobacconist
8 Cumberland St.
Toronto
416-481-6909

Tobacco Haven
595 Bay St.
P.O. Box 50
Toronto
416-593-6655

Walper Tobacco Shop Ltd.
15 King St. West
Kitchener
519-745-9984

MANITOBA

Thomas Hinds Tobacconist
96-185 Carlton St.
Winnipeg
800-790-7779

ALBERTA

Burlington on Whyte
10468 Whyte (82nd) Ave.
Edmunton
780-439-8519

Epicure Cigar & Pipe Ltd.
620 8th Ave SW
Suite #101
Calgary
403-269-2716

International Cigar & Pipe
203-530 8Th Ave South W
Western Gas Tower
Calgary
403-262-8286

La Tienda Cigars
8426 109 St.
Edmunton
780-439-5108

Zigarren
7112 Macleod Trail SE, #6
Calgary
403-532-2442

BRITISH COLUMBIA

2000 Cigars
881 Dunsmuir St.
Vancouver
604-647-6600

City Cigar Emporium
888 W. 6th Ave.
Vancouver
604-879-0208

Fidel's Cuban Cigar Store Ltd.
4-4433 Sundial Place
Whistler
604-905-4440

Goodfellas Cigar Shop
1441 Store St., Unit #1
Victoria
250-385-2772

La Casa Del Habano
402 Hornby St.
Vancouver
604-609-0511

Old Morris Tobacconists Ltd
1116 Government St.
Victoria
250-382-4811

Revolucion Cigars & Fine Gifts
1062 Mainland St.
Vancouver
604-662-4427

Whistler Cigar Co.
P.O. Box 1220
Whistler
604-905-2423

ASIA

HONG KONG (CHINA)

Stores

Cohiba Cigar Divan
Mandarin Oriental Hotel
5 Connaught Rd.
East Lobby
852-2825-4074

La Casa del Habano
Sheraton Hong Kong Hotel & Towers
20 Nathan Rd., Kowloon
852-2123-9952

Tabacalera Cigar Divan
Island Shangri-La Hotel
Supreme Court Rd.
852-2521-1734

SHANGHAI

Club

The Shanghai American Club
99 Huangpu Rd.
8621-6393-2850

BEIJING

Clubs/Lounges

The Cigar Lounge at the St. Regis
21 Jianguomenwai Dajie
(86) 10-6460-6688

CourtYard Restaurant
95 Donghuamen Ave.
(86) 10-6526-8883

Crystal Bar
The Ritz-Carlton Beijing, Financial Street
1 Jin Cheng Fang St. East,
Financial Street
(86) 10-6601-6666

Davidoff Cigar Lounge
The Ritz-Carlton Beijing
83A Jian Guo Rd.
(86) 10-5908-8888

LAN Club
4/F Twin Towers
B-12 Jianguomenwai Ave.
(86) 10-5109-6012

Redmoon
Grand Hyatt Beijing
1 East Chang An Ave.
(86) 10-8518-1234

EUROPE

MOSCOW

Stores

Davidoff of Moscow
Ul Tverskaya 23
7 (495) 200-57-00

Galereya Gradusov
5 Serpuhovskoi Val
7 (495) 952-05-42

Galereya Tabaka
Ul Tverskaya 16/2
7 (495) 935-89-31

Havana
17 Komsomolsky Prospekt
7 (495) 247-05-55

Tabachnaya Lavka
4 Prospekt Mira
7 (495) 608-99-12

Lounges

Ararat Park Hyatt
4 Neglinnaya
7 (495) 783 1234

Golden Ring Hotel
5 Smolenskaya
7 (495) 725-01-00

Wall St. Bar
9-1 Volkhonka
7 (495) 916-57-31

AMSTERDAM

Stores

P.G.C. HAJENIUS
Rokin 92-96
31-20-623-7494

Van Coeverden & Son
Leidsestraat 58
31-20-624-5150

PARIS

Stores

A la Civette
157 rue Saint Honoré
33 (0) 1 42 96 04 99

La Casa del Habano
169 Boulevard Saint Germain
33 (0) 1 45 49 24 30

La Cave à Cigars
Publicis Drugstore
133 Avenue des Champs Elysées
33 (0) 1 44 43 76 31

Maison Lemaire
59 Avenue Victor Hugo
33 (0) 1 45 00 75 63

Tabac George V
22 Avenue George V
33 (0) 1 45 01 81 41

LONDON

Stores

Alfred Dunhill
Bourdon House
2 Davies St.
44 (0) 845 458 0779

Alfred Dunhill
48 Jermyn St.
44 (0) 20 7290 8609

La Casa del Habano
100 Warbour St.
44 (0) 207 314 4001

Cigars Unlimited
129 Walham Green Ct.
44 (0) 77 7386 9000

Davidoff of London
35 St. James's St.
44 (0) 20 7930 3079

James's J. Fox & Robert Lewis
19 St. James's St.
44 (0) 20 7930 3787

Sautter of Mayfair
106 Mount St.
44 (0) 20 7499 4866

Hotels/Bars

Floridita
100 Wardour St.
44 (0) 20 7314 4001

The Lanesborough London
Garden Room/Cigar Patio
Hyde Park Corner
44 (0) 20 7259 5599

Maxibond Cigar Divan
63 Fairfax Rd.
44 (0) 20 7625 4490

CUBA

HAVANA

Stores

La Casa del Habano
Fábrica de Partagas
Calle Industria 520
Ciudad Habana (Vieja)
53.7.866 8060

La Casa del Habano
Hotel Melia Cohiba
1ra y 3ra
Ciudad Habana
53.7.835 2434

La Casa del Habano
Hotel Melia Habana.
Avenida 3ra e/76 y 80.
Miramar
53.7.204 5289

La Casa del Habano
Hotel Nacional
Calle 21 y O. Vedado
Ciudad Habana
53.7.866 3564 ext. 176

LA CASA DEL HABANO

For a complete list of La Casa del Habano locations, visit **www.lacasadelhabano.cu**. Be warned, however, that the site can be finicky.

SELECT CIGAR BRANDS BY COUNTRY A–Z

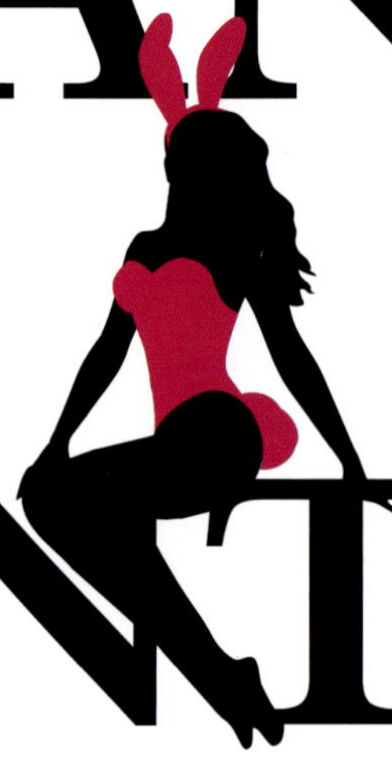

Cigars, like wine and other epicurean delights, are at their most fundamental level a subjective experience: Taste-wise, one man's Havana may be another's machine-made flavor-infused blunt (not that the latter smoke is bad . . . if that's your sort of thing). In that spirit, I've provided a short (actually, sort of long) list, subdivided by country, of the cigars that seem to enjoy broad popularity.

Hold on, you say: Why not just offer up a list of all the cigars on the market? Well, such a list would fill an entire book (actually, it does fill an entire book: *Perelman's Pocket Cyclopedia of Cigars*, now in its 15th edition, which exhaustively breaks down some 1,360 different brands)—and I have no interest in giving you, gentle reader, a hernia from trying to lift such a massive tome.

For the newbie, this short but extensive list will provide a reference for your exploration of cigars; for the connoisseur, at least some of the brands below may be ones you've never tried—and could very well be worth seeking out.

CUBA

Bolivar
12 sizes/formats

Cohiba Línea 1492 (Siglo)
6 sizes/formats

Cuaba
4 sizes/formats

Hoyo de Monterrey Epicure Range
3 sizes/formats

H. Upmann Magnum Range
2 sizes/formats

La Flor de Cana
2 sizes/formats

Montecrsto
15 sizes/formats

Partagas (Classic Line)
20 sizes/formats

Partagas Serie Connoisseur Range
3 sizes/formats

Por Larrañaga
3 sizes/formats

Ramón Allones
4 sizes/formats

Sancho Panza
6 sizes/formats

Edicion Limitadas
The Habanos Edicion Limitadas often (however, certainly not always) offer Cuba's best foot forward for any given year. As such, I am a big proponent of this unique collection of cigars. See the complete list of the Edicion Limitadas in the "Advanced" chapter.

DOMINICAN REPUBLIC

Arturo Fuente Don Carlos
7 sizes/formats

Ashton Heritage Puro Sol
5 sizes/formats

Ashton Virgin Sun Grown
10 sizes/formats

Aurora Barrel Aged
4 sizes/formats

Aurora Preferidos Cameroon Line
6 sizes/formats

Aurora Preferidos Connecticut line
3 sizes/formats

Aurora Preferidos Corojo line
3 sizes/formats

Bolivar
4 sizes/formats

Cohiba Puro Dominicana
4 sizes/formats

Davidoff Millennium Blend Series
8 sizes/formats

Davidoff Special Series
5 sizes/formats

Fonseca Cubano Limitado
6 sizes/formats

Fuente Fuente OpusX
size/format selection variable

La Flor Dominicana Cameroon Cabinet Series
4 sizes/formats

La Flor Dominicana Ligero
5 sizes/formats

Macanudo 1968
4 sizes/formats

Mi Dominicana
8 sizes/formats

Montecristo Cabinet Selección
5 sizes/formats

Onyx Reserve
8 sizes/formats

Paul Garmirian (PG)
15th Anniversary Series
10 sizes/formats

Playboy
4 sizes/formats

Seijas's Signature Series
7 sizes

Zino Platinum Crown
Ltd.-Edition Wrapper
2 sizes/formats

HONDURAS

Alec Bradley Tempus
5 sizes/formats

Punch Gran Cru
8 sizes/formats

Romeo y Julieta Habana Reserve
10 sizes/formats

Rocky Patel 1999 Vintage Connecticut
8 sizes/formats

Rocky Patel 1992 Vintage
8 sizes/formats

NICARAGUA

Don Pepin Garcia Serie JJ
4 sizes/formats

Dunhill Signed Range
6 sizes/formats

Joya de Nicaragua Celebracion
6 sizes/formats

La Riqueza
5 sizes/formats

Liga Privada No. 9 by Drew Estate
4 sizes/formats

Padrón 1964 Anniversary Series
10 sizes/formats

Padrón 1926 Series
7 sizes/formats

Tatuaje Havana VI
6 sizes/formats

Xikar HC (Havana Collection) Series
three blends
4 sizes/formats for each blend

OTHERS

A. Turrent Six Generations (Mexico)
4 sizes/formats

Cabaiguan (U.S.A.)
9 sizes/formats

Graycliff Chateau Grand Cru (Bahamas)
6 sizes/formats

La Gloria Cubana Artesanos de Miami (USA)
5 sizes/formats

Padilla Signature 1932 (U.S.A.)
6 sizes/formats

Tatuaje Miami (U.S.A.)
12 sizes/formats

SUGGESTED READINGS

The following books can further your cigar education as a lover of the leaf (or cigar geek, depending on your point of view):

The Cigar, by Barnaby Conrad III (Chronicle Books: 1996)
A classic that's out of print and worth hunting down

Cigars: Revised and Updated (Vol. 1), by Vahe Gerard (Flammarion: 2009)

The Cigar in Art, by Terence Conran (The Overlook Press: 1996)
Those who like both art and cigars would be well advised to find a copy

The Complete Guide to Cigars, by Steve Luck (Parragon Books Ltd.: 2008)

An Illustrated Encyclopedia of Post-Revolution Havana Cigars (Second Edition), by Min Ron Nee (2005)
Referred to in some circles as "the Cuban cigar Bible"

The Illustrated History of Cigars, by Bernard Le Roy and Maurice Szafran (Harold Starke Publishers, Ltd.: New Revised Edition 1999)
One of the few true coffee-table cigar tomes

Perelman's Pocket Cyclopedia of Cigars, by Richard B. Perelman (Perelman, Pioneer & Co.: 1995)
A new edition is released annually

Perelman's Pocket Cyclopedia of Havana Cigars, Third Edition, by Richard B. Perelman (Perelman, Pioneer & Co.: 2005)

The Ultimate Cigar Book, Third Edition, by Richard Carleton Hacker (Autumngold Publications: 2003)
A cigar-book classic

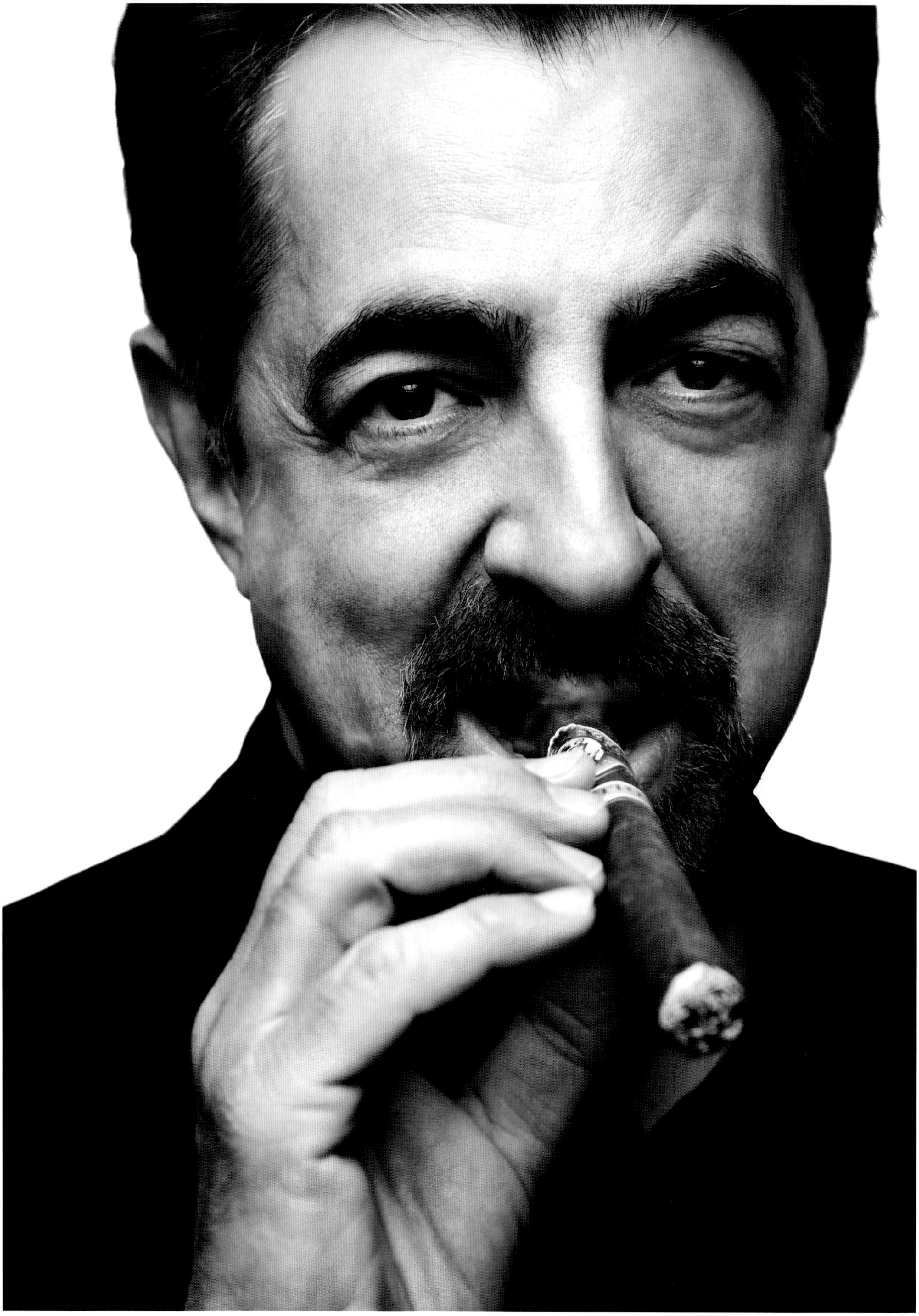

AFTERWORD >

By Joe Mantegna

I think it might have started with Edie Adams: my fascination with cigars, that is. Edie was married to the great comic Ernie Kovaks at the time, and one of the highlights of his television show was the occasional commercial Edie would do for a popular cigar company. Dressed in as sexy a costume as early-60's television would allow, she would sing in a sultry voice: "Why don't you light up a Muriel Coronella...anytime, anyplace, anywhere...look so handsome and debonair."

Now, if smoking a Muriel Coronella made me handsome and debonair enough to impress someone like Edie Adams, I was signing up. At that time, my only real association with cigar smoking was my uncle Danny, who would have me light the perpetual White Owl he had in his mouth while going over the *Daily Racing Form*. Needless to say, Ms. Adams made me understand that cigar smoking could be a lot more than that.

As a teenager, we all dabbled in the forbidden fruits of the time (as all teenagers have done and will do), and while all types of tobacco products had their moment in the sun, it was always the cigar that personified something more mysterious, more classy, more—need I say it—debonair. Pipe smoking seemed to carry elements of that, but being born and raised in Chicago, the pipe seemed more East Coast to me, while the cigar was the image of backroom politics, hardnosed cowboys, movie-star gangsters, and everything else that one associated with the City of the Big Shoulders. A few select friends and I experimented with all kinds of cigar smoking during those youthful times, confident in that Rat Pack era that smoking was probably good for you anyway.

As the years passed, my cigar habit ebbed and flowed with the times. Without opening the discussion as to the wisdom of putting burning leaves in one's mouth—at least with regard to health concerns—I would have to say my current status with cigar smoking falls under the axiom I long ago adopted as one of the maxims of my life: "Everything in moderation...including moderation." I have no doubt that excess—in cigar smoking as well as nearly everything else—is detrimental to one's health. Having too much of a good thing really is possible—but just enough of something is what gives life its meaning, its individuality, its style.

I remember reading once about a famous doctor who refused to give up his once-a-week cigar habit because he looked forward to that one smoke, and partaking of it at the end of a hard workweek was a greater comfort and medicine to him than all the therapies, pharmaceuticals or any other form of stress reliever one could imagine. Those who appreciate cigar smoking know what that means. Those who don't never will.

Finally, it's as much the society of cigar smoking that's the real pleasure, as opposed to the mere act itself. Some of the great friendships in my life have begun over the shared experience with a few men and/or women of sitting down and solving the world's problems over a beautiful hand-rolled smoke and an appropriate libation. Moments like that are the great equalizer, and that companionship has included world-famous actors, the neighborhood mailman, a local carpenter and the waitress from the diner next door. At this place and time, the occupations we partake in are secondary; we are drawn together by our common interest in this particular "forbidden fruit." Perhaps the fact that it's an activity that has become harder and harder to find places to practice it makes it all the more precious.

One doesn't smoke cigars casually anymore, and I gladly accept that. If it's that damn important to us, we'll find the time and place to do it...and we do. The list is too long to name all those who I now cherish as friends and colleagues due to this mutual interest, but you know who you are. It may well have been the Playboy image of the 1950's and 60's that introduced many of us to the world of cigar smoking, but what keeps us there are reasons that have grown and matured along with us. I'm not sure if it's actually made anyone handsome or debonair, but it certainly has provided endless enjoyment to a whole world of aficionados. I'm happy to be one of them.

A tip of the glass and a sip of the stogie to you, Edie.

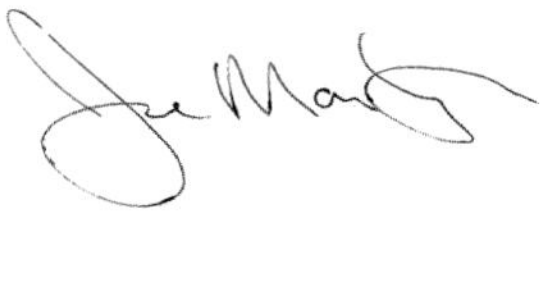

Bibliography

QUOTES BIBLIOGRAPHY/CITATION

Jay-Z: Snider, Mike. "Cigars: Celebs got 'em, and they smoke 'em." *USA Today. 24 July 2003, Life.*

James Coburn: Rhys, Timothy. "Quintessential Cool: A Conversation with James Coburn." *Moviemaker Magazine. Issue 33, April/May 1999.*

Johnny Depp: As told to the author

Samuel L. Jackson: Tarshis, Joan "101 Minutes With Samuel L. Jackson." *Smoke. Spring 1998: 131–141*

Michael Jordan: As told to the author

Sylvester Stallone: Mott, Gordon "Stallone II." *Cigar Aficionado. March/April 1998.* Quote reprinted with permission from Mr. Stallone.

SELECT BIBLIOGRAPHY

Maugham, W. Somerset. *The Summing Up.* New York: Penguin Classics, 1992.

Min Ron, Nee. *An Illustrated Encyclopedia of Post-Revolution Havana Cigars (Second Edition).* 2005.

Stevenson, Robert Louis. *Virginibus Puerisque and Other Papers.* New York: Adamant Media Corporation, 2000.

Tolstoy, Leo. *Anna Karenina.* New York: Signet Classics, 2002.

Wilde, Oscar. *The Importance of Being Earnest.* New York: Penguin Classics, 1995.

Acknowledgments

In the end no book is the work of a single individual; quite the contrary, it is very much a collaboration. As such, there are many who need to be thanked for their words of encouragement, insights, and contributions.

First and foremost, very special thanks to Christopher Napolitano and Leopold Froehlich of Playboy, Bill Wolfsthal, Abigail Gehring, and everyone at Skyhorse Publishing, and Jim Colucci and Janelle Rosenfeld of Altadis U.S.A. — this project would have never come to fruition without your collective support.

Special thanks to Warren Mason for his unflappable patience. And to Lucas Irwin, who was there from Day One.

An individual and gracious thank-you to Dr. Adrian Bartoli, my wine-and-spirits *consigliere personale*, who cowrote the "What a Pair—Smokes & Drinks" chapter and made great contributions to the "Cigars Advanced" chapter. He is indeed the maestro—*grazie!*

Others who deserve thanks for their generosity and kindness: A.J. Baime, George Brightman, Simon Chase, Claudia Chavez, Christina "CC" Citrola, Vivian Colon, Brian Dawson, Jemma Freeman, Liliana Guia, Michael Herklots, Earl Edward Hoyt III, Jimmy Jellinek, Ling Ma, Joe Mantegna, James Mauro Jr., LeRoy Neiman, Jimmy Nicol, Keith Park, Lynn Quayle, Dan Ramm, Matthew Scanlon, Nat Sherman International/The Sherman Family/Michael Holba, Edward Sahakian, Mark Stucklin, Lauren Weiss and, of course, Nick, Ian and Robert.

And last but not least, my heartfelt thanks to my wife Melissa Kaye and daughter Dashiell Eden, who don't let me smoke in the house, car or hotel rooms, but are always happy to go for a long walk with me while I puff away—as long as I'm downwind.

In making a list such as this, there are undoubtedly those who are erroneously omitted. To them I offer my sincere apologies and humble thanks.

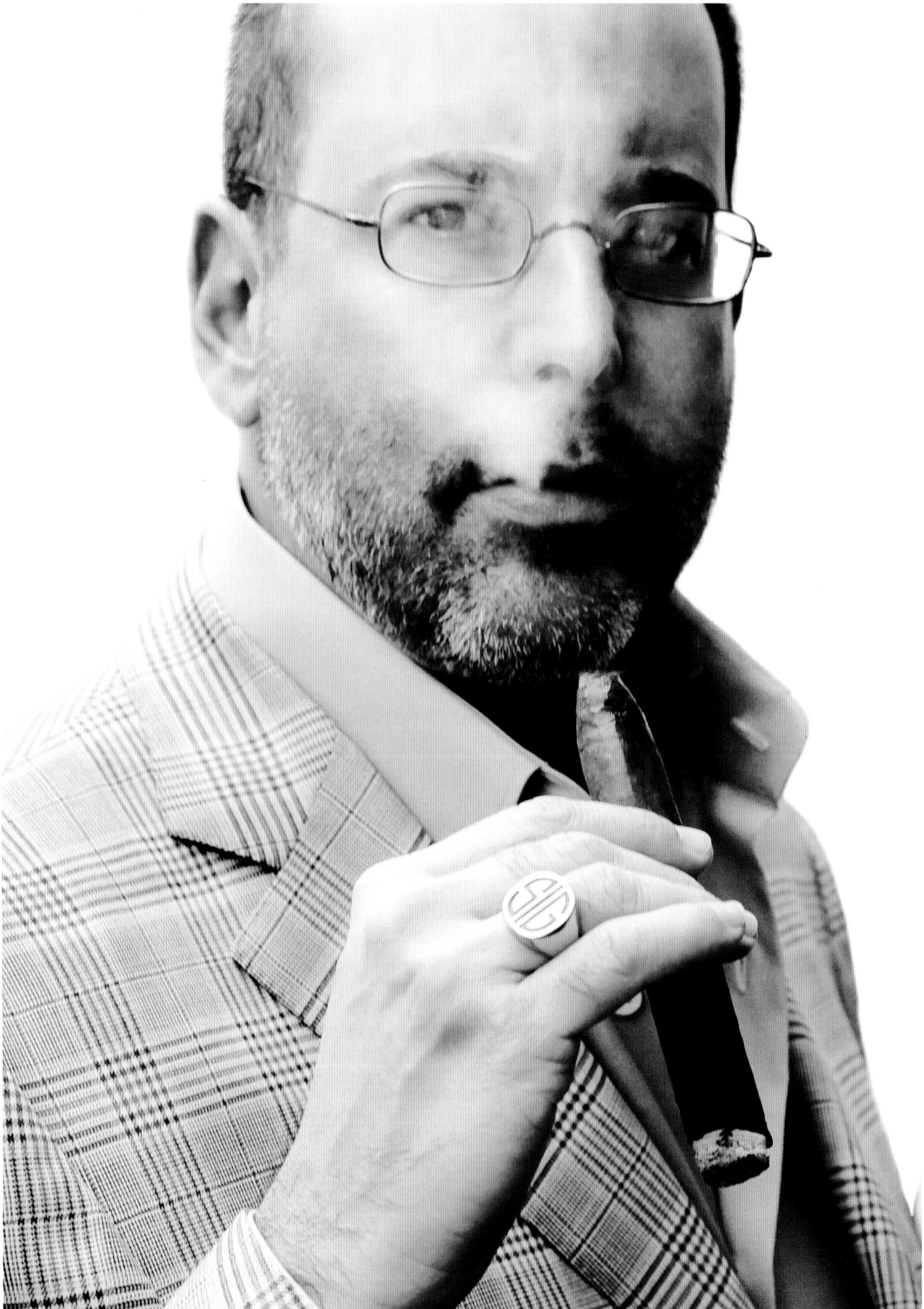

THE AUTHOR >

Aaron Sigmond is the founding editor of both *Smoke* magazine and *The Cigar Report*, a Doubledown Media publication, where he also served as Group Luxury Editor. Sigmond has written about cigars for *Playboy*, in addition to numerous other publications and websites. Sigmond has also written the forewords to "The Cigar Handbook" and "Cultivation Tradition: A Photographic Journey to Isla de Ometepe and San Agustin" respectively. He lives, works, and smokes in New York City.

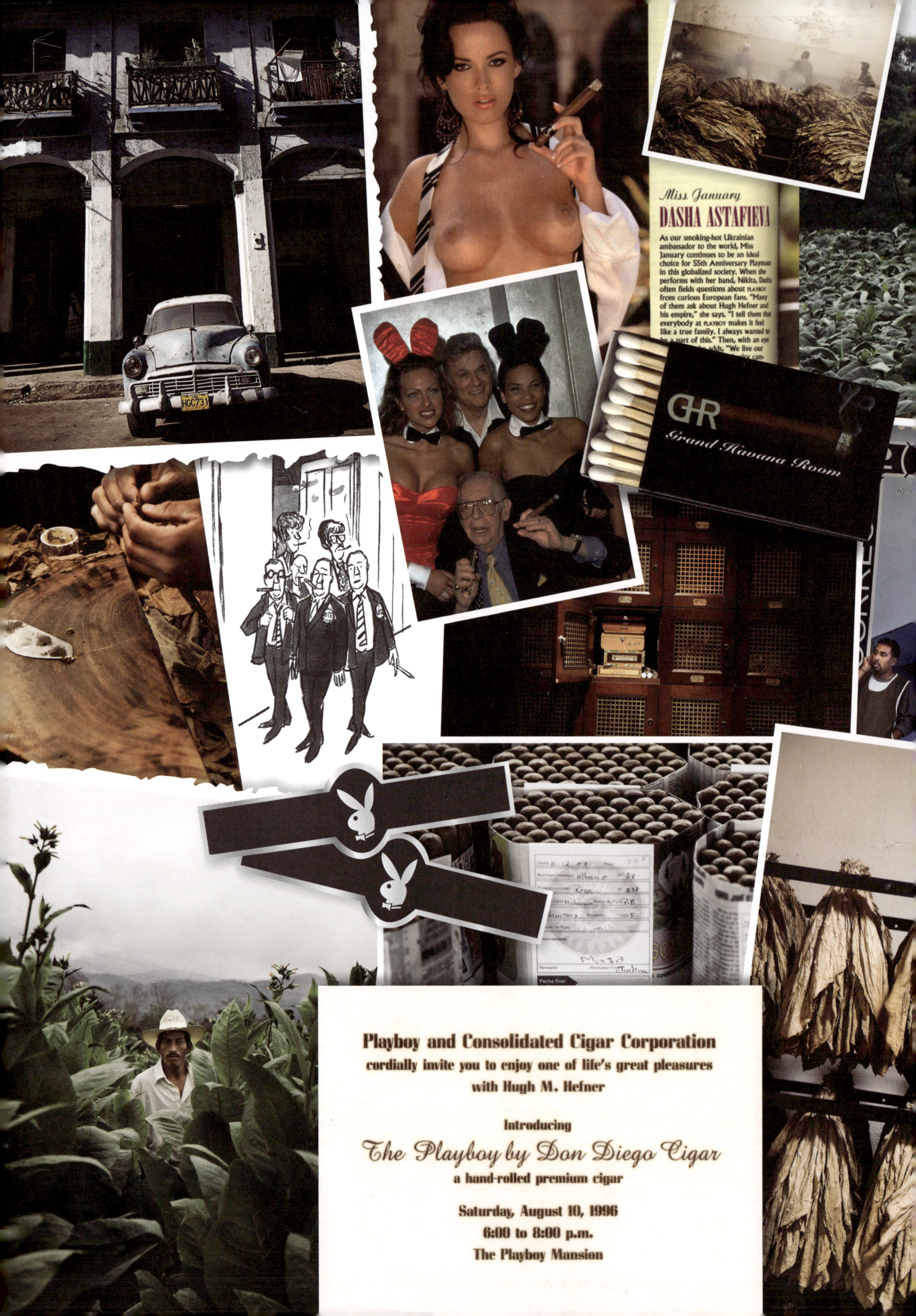
Miss January
DASHA ASTAFIEVA
As our smoking-hot Ukrainian ambassador to the world, Miss January continues to be an ideal choice for 55th Anniversary Playmate in this globalized society. When she performs with her band, Nikita, Dasha often fields questions about PLAYBOY from curious European fans. "Many of them ask about Hugh Hefner and his empire," she says. "I tell them that everybody at PLAYBOY makes it feel like a true family. I always wanted to
part of this." Then, with an eye
adds, "We live our
GHR
Grand Havana Room
HGC731
Playboy and Consolidated Cigar Corporation
cordially invite you to enjoy one of life's great pleasures
with Hugh M. Hefner
Introducing
The Playboy by Don Diego Cigar
a hand-rolled premium cigar
Saturday, August 10, 1996
6:00 to 8:00 p.m.
The Playboy Mansion